Advances in Child Health Nursing

1

Advances in Child Health Nursing

Edited by

Edward Alan Glasper BA RGN RSCN DipN(Lond) CertEd RNT
Professor of Nursing, University of Southampton
and
Ann Tucker MSc RSCN RGN PGCEA RNT DipN(Lond) RCNT
Head of Academic Affairs, The Nightingale and Guy's College of Health

618.92
GLA

First published 1993
Reprinted 1995

British Library Cataloguing in Publication Data

Advances in Child Health Nursing
  I. Glasper, Edward Alan   II. Tucker, Ann
  610.73

ISBN 1-871364-91-4

Typeset by Alden Multimedia
Printed and bound in Great Britain by Alden Press, Oxford

29/8/95

Acknowledgements

The poem 'Only a Sibling' by Tammy McGowan, a CanTeen member, is reproduced with permission of The Australian Teenage Cancer Patients Society (CanTeen).

The publishers wish to acknowledge the assistance given by Joan Smith of the University of Southampton in the preparation of this book.

Contents

Contributors

Helen Ainsworth, RGN RSCN DipN, Sister, Children's Neurosciences, University Hospital, Nottingham

Chris Betts, RGN RSCN DHSM, Hospital Manager, Tadworth Court Children's Hospital

Gosia Brykczyńska, RGN RSCN RNT BA BSc CertEd DipPH, Lecturer in Ethics/Philosophy and Paediatric Nursing at the Institute of Advanced Nursing Education, Royal College of Nursing

Janette Budd, RGN RSCN, Ward Sister, Plastic Surgery Dept, The Hospital for Sick Children, Great Ormond Street, London

Roberta Burton, RGN Cert in Research Methodology, Project Nurse for Quality Assurance and Research, Royal Belfast Hospital for Sick Children, Belfast

Brigid Carr, RGN RSCN, Clinical Nurse Specialist, Urology Department, Hospitals for Sick Children, Great Ormond Street, London

Anne Casey, RGN RSCN RNT DipN DipN Ed, Senior Nurse (Practice Development), The Hospital for Sick Children, Great Ormond Street, London

Virginia Colwell, RGN RSCN DMS, Clinical Nurse Manager, The Hospital for Sick Children, Great Ormond Street, London

Philip Darbyshire, RNMH RSCN DipN(Lond) RNT MN PhD, Lecturer in Health and Nursing Studies, Glasgow Caledonian University

Linda Davies, RGN RSCN, Senior Staff Nurse, Paediatric Ward, Glan Clwyd Hospital, Bodelwyddan, Clwyd

Sister Frances Dominica, RGN RSCN FRCN, Hon. Director of Helen House, Oxford

Nicola Eaton, RGN RSCN BSc(Hons Econ) PGCE, Lecturer in Nursing, Mid and West Wales College of Nursing and Midwifery, University College of Swansea

Margaret Evans, RGN RSCN FETC DipN(Lond) BSc(Hons) Nursing, Macmillan Lecturer in Cancer Nursing, Dept of Nursing Studies, Southampton University

Rachel Fretwell, RGN RSCN HV Cert, Health Visitor, Scarborough

Yvonne Fulton, RGN RSCN, Nurse Teacher in Child Health, Southampton University College of Nursing and Midwifery

Breda Gahan, RGN RSCN, Ward Sister, Queen Elizabeth Hospital for Children, London

Edward Alan Glasper, BA RGN RSCN DipN(Lond) CertEd RNT, Professor of Nursing, University of Southampton

Peggy Gow, RGN RSCN DN(Cert) NNEB Further Education City and Guilds 730, Co-ordinator Paediatric Community Nursing Services, Southampton Community Health Services

Anne Hunt, RGN RSCN Bsc(Hons), Nurse Member of Care Team, Helen House, Oxford

Lorraine Ireland, RGN RSCN RCNT RNT PGCEA, Clinical teacher, College of Nursing and Midwifery, Southampton

Noelle Llewellyn, SRN RSCN DPSN, Clinical Nurse Specialist, Acute Pain Service, The Hospital for Sick Children, Great Ormond Street, London

Gill Meyer, RGN RSCN, Business Manager, Tadworth Court Children's Hospital

Janet Mikkelsen, R(Comp)N RSCN Cert Paed (Melb) Adv. Dip. Child and Family Health (Auck), Charge Nurse, Auckland Children's Hospital, New Zealand

Jim Richardson, BA RGN RSCN PGCE, Lecturer in Nursing Studies, University of |Wales College of Medicine

Grethe Ridgway, RGN CMBI RSCN RHV CPT(HV), Director of Nursing Practice and Quality, Southampton Community Health Services

Margaret Rogers, BSc(Hons) RGN RSCN DipN(Lond), Facilitator, Nursing Development Unit, Hospitals for Sick Children, Great Ormond Street, London

Sharon Stower, RGN RSCN Cert MHS DMS IHMS, Senior Nurse Paediatrics, Nottingham Children's Unit

Rebecca Sury, RGN RSCN RCNT, Ward Sister, The Hospital for Sick Children, Great Ormond Street, London

Eileen Thomas, RGN RHV MA, Primary Care Development Manager, Southampton Community Health Services Unit

Margaret Thompson, MB CLB FRCP(Glasgow) MRCPsy DCH DRCOG, Consultant Child and Adolescent Psychiatrist, Paediatric Unit, Southampton General Hospital

Ann Tucker, MSc RSCN RGN PGCEA RNT DipN(Lond) RCNT, Head of Academic Affairs, The Nightingale and Guy's College of Health, London

Foreword

It is with particular pleasure that I write the foreword to this book, *Advances in Child Health Nursing*, for two reasons. First, because Jan Williams was both a loyal and respected colleague and family friend, and second, because I believe the care of sick children in the United Kingdom is not only good in itself, but is beginning to influence nursing care in other fields of nursing.

This book is a reflection of much that is innovative, exciting and challenging in the nursing care of children, and displays all the elements of professional practice that Jan so much enjoyed.

The book covers a variety of issues which demonstrate the complexity of caring for sick children in the 1990s, not only those related to high technology and powerful treatments, but also to the very ordinary demands on and expectations of the children and their families. Emphasis is laid on considering the child as a member of a family, who are all encouraged to participate in the care of the child, rather than in isolation.

We need to achieve more. This book will, I hope, enable you as practitioners to reflect on recent changes, and stimulate and encourage you to consider other ideas for the future.

Liz Fradd

Preface

Jan Williams, a well-known children's nurse and founder member of the Royal College of Nursing Society of Paediatric Nursing, died in September 1989 after a short illness. Her many colleagues in the United Kingdom, recognising her valuable contribution to the art and science of children's nursing, wanted to do something in her memory.

An opportunity presented itself in November 1989 when a group of children's nurses, attending the Society's Birthday Conference, decided to commission a publication. Since then, a number of experienced children's nurses have agreed to contribute to this publication. A trust fund has been created from the royalties of this book for the benefit of students studying to be children's nurses. The trust fund will enable students to apply for scholarships to attend conferences or other events which will enhance their learning.

The resulting book is a collection of essays reflecting advances in the art and science of children's nursing.

Edward Alan Glasper
Ann Tucker

Introduction

Children's nursing has advanced considerably over the last three decades. The opening of the Hospital for Sick Children in London in 1852 was a major step forward in establishing care for sick children, but the Nightingale tradition subtly changed the dynamics of this and other early institutions when military principles began to be applied. The growing professionalism of nursing ensured the gradual exclusion of parents from direct participation in care. The parental role continued to be denigrated and did not change for nearly a century, during which time nursing embraced the patriarchal model of medicine with its emphasis on protecting patients through the withholding of information. The *persona non grata* status of parents and the rigid barrier nursing techniques of the late nineteenth century, coupled with the dogma of prolonged and continuous bed rest, must have made life for children lonely and depressing. This is not to imply that care was callous; quite the contrary, care was meticulous, as was the attention paid to cleanliness on the wards in which children were nursed. However, parents were feared to be vectors of disease, as were other children, and this ensured a lonely existence for sick children in hospital.

Following the publication of the Platt Report in 1959, the emancipation of families began and today, in the 1990s, this process continues, with the emphasis on parental participation in care and partnership between families and professionals.

To date, the term paediatric nursing has always been used to describe the nursing care of children. However, with recent developments in health education and care in the community it is recognised that other terms such as 'children's nurse' and 'child health nurse' are used. This reflects the changing role of the nurse.

Advances in Child Health Nursing augments the concept of family-centred care and it is hoped that it will isnpire readers to greater innovations in practice.

1

Quality in Action

Alan Glasper and Ann Tucker

The term 'quality assurance' has become increasingly familiar to all nurses over recent years. Much is written about quality care and the setting of standards. The word 'quality', however, while greeted by some with interest and enthusiasm, is met by others with a degree of irritation and lack of understanding. Misconceptions abound; a common-sense approach, of which all nurses are capable, is needed in order to demystify the concept.

WHAT DOES QUALITY MEAN?

There are many definitions, from 'quality is the degree of excellence' to half-page definitions which use language which confuses rather than clarifies. Joseph Juran refers to quality as 'fitness for use'. The authors of this chapter prefer the statement issued by the Further Education Unit in July 1987. 'Quality is easy to recognise and much good quality already exists in the system. The definition of it is elusive and difficult.'

Yes, quality is easy to recognise. Nevertheless, it does mean different things to different people. In fact 'quality' can be almost anything you want it to be. As a result it is important to understand why quality is necessary.

WHY IS QUALITY NECESSARY?

Quality is not just a fashionable buzz-word; it is a necessity in today's world. Established professions regulate their practice and discipline. Nurses too need to demonstrate accountability, authority and responsibility; accountability being the key to the formation of professional standards.

Cost-effectiveness is sought within the National Health Service. Patient throughput is increasing, as this is one of the yardsticks by which general management measures success. But quantity does not necessarily equal quality. The number of experienced staff and establishment levels are being reduced as skill-mix exercises take place. The long-term effects of this are yet to be experienced.

The general public are now more aware of health care and their rights. Every family coming into hospital should be given, or should find displayed, the standards of care they can expect to receive. It is their right. This has implications for the paediatric nurse who must have a sound rationale for practice when participating in family-centred care. For example, when planning care with the family, the nurse needs to be able to give information to enable joint decisions to be made.

In law a nurse's performance is measured against that of a reasonably prudent nurse. How much better if performance were to be measured against standards, which act as guidelines for practice, and allow for deviations providing the nurse is prepared to be accountable. And on a personal level, it is rewarding to know that you are doing a job well.

REMOVING THE MYTHS

The concept of quality can be viewed as a continuum from excellent to bad. What constitutes 'good' care will differ for individuals according to their personal beliefs, attitudes, values and their beliefs about their rights. Everyone knows what quality is and feels secure with their own view of quality. Unfortunately, these views differ and are usually subjective.

There is a tendency in nursing to use the terms quality and standards as though they were the same thing. There is consequently the danger of treating them synony-mously. However, standards are a tool and as such contribute towards total quality improvement.

By reading the gurus of quality assurance, basic principles can be clearly identified.

Juran is a well-known and respected figure in the field of quality assurance. His approach is described in five stages:

1. *Breakthrough in attitude:* This involves providing a favourable climate for quality planning.
2. *Pareto:* Identifying the priorities by concentrating on the vital few and ignoring the trivial many.
3. *Organisation:* Co-ordinating the work.
4. Control at the new standard level performance.
5. Review and repeat.

(Cited in Vorley, 1991.)

Macdonald and Piggott (1990) describe six stages of quality improvement, which the present authors have adapted for use in nursing:

1. *Assessment and awareness:* Assessment of need for quality improvement of patient's satisfaction, of employee attitudes.
2. *Organising for quality improvement:* Establishing criteria and benchmarks to measure the process and resultant implementation. Setting standards.
3. *Education:* Providing education and training for all. Providing competence.
4. *Establishing stable processes:* Implementing a hospital-wide improvement system, so eliminating major problems.
5. *Total involvement of all employees:* The introduction of measurement by all. Audit.
6. *Continuous improvement:* Training for facilitators, managers and key employees. The whole organisation involved in the process of improvement. The Japanese

call this philosophy *Kaizen*, which translated means continuous, step-by-step improvement.

These basic principles can be applied to a ward, a department or an entire organisation.

HOW IS THIS PHILOSOPHY ACHIEVED?

Quality improvement must be planned. It is a pro-active exercise, which recognises that the culture of the organisation affects the behaviour of those working within it and hence affects quality. It depends on everyone being committed to providing quality. Total quality management is a motivational concept, aimed at motivating people for quality; it could be viewed as an agent for change (Collard, 1989).

To simplify what might appear to some to be nebulous, three key areas can be identified for action.

1. Participation and involvement of everyone.
2. Customer satisfaction.
3. Quality performance measures to assess current performance.

The first stage of the process is to involve everyone in selecting or designing their own definition of quality. From experience, the exercise of value clarification takes almost longer than writing the standard itself. It is important for everyone to come to a common understanding. If the attitude is wrong, sabotage will result and all efforts to set standards will be wasted. In reality this means communicating with each other, sharing ideas and agreeing on the common goals.

In doing this an assessment of the work area is essential. Are parents, carers and children satisfied with the care they receive? Are nurses gaining satisfaction from what they do? Is the climate right for the implementation of quality planning? Could the environment be improved to make work more enjoyable? It is futile imposing standards of care if the environment for those giving care is not considered.

The following questions can be given to individuals and used to assist in identifying areas for change within the environment.

1. Do I always know what is expected of me?
2. Am I satisfied that I am able to do my job to the best of my ability?
3. Do I always get agreement from the child/family about the care I give?
4. Does my manager want to know my problems in meeting the requirements of my job?
5. Do I always have the resources I need?
6. Is there a philosophy of clearly stated values, understood by everyone?
7. Can I recognise any barriers to communication in my clinical area?
8. Does conflict exist between ward objectives and what appears to me to be common sense?
9. Do I ever feel stress in my job?
10. Do I know what is going on in the hospital or do I always feel in the dark?
11. Have I ever asked other people what I can do to help them?

(Adapted from Macdonald and Piggott, 1990.)

Identifying topics which need to have written standards is an approach that can be used to clarify values and gives ownership to those who list them. This is described in the Dynamic Standard Setting System (DySSSy) (RCN, 1990).

The second stage is writing the standards. Many hospitals use the Donabedian model of structure, process, outcome, as used in DySSSy. However, it must be stressed that what is important is that a standard statement is agreed, and the criteria identified which will enable measurement to take place, i.e. What resources do I need to achieve the standard statement? What do I need to do? What will the outcomes be? DySSy applies the 'rumba technique': criteria should be Relevant, Understandable, Measurable, Behaviourally stated and Achievable. During this stage, education needs may be identified; and to provide competent care, education and training should be available to all. This follows the philosophy of continuing education, as identified in the Post Registration Education and Practice Project (PREPP).

To eliminate major problems a quality programme should be multi-disciplinary as no one exists in isolation. Gone is the day of the craftsman who saw a job through from start to finish. Within a hospital it takes many different disciplines to achieve a satisfactory outcome. There are many occasions, therefore, when standard setting should be multi-disciplinary.

At the same time as writing a standard the audit tool should be developed. This again involves asking questions: Can I observe this? Can I look at the care plan or the records to see if this has been achieved, or do I need to ask the child, the family and/or the nurse? From experience, if this is done at the same time as writing the standard, the criteria are often clarified, frequently reduced in number and the standard immediately becomes usable. If it is agreed that criteria from the structure, process and outcome sections are audited, the standard also becomes a flexible tool. It is not necessary to audit all criteria each time. A decision on which criteria to audit can be taken according to the identified need. The actual process for carrying out the audit must be agreed by all those involved. It is not an 'inspection'; rather, it is the study of actual practice against the concept of 'good practice' – in this case the standards set – in an attempt to improve the care offered to the child and family:

'If perfection could be achieved it would not be worth having.' (old Zen proverb)

Within a hospital these activities should be co-ordinated, so that problems and achievements can be shared. This frequently facilitates the 'aha' experience and so enables groups to learn from each other.

From experience in different settings it is possible to observe an improvement in morale and care, an identification of training needs, and areas where further research is required.

The case study that follows highlights the reality of quality in action.

THE PRECURSORS

Harris (1990) has stated that every experienced nurse has internalised standards. Irrespective of whether written standards of care exist in a unit, all practitioners are fully aware of what constitutes good, bad or indifferent practice, and, therefore, the current trend towards formal standard setting is merely a further step in the professional history of nursing. As a consequence, one must not be lulled into thinking that standard setting is merely a reflection of 'in vogue' attempts by nurses to maintain, improve and monitor standards of care.

Towards the end of 1987 morale on the paediatric unit at Southampton had plummeted. The staff were concerned that staff shortages were affecting standards of care and were not aware at that time of any tool that might help them to measure the effectiveness of their care. They felt that they were busier than usual and that the staff–patient ratios were greater than in previous years. But without sound empirical evidence, it was difficult for the senior nurses to present their case cogently to the management team of the paediatric unit.

A threefold situation existed: (1) an absence of formalised written standards, (2) no recognised method of measuring standards and their effectiveness in clinical practice, and (3) no method of measuring patient dependency or staff–patient ratios.

A PAEDIATRIC DEPENDENCY CLASSIFICATION SYSTEM

A system which is embodied within many 'off-the-shelf' quality assurance packages aims to determine the dependency of children based on the degree of nursing intervention received. The classification system may be used independently or in conjunction with the quality assurance Qualpaeds package.

This system attempts to measure the dependency of a child in hospital objectively, based on the amount of nursing intervention received. In this respect, the system differs from other, more traditional methods of assessing staffing levels, which in the past have concentrated on the number of beds occupied. Bed occupancy is at best a crude indicator of staffing levels. The paediatric dependency classification system places children into four categories:

Category I   Minimal care – relatively self-caring.
Category II Average care – here the child requires assistance and needs monitoring and treatment. The child is likely not to be in an acute stage of an illness or may be recovering from surgery etc.
Category III Above-average care. In this category the child requires an above-average amount of care. This would include a greater degree of care in the psycho-social domain and might be concerned with teaching a newly diagnosed child with diabetes or caring for children in the immediate post operative period.
Category IV Maximum care. In this category the child is subject to frequent nursing interventions. It might include children in all high-care situations.

Over 9 months, four acute paediatric wards at Southampton kept daily records of their patients' dependency levels. The information was subsequently collated and evaluated to assess its reliability and effectiveness as a measure of patient dependency.

The primary objective at the commencement of this survey was that staff believed it would lead to a greater ratio of skill-mix within the paediatric unit. From the onset, however, the staff using the dependency rating scale found it somewhat crude.

DIFFICULTIES AND DISADVANTAGES OF THE DEPENDENCY SYSTEM IN ACTION

1. Different trained staff perceptions of what constitutes a score on the dependency category inventory.
2. Ambiguity of the inventory schedule – some nurses found it difficult to categorise patients within particular modes of care.
3. The system does not easily differentiate between well dependent children and sick dependent children, i.e. a healthy baby who requires feeding, changing, bathing, etc., and a sick baby who may require sophisticated and constant nursing. These babies would receive the same dependency score using this classification system. Further work on dependency categories for sick children needs to be undertaken, although the existing model can be useful.
4. The design of the inventory schedule does not identify the number or skill-mix of staff on duty during the period (24 hr) of classification. This is a serious omission and therefore requires modification. The resulting numerical ward index using the existing scheme is, therefore, only partially useful when planning for peaks and troughs.
5. The numerical index in itself is meaningless and only becomes meaningful when looked at longitudinally, i.e. over a period of time. When looked at in this way it may be possible to plan future strategies for the staffing of a paediatric ward or unit.

During the period of the dependency study it was decided to undertake a parent satisfaction survey. A questionnaire based on a similar tool to that used at the Hospital for Sick Children, Toronto was designed to elicit parental perceptions and was administered to the families at the point of discharge (Ball, Glasper and Yerrell, 1988).

Quality is defined by Roberts (1975) as a grade of goodness, i.e. it is a measurement. Therefore, quality assurance is a process of looking at a given situation and appraising it against a measure, or set standard. In the nursing context this enables nurses to maintain a set standard of care. Naturally, the setting of standards is a vital part of this process. Although little work has been done on quality assurance in the paediatric field, Maddison (1979) has highlighted the importance of seeking the opinion of consumers – and families are consumers of health care. She believes that parental opinion accurately reflects the opinion of children in hospital and that seeking parents' opinion is, therefore, a valid exercise. She further states a desire to introduce a grading system (like a hotel star grade) into paediatric units and hospitals. How would this operate in hospital? (See Figure 1.1.)

Although parental opinion may well be a valid indicator of a child's perception of care while in hospital, paediatric nurses should not lose sight of the individuality of children. Children should be viewed as partners in care and further work to ascertain children's perceptions of their own care should be undertaken.

In view of the concerns expressed by the staff the pre-quality assurance exercise using the parental questionnaire was seen as a useful precursor to the more formal nursing audit. The questionnaire (Figure 1.2) consisted of a number of open-ended

*   Basic amenities. No rooming in facilities. Annex accommodation only. Some bedside chair accommodation. Some refreshment facilities. School and play facilities rudimentary only. Some visiting restricted. No unaccompanied visitors under 16 years. Minimal support services.

**   Some 'on ward facilities'. Full refreshment/meals available. Parents' recreation room. Open, unrestricted visiting. School and play facilities. Full-time play therapist. Washroom and laundry facilities. Adequate support services.

***   Good 'on ward facilities'. Extensive 'mother and baby cubicles'. Radio and television in all rooms. Tea and coffee facilities. Ward or dining room meal service. Some en-suite bathrooms. Large visitors' recreation room. Good school and play facilities. Full-time play therapist. Laundry facilities. Primary nursing programme. Good support services.

**** Full 'care by parent facilities' with large, well-equipped en-suite mother and baby cubicles. Radio and television in all rooms. Tea and coffee facilities. Ward or dining room meal service. Re-admission and parent education facilities. Plug-in mobile pay phones. Excellent school and play facilities. Parent support sister available office hours with on call facility.

New Town District General Paediatric Unit**
Lower Portman Street Children's Hospital, London***
Ashburn Children's Hospital**
The Royal Hospital for Sick Children, Brighton****

Figure 1.1 The National Institute of Consumers Guide to Children's Hospitals and Units.

questions and of forced choice Likent scale questions, in which parents were asked if they strongly agreed, agreed, disagreed or strongly disagreed with numerous statements. The questionnaire looks at many areas of paediatric nursing care and covers aspects of structure, process and outcome. Consumer satisfaction surveys represent one of many methodologies by which information related to quality can be obtained. Single criteria such as those used in commercial organisations are inadequate for measuring the effectiveness of a health care system.

The advent of the new management structure in the health service has concentrated on economy, efficiency and effectiveness. Thus consumer satisfaction represents one facet of this philosophy.

RESULTS OF THE SURVEY

Following a pilot study involving ten families on four wards a main study was undertaken using forty families from each ward. The ward clerks, whom we felt to be the best people to administer the questionnaires, did so to the first forty discharges from their wards. Total anonymity was guaranteed and completed questionnaires were placed in special posting boxes on a table away from the nurse's station.

Overall the results of the questionnaire demonstrated that parents were satisfied with the care they and their children received. Although one has to be aware of the inherent 'halo' effect of this type of consumer research, it is possible to gain much valuable data.

Parents in the sample enjoyed being able to stay with their children in hospital. Across the four wards overall, nursing care was rated as excellent by two-thirds of

For the following statements please check the response which most closely reflects your opinion.	1 *Strongly Disagree*	2 *Disagree*	3 *Agree*	4 *Strongly Agree*
1. I received consistent information/instructions from each nurse caring for my child during the hospital stay.				
2. I was given adequate information about my child's ward.				
3. I received no information about hospital rules and procedures that might have applied to my family and me.				
4. The nurses always responded to my requests promptly.				
5. The nurses and I discussed how my child's illness or hospitalisation would affect me and my family.				
6. The nurses always asked if I understood what the doctor told me.				
7. I always had trouble getting a nurse when I needed one.				
8. The nurses asked me what I would like to know about my child's illness or hospitalisation.				
9. I feel confident in the nurses caring for my child.				
10. The nurses protected my child's privacy.				
11. I feel confident that I can manage my child's care at home after discharge.				
12. All the nurses caring for my child were familiar with the care he/she needed.				
13. The nurses fully involved me in the planning of my child's nursing care and in the writing of the care plan.				
14. I had to answer a lot of the same questions about my child's needs many times.				
15. If my child was fearful or anxious during any procedures the nurse attempted to reassure, comfort and calm him/her.				
16. I feel the nurses would be willing to stay with my child if he/she was worried or upset about something.				
17. The nurses talked with me and my family about what we could expect to happen during my child's hospitalisation.				
18. I received adequate information about tests and procedures from my child's nurses.				
19. My child received explanation from the nurse that he/she could understand before any procedure was started.				
20. The nurses never asked me how I would prefer my child's care to be carried out.				
21. The nurses helped me feel comfortable in participating in my child's care.				
22. The nurses attended to my child's likes and dislikes as best they could.				
23. The nurses showed genuine interest and concern for my child.				
24. I felt comfortable asking the nurses any questions.				

25. Did you stay with your child during the hospital admission?   YES/NO

If Yes, was it: a) on the ward
                  b) in a cubicle
                  c) in Victoria House?

26. What in your opinion was most helpful to you during the period of time your child was in Hospital? Please comment:

27. What could have made the hospital stay better for you as a parent/guardian? Please comment:

28. How would you rate your child's nursing care on this ward?
     A   Excellent   C   Fair
     B   Good   D   Poor

29. Date today ....

Your additional comments would be most welcome. Thank you.

Figure 1.2 Parental Questionnaire.

the parents. Communication was perceived as problematic by some parents on all the children's wards. In particular, parents highlighted the problem of not receiving sufficient information about hospital rules and procedures.

Barbarin and Chesler (1984) have commented that in areas where staff–client relationships are good, quality of care was better than in those where interpersonal relationships were poor. Their study demonstrated that parents' respect for medical staff was strongly related to their interpersonal skills. Parents of children in hospital have an insatiable need for information. Attempts to provide information through improved communication may produce more co-operative families. Good communication helps minimise the disturbance caused by a child's admission to hospital, and any attempts to improve this should be explored.

Following the results of this pre-quality assurance exercise a pre-admission programme was introduced in order to address the parentally perceived problem of poor communication. Although parents on the whole appeared satisfied with the nursing care of their children, it was salutary to note that less than half the parents on all four wards were involved in any way with the planning of their children's care. Despite ten years of the nursing process, the idea that parents are equal partners in care is merely given lip-service. Parental involvement in the planning of care could have been greater, especially as all parents surveyed were involved to some degree in the provision of care.

These comments were fed back to the wards in a written report and it was hoped to reassess the principal issues following the first formal quality assurance exercise later that year.

It is important when undertaking surveys such as this that staff feel fully involved. A bottom-up approach will always be more successful than a top-down one. Where possible, quality assurance exercises should be undertaken by nurses who will not be perceived as pawns of 'management'. What should be fostered is a healthy peer review, which facilitates and augments the concept of reflective practice and highlights the desirability that paediatric units become fully self-evaluating.

The survey proved to be a useful precursor to the forthcoming quality assurance audit, as it helped prepare the staff, who naturally had some reservations. Many believed that the exercise would be a time-and-motion study; some believed it to be a form of staff appraisal; while others believed it to be a sinister tool of management designed to weed out less than perfect staff. Such an atmosphere, common in many units about to be audited, needs to be tackled head on before the exercise starts. Failure to spend time on this can only result in failure, for without staff co-operation any quality assurance exercise is doomed before it begins. The importance of peer review and reflective practice must be made clear to colleagues; so a number of workshops were held several months before the exercise. During these preliminary meetings the major fear (that the audit was just another type of staff appraisal) was discussed and dismissed to the satisfaction of all in attendance. Once this hurdle has been cleared, the serious work of planning an exercise can begin.

The path to full audit had commenced in late 1987, and in the spring of 1989 following the parent satisfaction survey, the first unit audit was undertaken. This was decided by the clinical nursing staff of the paediatric unit, and not the management team. The decisions may have come slowly but the investment in time paid dividends in that all clinical staff saw themselves as part of the initiation process.

PRE-FORMULATED AUDIT TOOLS

Pre-formulated audit tools can facilitate an assessment of the quality of nursing care on paediatric wards, one of which (Junior Monitor, derived from the Rush Medius system) was designed by Gallstone and Ball. There has been an increasing recognition in Britain of the need for work on quality. Of particular influence has been the implementation of Griffiths-style management, with an emphasis on cost-effectiveness. At the same time, the public have become more knowledgeable and have increasing expectations of the Health Service. Junior Monitor addresses these two developments.

Junior Monitor, in essence, seeks to establish minimum competences on a number of pre-stated standard statements.

One of the most frequently used frameworks for looking at quality of care was developed by Donabedian (1976). This is based on three distinct but interrelated factors: structure, process and outcome. Structure looks at the environmental and resource items and their organisation; process refers to the planning and delivery of interventions; and outcome is concerned with the result of care. Junior Monitor, and the standards embodied in it, are much vaguer than those suggested by Donabedian, but they can be considered as criteria for perhaps more specific standards which have the potential for being developed further at local level. Despite the vagueness, the criteria, which are expressed as questions to be asked during the audit/exercise, cover a lot of ground and can seem quite daunting at first. They are divided into the following:

Section A Planning nursing care. This includes the admission assessment.
Section B Meeting the child's physical needs. This includes protecting the child from accident and injury.

Section C Meeting the child's non-physical needs. This includes psycho-social and emotional needs.

Section D Evaluation of nursing care objectives.

The package is tied in with the nursing process and its use in areas where the nursing process is poorly done, if at all, would be a waste of time.

The underlying premise of Junior Monitor and most other audit tools is that all care is fully documented. Herein lies the drawback in the design of such packages in that they assume that all care will be documented. For unlike Britain, in North America care is recorded. (The high levels of litigation in North America may help explain this.)

So the interesting question posed by this concerns whether or not lack of documented care in Britain implies that no care is being given. The anti-intellectual and somewhat pragmatic stance of some clinical nurses in the United Kingdom would suggest that they are more interested in 'doing' nursing than writing about it. If the only valid care delivered is recorded care, then this is belied by the results of patient satisfaction questionnaires.

The numerical scoring system of Junior Monitor is entirely geared to documented care. In other words, if it is not documented it does not gain a score. This leads to an overall reduction in the total. It is thus possible for a ward renowned for its excellent nursing care to be awarded an overall low score using this system. This is the major flaw of the system. (See Figure 1.3.)

Dependency Category	Mean	Overall Mean
1. No patients	–	
2. 49%, 61%	55%	
3. 52%, 54.5%, 49%	52%	51%
4. 31%, 32%, 77%	46.5%	
A. Planning Nursing Care		24.175%
B. Meeting Child's Physiological Needs		63.8%
C. Psycho/Socio/Emotional Needs		69.3%
D. Evaluation		61.8%

Figure 1.3 Parental Questionnaire.

HOW TO USE PRE-FORMULATED AUDIT TOOLS

Once the staff consultation phase is complete, a number of novice auditors need to be selected and trained. The auditors should possess a recognised paediatric nursing qualification, and should not work on the ward to be audited. The ward should have no prior warning of the audit exercise. On the morning of the exercise a ward should be randomly chosen and the ward sister or charge nurse informed.

It is helpful for the auditors to be present during the early morning handover as the first task is to allocate each child to a dependency category. Once the children have been allocated, the auditors randomly select 50 per cent of the total for 20+ bedded wards. It is usually possible to audit a total of ten children in the course of a normal working day. The category containing the most children will command the greatest scrutiny, although all categories represented in the sample will be audited.

As mentioned earlier, much of the document measures written aspects of care. To enable the auditors to progress with reasonable speed, it is economical for them to collect as much written information as they can about the child they intend auditing. It should be highlighted at this stage that informed consent should be obtained from the parent and child where appropriate. When the admission documents, care plans, nursing records, drug charts, etc., have been collected, the audit can begin and the questions answered. Most auditors prefer answering the documentation-type questions first and the simple yes/no format facilitates a quick and easy rationale. Questions such as 'Is the child weighed on admission?' can easily be answered when all the documentation is to hand. Once the documentation-type questions have been answered, the auditors visit the clinical area to answer the remaining questions, some of which involve talking to the child and/or parent and the nurse responsible for that child's care. For ease of scoring, the auditor should group together all the questions for the nurse caring for a particular child.

The time taken with each patient audited will vary, but operators should allow at least $1\frac{1}{2}$–2 hours.

SCORING

Each of the four sections of the audit document is scored separately and generates subscores for each child. The majority of the questions have four possible responses: Yes/No/Not applicable/Not available. Responses which demand a 'yes always' or 'yes complete' response score 1, 'yes sometimes' and 'yes incomplete' score $\frac{1}{2}$. A 'no' response scores 0.

Scoring can be agonisingly slow for the novice auditor and each question will be dissected, examined and finally answered, but often at the expense of time. There is no doubt that a practice dummy-run is essential, as is the accrued wisdom of an experienced auditor. Despite the advice given in the audit document, it is important for the auditors to be registered children's nurses and have experience in the care of children. This will help ensure at least some degree of inter-rater reliability among the paediatric staff. Peer review and reflective practice will always be preferable to management reviews.

ANALYSIS OF DATA

It is important to score and analyse the data as quickly as possible as 'knowledge of result' is in itself a good motivator. First, the non-applicable responses should be subtracted from the total number of questions in each of the sub-sections. This allows the number of applicable responses to be calculated. The total score for each section will, therefore, be obtained by adding all 'yes' responses (score 1) and the other lesser value responses (score $\frac{1}{2}$). This total is divided by the number of applicable responses and multiplied by 100 to obtain a percentage index. This procedure is repeated for each child in each section to obtain a sum of scores which can then be computed to obtain the mathematical mean for each section. This computation can be further manipulated to obtain the mean scores for each dependency category. If all the children's scores used in the audit are added together, the mean of these scores gives the ward index. The instructions contained in the audit document are clear, and easy to follow.

PRESENTATION OF DATA AND THE CONSTRUCTION OF THE ANNUAL REPORT

The ward index in itself is merely a figure. This can be presented as a summation of all children audited, or of each individual dependency group. Expressing nursing care in numbers is always dangerous and it should never be assumed that it is possible to do so. Pollitt (1984) describes the use of blunt tools in the measurement of health care performance, and certainly Qualpaeds is a relatively crude instrument. That does not mean that it has no place in clinical practice, but rather that it is not an end in itself. The accompanying report, which augments the ward index, is extremely valuable to the nurses working on the audited ward, especially if it is constructed by peers. The written report allows flesh to be put on the bones of the rather stark list of figures and percentages.

In compiling the written report, the auditors should examine the means of each section of the Qualpaeds document. The report should describe the data accurately and should offer both praise and constructive criticism. Subsections can be explored and, where there is a lot of 'no' scores, this can be addressed heading by heading. The strength of the accompanying report lies in its ability to inform wards of their strengths and weaknesses. It must be remembered that the tool measures overall performance, not individual nursing actions. Quality assurance should never be used and has no place in staff appraisal. If full co-operation of staff is to be anticipated, this must be fully explained. Ward sisters and charge nurses deserve to have more information about the outcome of the audit than the simple breakdown of figures. It may well be that the ward index is a prelude to the audit report, which should be rich in detail where appropriate. The total package of the ward audit should assist practitioners in their quest for excellence; it should not hinder them. It is possible that certain clinical areas will be good at certain aspects of nursing, but fail in others (e.g. wards may demonstrate excellent standards of physical care but score less in areas of psycho/social care). Such discrepancies need to be highlighted in the report. Overall the report should be clear and concise and leave the reader in no doubt about the steps to be taken in order to achieve greater scores in a subsequent audit.

ACTING ON THE ANNUAL AUDIT

The ward indices and accompanying report should be written as soon after the audit as possible. Failure to do so will result in an unacceptable delay in the debriefing exercise, which is essential to the degree of success of any quality assurance exercise.

The language used in the construction of the report should be moderate. It is very easy to appear over-critical. Full co-operation of the ward staff is essential, and harsh criticism will not endear the auditors to the staff. Any areas of concern should be handled sensitively.

The object of the exercise is to allow ward staff to gain greater insight into their care practices, i.e. to facilitate reflective practice. A meeting should be arranged between the auditors and the ward staff to examine the ramifications of the audit report and ward index. Full and frank discussion should be encouraged and this will facilitate the formation of objectives to be achieved prior to the following year's audit.

CONCLUSION

As an audit tool 'off-the-shelf' packages leave a lot to be desired but they represent a genuine attempt to measure the quality of nursing care in children's wards. However, nurses who identify their own values, write their own standards and then acknowledge their professional accountability by using their own audit tools, will derive greater satisfaction and enhance the care they give.

REFERENCES

Ball M, Glasper A and Yerrell P (1988) How well do we perform? Parents' perceptions of pae-
diatric care. *Professional Nurse*, **4**(3), December.
Barbarin O and Chesler M A (1984) Relationships with medical staff and aspects of satisfaction
with care expressed by parents of children with cancer. *Journal of Community Health*, **9**(4),
302–13.
Collard R (1989) *Total Quality: Success through People*. London: Institute of Personnel
Management.
Donabedian A (1976) Measures of quality of care. *American Journal of Nursing*, **70**(2), 186.
Harris I (1990) Quality assurance makes sense. *Nursing Times*, **86**(8), 21 February.
Macdonald J and Piggott J (1990) *Global Quality: The New Management Culture*. London:
Gold Arrow Publications.
Maddison M (1977) Consumer survey of paediatric wards. *Australian Nurses Journal*, **6**(1),
27–8.
Pollitt C (1984) Blunt tools: performance measurement in policies for health care. *Journal of
Management Science*, **12**(2), 131–40.
Roberts I (1975) *Discharged from Hospital*. London: RCN.
Royal College of Nursing (1990) Quality Patient Care – *The Dynamic Standard Setting System*.
London: RCN.
Vorley G (1991) *Quality Assurance Management*. Kent: George Over Ltd.

2

A Play Programme

Nicola Eaton

INTRODUCTION

Play is often claimed to be the work of the child. All children play; it is a vital part of their development. Play can strengthen personality, encourage interpersonal relations, further creativity and increase learning (Caplan and Caplan, 1973). The concept of play is familiar but difficult to define. Garvey (1977) lists the criteria that most observers use to define play:

1. Play is pleasurable and enjoyable.
2. Play has no extrinsic goals, the child's motivations are subjective and serve no practical purpose.
3. Play is spontaneous and voluntary and chosen by the player.
4. Play involves some active engagement on the part of the player.

This chapter discusses the play needs of children and the provision of play in hospital. It then describes a computer program developed to help nurses to decide on and meet the play needs of children in their care.

PLAY AS A GENERAL TOPIC

Play is about discovery, acquiring and perfecting new skills, both social and motor skills, expressing personality. It can be work or relaxation, fun or serious, and is a natural way of learning and interacting with the environment.

All children need to play; it is an essential part of their intellectual, social and emotional development and not a purposeless activity merely to pass the time (Platt Report, 1959). This is how they discover the world and their own capabilities. Play can be divided into categories such as creative, imaginative, therapeutic, social, and rough-and-tumble play.

The play of boys and girls is similar, but boys are more likely to engage in more rough-and-tumble play, which is vigorous and often aggressive. Girls are more likely to engage in play with social themes.

TYPES OF PLAY

Physical play involves activity and using energy to move and control the head, limbs and body. Such activities as bicycle riding, climbing, running and jumping are all physical types of play.

Intellectual play, also called educational or cognitive play, involves problem-solving through trial and error. Construction kits, jigsaws and computer games all feature in intellectual play.

In exploratory play children practise hand skills, often through repetition. They use their senses to discover new things and reinforce knowledge. It is widely thought that exploratory behaviours reflect the infant's early interest in mastering its environment and is considered a vehicle of cognitive development (Jennings et al., 1979).

Creative play can be messy as the child explores new substances and creates some-thing real or from fantasy. It may utilise paint, dough, sand, water or mud, and involve cutting and sticking as in model-making or collage. Constructive play is prob-ably the most common form of activity during the preschool and kindergarten years. Up to 40 per cent of all activity at $3\frac{1}{2}$ years and 51 per cent at 4, 5 and 6 years is in constructive play (Rubin et al., 1983).

Imaginative play may involve imitation and make-believe, and involves looking, listening and remembering. Communication and creativity are also involved. Small figures, cars, trains and animals may be used in imaginative play, or the child takes on a particular role, such as the mother, soldier or train driver, and acts this out. The imaginative play world is made by the child for the child and as such gives him a sense of mastery. Some children go so far as to invent an imaginary friend. Usually this imaginary friend is another child but sometimes is an animal. In a study at Yale involving 210 children, 41 had imaginary friends, 30 of which were human and 11 animal. Most of the children were aged 3 or 4 years (with 50 per cent being under 5) and half were only children. Imaginary friends are usually thought to be the compa-nions of only children but seem to depend more on the imagination of the child rather than on his being lonely or dissatisfied. Most 'friends' were companions, but in a few cases the 'friend' was allowed to do things which the child was not; they were weak and either bossed or cared for by the child. The interpretation given to this behaviour was that the imaginary friend gave the child the opportunity to express impulses maturing at the time. Terman, in his study of gifted children (554, aged from 6 to 13), found that 85 per cent of the girls and 51 per cent of the boys had had imaginary playmates at some time (cited in Valentine, 1975).

Wolf and Grollman (1982) categorised children into dramatists and patterners. Children who use toys to act out scenes in which they play the role of another are categorised as dramatists. Patterners are those children who use their toys to form patterns or designs.

HISTORY OF PLAY

Throughout history play has been recognised as an activity which children indulge in and it has been at various times promoted or discouraged. Plato advised against forced learning and encouraged play instead. Aristotle thought that children should play at what they would do seriously as an adult, e.g. play at being a farmer or a carpenter. Various writers during the eighteenth and nineteenth centuries looked on play as restoring or utilising excess energy. The German Froebel, known as the 'apostle of play', was the founder of the kindergarten movement. He insisted that children learn through spontaneous play. Hall, an American working in the nineteenth century, evolved capitulation theory, which states that from conception to adulthood children re-enact in play the interests and occupations in the sequence in which they occurred in prehistoric and primitive man. Groos thought that play was biologically valuable for children and young animals as a preparation for more serious activities later in life (Valentine, 1975).

THEORIES OF PLAY

Play helps a child to develop physically, socially, emotionally and intellectually, and can be solitary, in parallel with other children, or a group activity. During the twentieth century theories regarding the role of play in the physical and mental development of children have been put forward. There is general agreement about the importance of play. If the child's development is abnormal, play therapy is viewed as a tool for correcting maladjustment.

Sigmund Freud's *psychoanalytic theory* of play was posited from the belief that behaviour is motivated by the subconscious. In children play is the acting out of conflicts or unpleasant events in order to overcome the anxiety and fear these produce. Thus play can be studied as revealing something about the 'inner life' and motivations of the individual. Projective techniques such as making up stories to inkblots or pictures have been used for this purpose.

Melanie Klein (1930) adapted Freud's theories to play therapy when working with children. She initiated the use of a playroom at her clinic. She equated the free play of children with the free association of adults and looked for symbolic meanings within it. With direct and often deep interpretations, she tried to provide insight into the child/parent relationship. Klein suggested that play could be used from an early age to understand the child's traumas and perhaps resolve them. The children were viewed as problems to be solved.

This early play therapy is still closely tied to the conventional verbal relationship between the patient and therapist. This form of therapy has since been criticised, as understanding and interpretation are both difficult and sometimes dangerous; attributing deeper meaning to play needs care.

Cohen (1987) believes that from her work, 'we know all about the stages of "emotional" play in abnormal children, far more than we do about the normal child.'

Anna Freud (1946) questioned Kleinian play and suggested that it was inappropriate to look for the symbolic significance underlying all the child's actions. The therapist's behaviour and choice of toys would also influence the child's behaviour. Instead, Freud emphasised the importance of the child's environment outside the therapeutic setting; she felt that the child was reacting to the present rather than transferring to the analyst experiences from the past. For Anna Freud the target for change was the child's inappropriate behaviour, rather than his inner psyche. Emphasis was put on the quality of the relationship between the child and the therapist, an atmosphere of acceptance and warmth created. But the therapist was still using play as a diagnostic tool.

Cognitive theorists see play as an extension of the theory of intellectual development. It is seen as a window on the workings of the child's mind, an external manifestation of his cognitive processes. Piaget (1951) used play to indicate the thought processes of the child in his four stages of development:

1. Sensori-motor (0–2 years): children engage in mastery and practice play, they must master limb control to attract the attention of their care-giver.
2. Pre-operational (2–7 years): symbolic or make-believe play reflects the child's increasing experience and imagination. Children are also learning to communicate symbolically through language.
3. Concrete operational (7–12 years): in this stage children learn how to play within rules imposed by others, they are now more sociable, learning about give-and-take and rights and responsibilities.
4. Abstract thought (12 years to adult): mental operations can now be logical, abstract and formal, philosophical arguments to which facts are not relevant are possible, competitiveness is increased in this stage.

Later work has suggested that some of the tests Piaget (1962) used to demonstrate these stages and concept development within them were too abstract and were misunderstood by the children. Cohen suggests that 'after Piaget's pioneering work, too much effort has been devoted to isolating the cognitive aspects of play, without any consideration of the actual environment it blossoms in' (Cohen, 1987, p. 59).

Another criticism of the cognitive theory of play is that it does not take account of the active way in which the child uses his own model of the world to make sense of his experience. However, children who engage in a lot of fantasy play have been shown to be more socially competent, assertive and skilled in understanding other people's perspectives than children of comparable intelligence and sociability who indulge in less fantasy play (Connelly, Doyle and Ceschin, 1983).

Kelly's construct theory views the child as a problem-solver. The child tries things out and learns from experience; he is constantly generating new hypotheses about the environment and trying them out. These hypotheses are bipolar entities called constructs, which are developed according to individual experience (Kelly, 1955). This differs from Piaget's view in that there can be no absolute reality, as everyone experiences and makes sense of the world in their own way. The child has the potential to develop further at his own rate as the constructs become invalidated and have to be reconstrued. Thus children can be seen as problem-solvers and not immature thinkers. Emotional problems are not so much reactive as active attempts to solve problems with the available tools. Their behaviour reflects strategies that they adopt in order to make sense of the world.

STAGES OF PLAY

In the course of their development children usually pass through the following stages in their play activity:

1. symbolic or make-believe play;
2. solitary play;
3. parallel play; children under 3 tend to concentrate on parallel play. This is where

two or three children may be using the same toys in the same area but they are playing independently alongside each other.

4. Play with rules.

'Free play' is the ideal form of play for most children. They are free to play with what they want how they want, for as long as they want, with the minimum of adult interference. This type of play gives the child confidence, encourages concentration and mental development, and allows the child to follow through ideas. The role of the adult in free play is to provide a safe environment and facilities, to respect the child and the play, allow the child to play without interference, encourage the slow or shy child, and help language development by talking to the child.

Work by anthropologists and psychologists suggests that play promotes cognitive development. Studies appear to indicate that children who have no toys and little opportunity to play have delayed cognitive development. Children from economically disadvantaged families engage in less pretend play at playschool than middle-class children. Anthropologists also suggest that there are important cultural and class differences in the extent that children play (Mussen *et al.*, 1990).

PLAY FOR SICK CHILDREN

When a child is admitted to hospital he is removed from all that is familiar – his family, pets, friends and his normal environment and routine. He may also be afraid and in pain. To help the child to cope with this new experience, links need to be made between the new experience of hospital and the normal experience of home. While the medical staff prescribe treatment to aid his recovery, the nurses, play staff and teachers help him to make sense of these new experiences. Having familiar objects and toys and playing with domestic pets will help.

In 1972 the DHSS set up an expert group to determine how to meet the needs of the child for play in hospital. One third of the group were nurses, and the rest doctors, teachers, psychologists, administrators and others. The group was unanimous that a new discipline of 'play workers' should be formed and that neither nurses nor volunteers on their own could carry out this work. The initial target should be one play worker for each children's ward and one for each children's outpatient session to help the children in the waiting area. This does not reject the skill of, or the necessity for, the nurse in these areas to play with the children (Jolly, 1976). When the report was first published it was accompanied by a circular which disputed the recommendations – the reason given was lack of finance. Later, a further circular from the government accepted the recommendations of the report.

One way in which hospitalised children can maintain some normality is to continue to play. As the child is less likely to be his normal lively self there will probably be less energetic, rough-and-tumble play, but more activities such as creative and problem-solving play, especially if pretend play is encouraged. The child may have more time on his hands for skilful play or hobbies. However, the activities of the ward may be a distraction to the child and his concentration span may be limited. Also, the effects of an illness or treatment (such as an intravenous infusion) may limit his motor capabilities. Play which involves emotions is important in hospital as it allows the expression of frustration or anger. Clay or dough or wooden hammering toys are good for helping to express this. Musical instruments too can help the child to express feelings through objects rather than taking them out on people. Also during hospital play children are able to work through some of their deeper fears and anxieties about illness and dying.

Harvey and Hales-Tooke (1972) identify some ways in which play can help hospitalised children to deal with the distress, pain, anxiety and even boredom which they will encounter:

1. Through play children can give expression to their fears, worries and aggressive feelings, their hopes and their efforts to overcome disabilities.
2. Children can keep alive their warm and loving feelings for their families and friends.
3. They can continue to grow and develop normally while in hospital.
4. Play can promote health and happiness and combat boredom.
5. Confidence can be built up that the hospital is not merely a place of pain and misery. Play helps to make the hospital seem a more friendly, relaxed and homely place.
6. Play is an antidote to the atmosphere of cleanliness and orderliness in the hospital.
7. Play helps children to confirm that they are in 'working order' after operations and illnesses, and not permanently damaged.
8. In play friendships are formed and problems shared. Older children take pleasure from caring for babies and toddlers.
9. Play can promote concentration and provide opportunities for learning through exploration and experiment.
10. Play can take place wherever the child is, in bed or up, and whether sick or well, of whatever age group.

HOSPITAL PLAY

Hospital dressing-up clothes, such as nurses' uniforms and doctors' white coats, and equipment such as syringes (without needles) and stethoscopes, are often a part of the play provision on wards. However, an adult needs to be nearby to correct misinterpretations and answer questions. Even children up to 10 or 11 years need truthful but simple explanations, which may need to be repeated or put into a story.

Play can be used to prepare a child for investigations such as blood tests, intravenous therapy, surgery and plaster of paris application.

Nursing students may have difficulty in talking to children, and often do not know how to play with them. Is playing with a child work? Student nurses may also have difficulty choosing appropriate toys for children of different ages and conditions. The program developed and explained later (pp. 22–5) was an attempt to address this problem.

A vital part of a nurse's duty on the children's ward is playing with children, and it has been observed that they play more when the ward has a play specialist (Jolly,

1976). However, the nurses cannot be the sole players, and when they have to care for many children, play suffers.

PRE-HOSPITAL VISITS

It has been estimated that 25 per cent of all children have had a stay in hospital before they are 5 (Butler, 1980). For this reason many hospitals have developed pre-hospital admission visits, when parents and children visit the hospital, perhaps to watch a video about preparation for surgery or the daily workings of the ward. The children may also experience riding on a theatre trolley, playing with hospital equipment (made safe if necessary) and dressing up in a nurse's uniform or doctor's white coat. These sessions, often organised by ward staff and play leaders, are an important way to give children and parents information and to equip parents with knowledge so that they can continue to prepare their child appropriately. Work by Jessner et al. (1952) showed that if the parents were prepared, their children's post-operative anxiety was reduced. The preparation must be appropriate to the age, developmental stage and reason for admission of the child. Many children's books and cassette tapes are now available telling stories of favourite characters and their reactions to hospital visits and procedures. These, combined with a visit to the ward, make it easier for the child to anticipate the experience and begin to work through some of their anxieties.

Children's psychological growth and development may be adversely affected by hospitalisation (Golden, 1983) and they therefore need opportunities when they are hospitalised to ventilate their emotional stress. This is usually done through play, which may need to be guided. In hospital therapeutic play is thought to help children regain control, express feelings of anxiety and transform children from passive to active participants in their care (Thompson, 1988).

Phillips (1988), however, reported that the benefits of play therapy in hospital were overestimated. He reviewed work which looked at four categories of benefits of play therapy:

1. mastery, autonomy and control;
2. co-operation and communication;
3. coping with anxiety and fear;
4. learning and information giving.

He concluded that play therapy for hospitalised children has yet to be shown to be effective in practice. However, research since then has started to show that in areas such as information-giving and dealing with anxiety, play therapy may have a role to play. Research by Rae et al. (1988) compared the psychosocial adjustment of a group of hospitalised children. They were placed in one of four groups: (1) therapeutic play, (2) diversionary play, (3) verbal support, or (4) no intervention. After using at least five different data-collecting tools and rating scales, the researchers concluded that there was a reduction in the reported hospital-related fears of the children in the therapeutic play group. However, there appeared to be a difference between the self-reportings of the children's fears and their parents' rating of the same children's fears.

The conclusions to be drawn here about the role of play in hospital remain unclear; most research defines play, especially therapeutic play, in a different way and measures the outcomes in different ways.

PLAY THERAPY

True play therapy is not an area for the amateur. It is used with problem children, those with difficulties after divorce, behaviour problems or victims of abuse.

Play therapy is based on the idea that play is the child's natural medium of self-expression (Axline, 1947). It can be directive or non-directive. Non-directive therapy is based on the idea that the individual has within himself the ability to solve his own problems. A growth impulse makes mature behaviour more satisfying than immature behaviour. Non-directive therapy starts where the person is, and allows him to be himself. It does not seek to explain or interpret past behaviour, only to understand motivations for present behaviour. Non-directive play therapy, based on the work of Carl Rogers (1942), accepts the person as he is without pressure to change, recognises attitudes and emotions by reflecting what the client expresses; it offers the individual the opportunity to come to know himself and create a more satisfactory design for living. Non-directive play allows the child to have the opportunity through play to experience growth under favourable conditions. The child plays and his accumulated feelings of tension, frustration, insecurity, aggression, fear, bewilderment and confusion emerge. By playing the child brings these feelings to the surface, faces them, learns to control or abandon them. This leads to emotional relaxation. The child realises the power in himself and thinks for himself, makes his own decisions and in the process, matures. The therapist accepts the child as he is and does not rebuke, restrain, criticise or direct the child in his play or expressions. Play therapy can be in a group or individual situation.

Saucier (1989) studied abused children to examine the relationship between abuse, developmental achievement and play therapy. Twenty abused children, between 1 and 7 years, were given play therapy over an 8-week period. The results indicated a significant difference between abused children receiving play therapy and abused children not receiving play therapy in personal-social development (1 of 8 behaviour domains identified using the Minnesota Child Development Inventory (MCDI)). This study suggests that children who have been abused can benefit in the development of personal and social behaviour through therapeutic play.

DEVELOPMENT OF A PLAY PROGRAM

The next section of this chapter describes the development of a computer program designed to help nurses encourage children in hospital to play according to their needs and abilities. The author of this chapter is a paediatric nurse in an educational setting and also has an interest in the use of computers as a teaching medium.

Prompted by an interest in the development of an expert system and the topic of play for sick children a project was undertaken to marry the two together. The following section describes what an expert system is, explains the need for a program on play, how the program was developed and its envisaged future use.

EXPERTS AND EXPERT SYSTEMS

An expert is a person who has considerable knowledge of a particular field gained through formal and informal learning as well as experience (Frenzel, 1987). Experts use their knowledge widely to solve a variety of problems. Their extensive experience makes them extremely valuable to their employers and colleagues; experts can solve problems and make good decisions quickly. Experts are a rare commodity and consequently are much in demand. As everyone cannot be an expert in every topic an expert's knowledge and ability needs to be acquired in some other way. One way to resolve this problem would be to have more experts. When this is not possible, an expert must be 'cloned'. An expert system computer program can become a clone of an expert.

An expert system packages the knowledge of one or more experts in a specific domain into software that can operate on a computer. When an expert is needed the software is activated and problems put to it. There are many benefits to expert systems. These include:

1. Improved productivity: knowledge is available when needed to get the job done more quickly or accomplish more in the same time.
2. The preservation of knowledge: the expert is the prime resource in developing an expert system which embodies his or her knowledge. Should the expert be unavailable, his or her knowledge can still be used if it has been acquired and appropriately packaged into a useable expert system.
3. Improved understanding and learning: expert systems also help to understand how an expert goes about solving a problem or otherwise applying knowledge. Experts often take their knowledge for granted and never analyse the way they apply it. The developer of an expert system must interrogate the expert to discover how he or she uses the knowledge; this interrogation in turn helps to understand how the human mind reasons. An individual using the expert system to solve problems regularly is likely to increase his or her expertise and eventually become more like the expert. The expert system can be interrogated for the reasoning behind the advice given.

THE NEED FOR AN EXPERT SYSTEM FOR SICK CHILDREN

Play for the sick child is an often overlooked part of his care. The sick child's environment, age, abilities, developmental stage and illness or therapy all need to be taken into account when planning play. An experienced sick children's nurse will have the skills to encourage the child to play. These nurses will take all the above factors into account (often assessing the child intuitively) and choose play activities with the child. For example, a child with asthma may need to have a play scheme developed, which encourages the expansion of his chest. Games here may involve blowing bubbles or balloons or feather games. A child who has a leg in traction may be encouraged to throw bean bags at a target as a method of releasing frustrations and energy.

It was decided to develop an expert system which can advise the less experienced nurse about the play needs of sick or handicapped children. The expert system was also envisaged as a teaching aid for student nurses.

THE DEVELOPMENT OF THE SYSTEM

Many of the above descriptions of expert systems involved the developers in writing the expert systems from scratch. However, recently, Expert System Shells have been developed. An Expert System Shell is a collection of programs which enable an expert system to be developed without using a programming language.

The shell used for the play program was Crystal. It was chosen because it was available on both a mainframe and a microcomputer, and the author and the computer scientist involved had access to one or both of these. The Crystal Expert System builder lets the user build systems using rule-based programming. It is for personal computers and has many useful facilities for program development. The development rules are highly structured, and the conclusions and actions are described together with the conditions which lead to them or the commands which carry them out. Editing facilities like the dictionary speed up the finding, copying and moving of sets of rules.

Development of the program started in October 1989 and irregular meetings went on over the next six months between two or all the three members of the team. Developing the program took many hours as the two experts (both qualified paediatric nurses with a special interest in play) needed to be interrogated in such a way that their knowledge was incorporated in the expert system shell. Initially, the thought processes of the experts were investigated to determine how they decide on a play activity for a sick child. They took such things as the ability of the child, his age, his need for activity or his therapy into account. They also discussed why they would rule out some play topics and how they would discard some topics as being outside the child's capabilities.

Lists were drawn up to put into the shell. These included: 'type of game', 'general purpose', 'psychological purpose', 'physical purpose', 'social purpose', 'intellectual purpose', 'constraints', 'treatment constraints' and 'other constraints'. A maximum of 22 items was allowed in each list. For example, treatment constraints included none, intravenous infusion, plaster of paris, dressings, in bed, etc.

The program, when run, asks for basic details such as the name and age of the child, then goes on to ask questions relating to each list it has stored. If the answer to a question is negative to the initial list question, the program goes to the next list. If the answer is positive, the program asks more questions until it can start to match its lists and output a suggested list of play activities for the specific child. At any stage in the proceedings the program can be asked 'why' by the user, and it will explain why a particular question was asked and how it relates to the present hypothesis being followed. The output can also contain a list of play activities discarded and explain why.

The system has not yet been evaluated, but it is intended as both a teaching aid and as a ward-based tool. The lists are still under-developed due to time constraints. This is an exciting new development in the use of expert systems for nursing and further development and evaluation is to continue.

CONCLUSIONS

The purpose of this chapter has been to present a selected literature review of play of normal and sick children, outline play therapy, define an expert system and describe the early development of an expert system on play for sick children. The literature on expert systems and the discussion of the early nursing systems show that they have the potential to aid in medical and nursing diagnosis. It is not intended that they should take over the skilled parts of the work but should be used as knowledge aids to help in decision-making, and as teaching tools. The human experts are still needed to develop more programs and in so doing stay one step ahead of the machines. Computers cannot yet be programmed for 'common sense', so there will always be a need for the human element.

The expert system on play for sick children, although still in the early stages, promises to be an area of fruitful research in paediatric nursing in the future.

REFERENCES

Axline V (1947) *Play Therapy*. London: Churchill Livingstone.
Butler N (1980) Child health and education in the seventies: Some results on the five-year follow-up of the 1970 British birth cohorts. *Health Visitor*, **53**, 81.
Caplan F and Caplan T (1973) *The Power of Play*. New York: Anchor Press/Doubleday.
Cohen D (1987) *The Development of Play*. London: Croom Helm.
Connelly J, Doyle A B and Ceschin F (1983) Forms and functions of social fantasy play in preschoolers. In Liss M B (Ed.) *Social and Cognitive Skills: Sex Roles and Children's Play*. New York: Academic Press.
Frenzel L E (1987) *Understanding Expert Systems*. Indiana: Howard Sams & Co.
Freud A (1946) *The Psychoanalytic Treatment of Children*. London: Imago.
Garvey C (1977) *Play*. London: Fontana.
Golden D B (1983) Play therapy for hospitalised children. In Schaefer C and O'Connor K (Eds) *Handbook of Play Therapy*. New York: Wiley.
Harvey S and Hales-Tooke A (1972) *Play in Hospital*. London: Faber.
Jennings K D, Harmon R J, Morgan G A, Gaiter J L and Yarrow L J (1979) Exploratory play as an index of motivation: Relationships to persistence, cognitive functioning, and environmental measures. *Developmental Psychology*, **15**, 386–94.
Jessner L, Blom G E and Waldfogel S (1952) Emotional implications of tonsillectomy and adenoidectomy in children. In Eissler R S, Hartmann H, Freud A and Ketis E (Eds) *The Psychoanalytic Study of the Child* (7). New York: International Universities Press.
Jolly J (1976) Why children must be allowed to play in hospital. *The Times*, 21 April.

Kelly G (1955) *The Psychology of Personal Constructs*. New York: W W Norton.

Klein M (1930) *The Psychoanalysis of Children*. London: Hogarth Press.

Mussen P H, Conger J J, Kagan J and Huston A C (1990) *Child Development and Personality* (7th edn). London: Harper & Row.

Phillips R D (1988) Play therapy in health care settings: Promises never kept? *Children's Health Care* **16**, 182–7.

Piaget J (1951) *Play, Dreams and Imitation in Childhood*. London: Routledge & Kegan Paul.

Piaget J (1962) *Play, Dreams and Imitation*. Norton: New York.

Platt Report (1959) *The Welfare of Children in Hospital*. London: HMSO.

Rae W A, Worchel F F, Upchurch J, Scanner J H and Daniel C A (1988) The psychosocial impact of play on hospitalised children. *Journal of Paediatric Psychology*, **14**(4), 617–27.

Rogers C (1942) *Counselling and Psychotherapy: Newer Concepts in Practice*. Boston: Houghton.

Rubin K, Fein G and Vandenberg B (1983) Play. In Mussen P *Handbook of Child Psychology*, **4**. New York: John Wiley.

Saucier B (1989) The effects of play therapy on developmental achievement levels of abused children. *Pediatric Nursing* Jan/Feb, **15**(1).

Thompson R H (1988) From questions to answers: Approaches to studying play in health care settings. *Children's Health Care*, **16**, 188–94.

Valentine C W (1975) *The Normal Child and Some of His Abnormalities*. Harmondsworth: Penguin.

Wolf D P and Grollman S H (1982) Ways of playing. *Contributions to Human Development*, **6**, 46–63.

ORGANISATIONS INVOLVED WITH PLAY AND CHILDREN

NAHPS   National Association of Hospital Play Staff, Thomas Coram Foundation, 40 Brunswick Square, London WC1N 1AU

NAWCH   *Now* Action for Sick Children, *formerly* National Association for the Welfare of Children in Hospital, Argyle House, 29–31 Euston Road, London NW1 2SD

NCB   National Children's Bureau, 8 Wakley Street, London EC1V 7QE

PPA   Pre-School Playgroups Association, 61 Kings Cross Road, London WC1X 9LN

SCF   Save the Children Fund, 17 Grove Lane, London SE5 8SP

3

Children's Hospices

Sister Frances Dominica and Ann Hunt

HELEN

Sister Frances Dominica

In order to describe the innovation of hospice care in paediatrics it seems important to tell the story of one child in some detail. It is fourteen years since the mother of a critically ill child telephoned to ask if she could talk to me. I drove to the hospital and she introduced herself as Helen's mother. The friendship which ensued resulted in the opening of Helen House, the first known children's hospice, some four years later. All that I learnt from Helen and her family was, and continues to be, fundamental to our understanding of families whose child or children suffer from a life-threatening or life-limiting illness. It is thanks to them that we began to see ways of supporting such families through the devastation and tragedy they experience.

Helen was $2\frac{1}{2}$ years old when I first met her. Having been a happy, healthy, intelligent and loving little girl, she had suddenly become unwell. At first the family doctor had thought she was suffering from a mild infection which was prevalent in the neighbourhood. Then one day she was abnormally drowsy. Within hours she was diagnosed as having a massive cerebral tumour. She had major surgery the following day. By the time I met her, ten days later, she was out of the intensive care unit but remained unresponsive and critically ill.

In the months that followed I visited Helen and her parents in the hospital frequently. As a nurse I had much to learn; I was not there in a professional capacity but as a new friend. I quickly learnt that however articulate, skilled and self-assured you may feel in the normal course of events, once you are in hospital, either as a patient or someone close to that patient, you often feel inarticulate, deskilled and at the mercy of the professionals. I learnt that the moment in which a diagnosis with a poor prognosis is imparted is a moment forever impressed on the memory of patient or relative, and that the way in which it is imparted is of crucial importance. I learnt how essential it is that there are people on the team who care about the sick person as an individual even when that sick person is too ill to communicate or respond, and there were some such people there. I felt keenly for those on the ward team for whom 'failure' in terms of response to treatment was too painful to bear and yet it hurt when they failed to make eye contact with Helen's parents any more, or passed by the end of Helen's cot without pausing on a ward round, or resorted to superficial conversation when confrontation was inevitable. Waiting to be told the result of tests, I soon discovered, was often excruciating, and hours seemed like days and days like weeks.

Six months post-operatively brain scans showed severe, irreversible damage due to haemorrhage, and Helen's parents were told that there was nothing that could be done to promote their daughter's recovery. They had trusted in the skills and support of the hospital team during the acute phase of Helen's illness and they were very grateful. But now the situation was changing. They were convinced then, as now thirteen years later, that home is the ideal place for a child who cannot benefit from treatment aimed at recovery. They took her home two months after her third birthday. She is now sixteen and remains very frail, with no voluntary movement, no means of communication and minimal awareness. Seizures are only partially controlled by medication.

No child could be more greatly loved or more tenderly cared for than Helen is by her parents, helped by her two sisters who are three and five years younger than Helen. But the strain was, and is, immense. Night after night of broken sleep, days of anxiety and anguish, and the exhaustion resulting from long drawn out, unresolvable grief, all take their toll. Almost any parent who lives with the chronic life-limiting or life-threatening illness of their child will have the bitter experience of feeling isolated and lonely. Neighbours, friends, and even sometimes relatives, are less and less in evidence. They seem to cross the road to avoid encounter or disappear round the other side of the shelves in the supermarket. Neighbours who used to drop in casually no longer do so. People may sometimes ask how the child is – or how you are – but do not often stay long enough to hear the honest answer. The rational mind may recognise that such behaviour is not usually because people are uncaring but because they are embarrassed or fearful of saying or doing the wrong thing. In any age of heavy reliance on experts and specialists there is a tendency in most of us to make ourselves scarce in the face of extreme suffering or grief – we feel so painfully inadequate. The other side of that coin is that the privacy of one's home may often seem to be invaded by representatives of the various agencies involved in supporting families of very sick children at home. Grief has a way of rendering its victims hypersensitive and those in supporting roles need to develop a proportionate sensitivity in their relationships with such families.

Several months after Helen's return home I became so concerned about her parents' tiredness that I plucked up courage to ask them if they would trust me enough to 'lend' her to me from time to time in order that they could have a break. There is a tendency in any parent to feel guilty if their child becomes ill, as if by some means they should have been able to protect the child and prevent the illness. When the illness is very serious the sense of guilt is often correspondingly great. Perhaps partly for this reason and partly because death brings enforced and irreversible separation, many parents are reluctant to allow anyone else to care for their child. All around them well-meaning friends and relatives may be urging them to take a break to care for themselves, if only in order that they are able to take on again the long-term care of their child. Rationally, the parents probably see the sense of this, but emotionally their response may be very different.

Helen's parents said that it was because they believed I knew and loved Helen as a person, even though I had not known her before she was ill, that they felt able to entrust her into my care for a brief period from time to time. It was because I knew the song she had loved most before she was ill and that they continued to sing to her at bedtime since her illness; because I knew that she had hated baked beans and, even liquidised, they still taste of baked beans; because I knew the little cat who had been, and continued to be, her constant companion; because of these and so many other seemingly trivial things, it felt safe to leave her with me.

She would come for a few days at a time several times a year. This gave her parents an opportunity to catch up on sleep, to take a short holiday, to focus special attention on the other children or do things that were difficult or impossible to do when Helen was at home needing so much care and attention, albeit so willingly and lovingly given.

Between Helen's visits I would often call on her and her family at home. Many, many times we talked of Helen as she had been, of Helen as she might have become if she had remained well, and of the cruel reality of the present and the dreadful uncertainty of the future. I learnt so much from Helen's parents as they lived through the unremitting pain of adjusting to the fact that their beloved child would not get well and might die at any time. I learnt that, however close a relationship a couple may share, they will react not only as a couple, but as individuals. Sometimes one is too spent to speak while the other needs to find relief in discussion. When one is surviving by focusing on the business of everyday, the other cannot stop crying. One falls into deep exhausted sleep, the other suffers with insomnia. Those who grieve often feel out of step with everyone, even those closest. For a long time the whole situation seems too terrible to be true, like some long drawn out nightmare from which one will surely awaken.

Meanwhile there may well be other children in the family who need the love and care and attention of their parents and who may understandably feel left out and second best. The couple may feel the need to consider whether to risk further pregnancies. Grandparents, other relatives, close friends and other children who have known the sick child will all have their personal grief to live with. In many ways it becomes harder rather than easier for those closest to the sick child as the weeks of illness become months and the months, years. The loneliness often becomes more accentuated because those on the periphery find it so hard to stay alongside the chronic grief brought about by long drawn out life-limiting illness, especially that of a child.

As I reflected on the lessons I was learning from Helen and her family I realised that one of the things they valued most was friendship. They knew that I loved Helen as the unique and cherished child that she is and they trusted my love for her. They knew too that when they 'lent' her to me from time to time I would model the care I gave her on theirs – her daily routine, the way she was fed, her most comfortable positions, the music she loved, and not just her physical and environmental needs. It was important to them, too, that I recognised and respected that which animated Helen, her spirit which lived on inside her frail little body.

One day, as I sat with Helen in my arms while her family was away for a short break, I began to wonder about other families with children who suffer with chronic life-limiting illness, and whether the same concept of friendship might be useful to them. At a time and in a culture where the extended family has almost ceased to exist I wondered about an alternative extended 'family'. And so the idea of Helen House was born. It was and is a friendship with one gravely ill child and her family developed to include other sick children and their families.

FROM IDEA TO REALITY
Sister Frances Dominica and Ann Hunt

In the planning of Helen House we learnt much from the philosophy of the adult hospice movement. But we quickly realised that the practical application would differ considerably. There was, it seemed, no residential hospice for children yet in existence in this or any other country, so the people on whom we relied most heavily for advice and guidance were the parents of sick children themselves. Helen's parents had prepared us well. As we listened to others they so often echoed their experiences, reactions and needs, but despite this, each family and each child was different. Flexibility ranked next most important after friendship. As a father of two children with Sanfilippo disease (one of the mucopolysaccharide storage disorders) was to express it later, 'a take-it-or-leave-it care package' would have been unacceptable.

'We realise we can't grow away from our children or they from us: in fact because of their increasing dependency the bond between us grows stronger and the responsibility towards Emma and William increases. This leads to:

1. Phenomenal degrees of tiredness.
2. No time for one another.
3. Little time to relax.
4. Social isolation and loneliness.
5. Feelings that you are on your own with your children.
6. A knowledge that your friends have their life to lead and cannot help you very much.
7. Almost total self-denial.
8. Feelings of guilt that you always fail in your attempts to do your best by all family members.

Traditional forms of help offered tend to emphasise the need to separate your child from you. Emma and William are part of us – separation and institutionalised care are out of the question. The ethos of hospice acknowledges our family dynamics and deals with them where we are. We are not offered a take-it-or-leave-it care package but one which understands our closeness to Emma and William and which meets our ability to 'let go'. The important thing for us is that the staff realise that they can't offer us, the parents, any respite unless they can demonstrate that Emma and William are special people for them too. Helen House has become very much a second home. There, because of the love, we glimpse normality – the normality of sleep, physical and mental relaxation and being able to spend time with each other recharging our marriage. The hospice is a place where people understand what it is like to care for a dying child. We don't get asked foolish questions about the illness; rather, we are given information and support by people who are experts. We know that despite living 180 miles from Oxford the friends we have made there will help sustain us through the dark days which lie ahead. Emma and William's deaths will be a traumatic separation for us but we know that these friends will be grieving with us for they also love Emma and William. The hospice provides us with the best of all worlds enabling us for a short while to put aside the worst excesses of caring for two very dependent children and engage in a little self-indulgence rather than self-denial.'

In eight years the family, always together, has visited thirty-four times. Emma died in Helen House in November 1992.

The Building

Helen House was built in the grounds of All Saints Convent, Oxford, and completed in November 1982. The garden gives the feel of being in the country and is in constant use in fine weather, but just round the corner are busy small shops and all the activity of local town life, and a little further away the beauty of the City and University.

It was Helen's parents who said that Helen House should be family sized and that eight children was the maximum number they could conceive of within that limit. So, contrary to recommendations on cost-effectiveness and the fear of demand exceeding supply, Helen House was designed with eight beds for sick children and we have no intention of expanding. There is accommodation, too, for members of the children's families to stay. Each child has his or her own bedroom and these, and the various living rooms, are designed to be as homely, light and attractive as possible.

Ten Years On

When Helen House opened in 1982 there was much uncertainty in many quarters about the role of the children's hospice and what patterns of care would evolve (Burne, 1982; Dominica, 1983; Chambers, 1987; Goodman, 1987; Wilkinson, 1987; Goldman *et al.*, 1990). Nearly ten years later, and with the opening of several more hospices for children, their role has become more clear. Hospice has been described as 'holistic care for patient and family units, intended to maximise present quality of life whenever there is no reasonable expectation of cure' (Corr and Corr, 1985). While it is apparent that Helen House, as a children's hospice, has evolved as a very different establishment from an adult hospice, its designation as a hospice remains as valid.

Staffing Helen House

Day-to-day care of the children is provided by a team of multidisciplinary staff, who as well as caring for the child and family look after the housekeeping and catering aspects of the house. Helen House is registered as a nursing home, so, while there is minimal emphasis on hierarchy, one of the registered nurses takes overall responsibility for co-ordinating each shift, with the varied skills and experience of all members being used and valued. Many of the staff have paediatric nursing backgrounds, while others have experience in different aspects of child and family care, including nursery nursing, play, teaching, physiotherapy and social work. A high ratio of staff to children is maintained. Children and families have a member of the team allocated to them for each shift, with greater emphasis on compatibility than on particular qualification. Each family will have two key workers from among the staff, who will maintain contact between visits and where possible care for the child when he or she is staying. Medical care is provided by three local general practitioners who have become experienced in paediatric palliative care. The common qualifications we look for in appointing team members are love and concern for children, a willingness to listen and to learn from the families who are the true experts, a sense of humour, and the attitude of being happy to be a paid-up, card-carrying member of the human race. Both informal and formal staff support systems operate (Woolley *et al.*, 1989) and help to ensure a low staff turnover.

Working with the Families

It is essential that team members recognise and respect the parents' wishes in sharing the care of their sick child. This will vary from the parents caring for their child in Helen House with virtually no assistance, to leaving the child in our care for a period of time. No pressure is put on them to alter their pattern of care unless or until they are ready. Discussions regarding any change in treatment are only made after honest consultation with them and with their full agreement. There are sometimes differences of opinion or serious divisions within the family and it is not our role to take sides but rather to try to be aware of the stress and grief each one is experiencing and to offer sensitive support. The immediate family members are the key people in the caring team, with the rest of us alongside to support, to enable and to encourage in whatever ways seem most helpful. The relationship is not so much professional to patient and relatives, as that of friendship backed up by practical skills.

In our attempt to support the children and their families it is vital that we work in co-operation with any other individuals or agencies involved. Indeed 'hospice' can be seen as a whole spectrum of care, community-based and hospital-based as well as hospice facility-based. It is in the interest of child and family that we work together for their greatest well-being.

The Children

Of the 275 children who had stayed at Helen House up to the end of 1991 27 per cent suffered from a progressive neurological disease, mainly of genetic origin, and another 21 per cent from other inborn errors of metabolism, two-thirds of whom had one of the mucopolysaccharide storage disorders. Sixteen per cent of the children had a malignant disease, with nearly half of these having a cerebral tumour. A further 15 per cent of children had a non-progressive neurological disease such as cerebral palsy. Twelve per cent had an inherited neuromuscular disease such as Duchenne muscular dystrophy, or spinal muscular atrophy and 8 per cent had a congenital abnormality, such as congenital heart disease, or chromosome disorder (Table 3.1). Overall, more than 60 per cent of children had disease of genetic origin and 12 per cent of families had more than one child with the same disease. Of 73 families (87 children) who came to stay in 1991, 25 per cent had at one time two or more children with the same disease including 19 per cent who were still caring for two sick children.

Time Span

While a high proportion of children suffered from a chronic life-threatening disease, 15 per cent of children died within a month of their first admission, 21 per cent within 6 months and 30 per cent within a year of their first admission. Reflecting the chronicity of many of the conditions, however, 50 per cent of the children were still living 4 years after their first admission, 15 per cent after 5 years, and 5 per cent of the children were alive more than 7 years after their first admission. Such a trend

Table 3.1 Diagnoses of 275 children admitted to Helen House from 1982 to end-1991

CNS progressive			
Juvenile Battens disease	9		
Infantile Battens disease	9		
Adrenoleucodystrophy	7		
Metachromatic leucodystrophy	5		
Subacute sclerosing panencephalitis	4		
Leigh's encephalomyelopathy	4		
Other neurodegenerative	39		
		77	28%
Inborn errors of metabolism			
Mucopolysaccharidoses			
Sanfilippo syndrome	27		
Hurler's syndrome	6		
Hunter's syndrome	5		
Epidermolysis bullosa	4		
Other metabolic disease	18		
		60	22%
Neoplastic disease			
Cerebral tumours	21		
Neuroblastoma	7		
Rhabdomyosarcoma	4		
Leukaemia	4		
Other neoplastic disease	8		
		44	16%
Non-progressive CNS			
Cerebral palsy/brain damage	29		
Cerebral malformation	7		
Encephalitis	1		
		37	13%
Neuromuscular			
Duchenne MD	23		
Spinal Muscular Atrophy	11		
		34	12%
Congenital			
Congenital heart disease	9		
Other	12		
		21	8%
Other		2	1%
Total		275	100%

has meant that after nine years of opening the number of new children being admitted each year is now much reduced in relation to the early years.

James, who suffered from Duchenne muscular dystrophy first came to stay at the age of 10 years when he lost his walking ability. From then until his death in Helen House aged 18 years he visited frequently for respite and at times of chest infections. He became much loved and respected by us, and Helen House became a trusted extension of his family. This was important as in addition to happy times he also shared with staff many problems both physical and emotional. This stood us in good stead when his disabilities and problems became very severe.

Age

At referral the age of the children ranged from a few days to 19 years. Of 87 children who stayed during 1991 7 per cent were under 4 years of age, 27 per cent between 4 and 9 years, 46 per cent between 10 and 16 years, and 20 per cent over 17 years of age. Providing the condition of the child continues to be life-threatening Helen House has continued to offer care to families to whom it has made that commitment if the child lives on into adult life and Helen House remains the most appropriate option for the young person.

John has been coming to Helen House regularly since he was a young man of 14 years. The Batten's Disease that took his sight, and from which his sister died at 18 years of age nearly 6 years ago, has slowly enfeebled him physically, but mentally he remains the charming courteous person we have grown to know so well. At 23 he seems happy to return often to stay with friends in whose lives and events he shows great interest.

Referral

The families have been referred by several agencies with 34 per cent being first referred by the families themselves. Twenty-two per cent were referred by their hospital consultants and 15 per cent by their social worker. Only a relatively small proportion (6 per cent) were referred by their general practitioner and a further 6 per cent by their health visitor. A study of the early families using Helen House demonstrated that the parents' needs and expectations from Helen House were a desire for care in a supportive, non-hospital environment, with an emphasis on symptom control rather than on active intervention, and the need for respite care (Stein et al., 1989). For most families who have been referred the prime reason stated for referral to Helen House has been the need for respite care. The great majority of the children were very disabled and highly dependent, making great demands on the time and energy of their parents. Parents wanted to be able to give time to their well children also, and to recharge their own batteries.

Unlike some of the children's hospices Helen House has no specific catchment area, taking children from all over the country, though we would now suggest one of the other hospices if it might be more conveniently placed for the family. At present more than half the families travel over 50 miles to Helen House, with 16 per cent travelling over 100 miles.

Admissions

Over the past 9 years the mean number of admissions has been 300 per year, with a mean stay of 5 days per admission and an average number of stays of 4–5 a year. On average each child stayed 20 days per year, but overall variation was from 1 day to more than 100 days in the year. Bed occupancy now runs at about 61–65 per cent.

So that it is possible to admit children in an emergency, only 6 of the 8 beds are routinely booked for respite care provision. Over the years some 90 per cent of admissions have been for booked respite, 5 per cent for emergency respite, for instance when a parent has been taken ill, and 3 per cent specifically for symptom control or for terminal care.

The bulk of Helen House's work has evolved therefore as the provision of respite care for families with children who require skilled and time-consuming day-to-day care, together with the management of difficult symptoms when they arise (Hunt, 1986, 1990), and the provision of terminal care for those children if the parents wish them to be at Helen House rather than at home or in hospital at the time of death. The care of children with malignant disease has tended to make rather different demands. The children are often referred later in their disease at a point when treatment aimed at cure has ceased. Many children with cancers have by this time developed close relationships with both their local and tertiary referral centres, and many of these centres now provide very good domiciliary care and support, which enables the parents to continue to care for their child at home (Chambers *et al.*, 1989; Beardsmore, 1990; Goldman *et al.*, 1990). This may be less true for some of the children with brain tumours who in some areas are cared for by adult neurosurgical teams, and who may also have a more chronic and disabling terminal phase to their illness. Referral to Helen House for children with malignant disease has tended to be more usual where the required support at home has been unavailable, or where provision of home care may be particularly difficult, for instance for some separated or single parent families.

Mark, whose mother was unwell and whose father was under stress looking after Mark and two younger children, had a cerebral tumour. He came to stay at Helen House for terminal care in liaison with his local hospital and community services so that care for the whole family could be provided in a homelike atmosphere. Whilst pain control was not easy to establish at times, an equally important role was to offer support to Mark and his family as they explored their many anxieties.

Half-way House

Helen House has also occasionally played a role in bridging the gap between hospital and home, providing a supportive, home-like environment in which a family may adapt to a new diagnosis or stage in their child's illness, giving them time to develop the new skills necessary for caring for their child.

Daniel's sudden onset of the symptoms of subacute sclerosing panencephalitis and his rapid physical deterioration left his family shocked and feeling inadequate to face the difficult nursing and feeding programmes instituted in hospital. A period of care for Daniel and his family at Helen House allowed them time to learn the nursing skills and to gain confidence sufficient to return home and cope extremely competently with Daniel for a considerable time. Daniel died at Helen House last year.

Sharing

Parents have expressed a need to share with other parents facing similar problems, and staff have played a role in passing on from one family to another those skills which each family learn and share with the staff. Many of the children's diseases are individually rare, but at Helen House the staff have an opportunity to develop an expertise in managing some of the problems, as they may over time see several children with the same rare conditions. Members of staff, for example, who have worked at Helen House since it opened will have cared for nearly thirty children with Sanfilippo Syndrome (one of the mucopolysaccharide storage disorders), and eight children with Infantile Batten's Disease (ceroid lipofuscinosis).

The Price family had two children with Infantile Battens Disease and had made several long dashes from the West Country to Helen House when either Kim or Mary were in difficulty with seizures or the chest infections which were exacerbated by the girls' difficulty in swallowing oral secretions. The prescription of hyoscine patches (Scopaderm), whose use in this context we had learnt through another child visiting us, has proved invaluable in reducing the excess secretions which caused so much distress for the girls.

Symptoms and Problems

An analysis of the symptoms and problems suffered by the children on their admissions has shown these to be multiple and persistent. The symptoms themselves are not placed in any order of severity for all may be equally distressing from drowning in saliva, or dyspnoea, to fitting, or pain.

Feeding problems

Fifty-eight per cent of children had feeding and swallowing difficulties, including 20 per cent who were fed via nasogastric tube or gastrostomy. For some children mashed or liquidised food is manageable. As swallowing becomes more impaired liquids become more difficult than solids, and thickening of liquids with agents such as Carobel is useful in maintaining oral hydration as long as possible. The decision whether or not to tube-feed their child is a difficult one for many families but must be uniquely that of the family, with the professional explaining the options but not presenting what may be their own bias. What we do hope to offer is a particular expertise gained through caring for many such children.

Respiratory problems

Fifty per cent of children had symptoms from respiratory disease, with 38 per cent having had a chest infection at some time during the year. Forty-three per cent of children received antibiotics, most of these prescriptions being for chest infections. Eleven per cent of children suffered from dyspnoea at some time. Respiratory distress occurred in children with neurological disease in the terminal phase of their illness and here the use of diamorphine subcutaneously via a syringe driver has proved useful.

Pain

On average, 32 per cent of children had some degree of pain. Virtually all children with cancers had pain requiring strong opioids (Burne and Hunt, 1987; Hunt, 1990). Morphine sulphate administered orally on a regular basis has been the drug and route of choice with the dose being titrated against the pain until pain relief is achieved. When a stable dose is achieved it can be more convenient to change to a controlled release preparation. Where morphine could not be taken by mouth and more than a single injection is likely to be required, we have administered dia-morphine subcutaneously using a syringe driver. In 1991 five children (6 per cent) received strong opioid analgesia for control of pain or respiratory distress.

In children with neurological disease pain due to muscle spasm and to immobility was a more chronic problem. Children with the leucodystrophies and with Sanfilippo syndrome were particularly prone to severe muscle spasm. Muscle relaxant drugs such as diazepam and baclofen have been used regularly to relieve the spasticity. Twenty-one per cent of children received muscle relaxants. Where muscle spasm is poorly controlled dislocation of one or both hip joints is not unusual and creates its own source of pain. For some children, especially those with mucopolysacchari-doses, joint pain was common. The use here of the non-steroidal anti-inflammatory drugs such as naproxen and ibuprofen seems to have been helpful. Forty-four per cent of children received non-opioid analgesics such as paracetamol and the non-steroidal anti-inflammatory drugs.

Other problems

Sixty-five per cent of children were immobile to a degree that they could not turn in bed, and a further 32 per cent had restricted mobility. Nearly 80 per cent of the children were incontinent of urine and 70 per cent incontinent of faeces. Forty per cent suffered from constipation and 47 per cent received laxatives. Nearly 70 per cent of children had no speech, and a further 13 per cent had impaired speech. Forty-two per cent regularly had epileptic seizures with 54 per cent of children receiving anticonvulsants. Nearly 30 per cent of children were blind or had impaired vision, while nearly 20 per cent had a hearing deficit. Twenty per cent had very dis-turbed sleep at night. Boys in the later stages of Duchenne muscular dystrophy would sometimes require their parents to turn them up to ten times a night, and young children with Sanfilippo syndrome would be hyperactive and might not sleep for days and nights on end.

Most of the children are therefore highly dependent and also have difficulty in communicating. The management of their physical problems and the provision of emotional support and play can present both parents and professionals with great challenges. Nurses and other staff working at Helen House need to develop skills of observation, intuition, patience and stamina. A sense of fun can be a great asset to both children, parents and colleagues.

Bereavement Follow-up

Of the 155 children who had died by the end of 1991 41 per cent died at home, 32 per cent at Helen House, 22 per cent in hospital and the remaining 5 per cent at various other places. Following the death of the child, staff from Helen House maintain con-tact according to the parents' wishes, and two bereavement visitors follow up the families by visits or by phone. Approximately twenty-five families are currently being actively followed up by the bereavement visitors.

Many children who die at Helen House will remain in a small, simple, cooled room in the House for several days, often up to the time of funeral, where the parents, brothers and sisters, grandparents and family friends may spend as much time with the child's body as the parents wish so that they may take their time in saying their goodbyes (Dominica, 1987). This service has also been used by families who have visited Helen House and whose children died at home or in hospital, as well as by several local families whose child was not previously known to Helen House. Staff are available to support the family and to help with funeral arrangements where appropriate.

Defining the Need

It is suggested that the children's hospice can offer a service which was hitherto provided in less adequate form and quantity for many families (Wilkinson, 1987). Even with the existence of several other children's hospices the demand for this form of care is far from satisfied. Helen House has found that with approximately 85 children currently receiving care its respite facilities are insufficient to take on more children and a waiting list now operates, though children referred for symptom control or terminal care are still seen at very short notice. New children accepted for respite care tend now to be sicker and more vulnerable than they were in the earlier years, and the children who have been visiting since the early years are now more frail and dependent. In spite of this, for most children and their families Helen House retains a light-hearted atmosphere and remains a place of relaxation.

Sarah, aged 11 years, who accompanies her two brothers who have Leigh's Disease when they come to stay at Helen House, recently asked a member of staff why they need to have days off when they work in such a fun place as this.

Perhaps it is the fun and enjoyment that the respite focus of the children's hospice provides which, in balancing the inevitable times of sadness, death and mourning, sustains the staff in their work with the children and their families.

CONCLUSION

There can be few experiences in life more devastating than the illness and death of your child. To be alongside offering friendship and support requires the very best that a nurse has to give both as a professional and as a fellow human being. We do not help as long as we hide behind professional status. We cannot but become emotionally involved, and that is costly. But we believe that this is one of the most rewarding jobs a nurse can do. It is about caring for the child as a whole person, body, mind and spirit, helping that child to live fully until he or she dies. It is also about caring for the child's whole family. Over the years we have come to believe that there is the potential in every man, woman and child to meet tragedy with courage, strength, nobility and love. Yet on our side we have so little to offer. By the very nature of the families we meet it is not possible to restore health and life to their child; we are unable to answer the question 'Why' in all its agonising forms; we can at least stay alongside the family through all the length and breadth of their personal hell for as long as we are wanted.

REFERENCES

Beardsmore S (1990) Symptom care of the child with cancer. *Nursing Times*, **86,** 72–4.

Burne R (1982) Hospice care for children. *British Medical Journal*, **284,** 1400.

Burne R and Hunt A (1987) Use of opiates in terminally ill children. *Palliative Medicine*, **1,** 27–30.

Chambers E J O A, Cornish J M and Cusnick S (1989) Terminal care at home for children with cancer. *British Medical Journal*, **298,** 937–40.

Chambers T L (1987) Hospices for children? *British Medical Journal*, **294,** 1309–10.

Corr C A and Corr D M (1985) Pediatric hospice care. *Pediatrics*, **76,** 774–80.

Dominica F (1983) The dying child. *The Lancet*, 1107.

Dominica F (1987) Reflections on death in childhood. *British Medical Journal*, **294,** 108–10.

Goldman A, Beardsmore S and Hunt J (1990) Palliative care for children with cancer – home, hospital, or hospice? *Archives of Disease in Childhood*, **65,** 641–3.

Goodman S L (1987) Hospice for children? *British Medical Journal*, **295,** 122.

Hunt A (1986) Open house (Caring for the terminally ill child. Helen House – a review). *Nursing Times*, **82,** 53–7.

Hunt A (1990) A survey of signs, symptoms and symptom control in 30 terminally ill children. *Developmental Medicine and Child Neurology*, **32,** 341–6.

Stein A, Forrest G C, Woolley H and Baum J D (1989) Life threatening illness and hospice care. *Archives of Disease in Childhood*, **64,** 697–702.

Wilkinson J M (1987) Hospices for children? *British Medical Journal*, **295,** 210.

Woolley H, Stein A, Forrest G C and Baum J D (1989) Staff stress and job satisfaction at a childrens hospice. *Archives of Disease in Childhood*, **64,** 114–18.

4

Innovative Practice in the Out-Patient Setting

Sharon Stower

INTRODUCTION

Care of children in the out-patient department is often seen as mundane and uninteresting – a view held by many nurses who do not work there and strongly opposed by those that do.

This chapter reflects on out-patient care of the past, where it currently stands and the direction it is sure to go in the future. In order to look at past paediatric out-patient services a literature search was necessary. It was disappointing, but not surprising, to find that little has been previously documented on this subject. Aspects such as waiting lists, poor out-patient department (OPD) attendance and clinic waiting times have been previously mentioned, if only fleetingly.

There has been little written on innovative practice and high-profile out-patient care. Indeed out-patient care has never been given much credence at all – but this is slowly changing and needs to change in order to meet the complete needs of children and their families.

The NHS Management Executive Report entitled *The Role of Nurses and Other Non-Medical Staff in the Out-Patients Department* (NHS, 1990) has had some effect on the management and practice in OPDs. This document looks at skill-mix and role content of nurses and other non-medical staff in the out-patient setting. This is the beginning of observing OPDs in a new light – looking at practice which takes place and looking at the question of quality of service. The future of paediatric nursing will be increasingly centred on the services provided for those families attending as out-patients, as this fits comfortably with the culture of nursing children in their own homes for as long and as often as possible.

A LOOK TO THE PAST

Historically, out-patient departments have been the poor relation in hospitals, often situated in a remote corner and the place where medical staff can be contacted if not on the wards or in theatre. Often this is the most importance out-patient departments are afforded.

In the past, out-patients had their treatments on busy wards if at all, and when this became unmanageable, clinics were established in a crude way. Patients could be seen lined up along the lengthy corridors of the old Victorian workhouses, and the attending physician would start at one end and work his way through to the other. Those who required privacy were not given such a courtesy because it did not exist until later, when screens were provided in a fairly makeshift way to separate patients from each other.

THE PRESENT

Fortunately, things have improved quite considerably since then, but many aspects of out-patient care in some hospitals are still of a relatively low standard and this is often attributed to the unimportance placed upon its function.

The usual image of children's out-patient services is a matter for concern. The theory of the work is often considered to be that of a low-profile, non-acute area where standards of care are unimportant, staffed with nurses and care assistants who have a reputation for wanting an easy life and not have to work any unsocial hours, or it is often referred to as the backwater where nurses are sent to work when a back injury demands a lighter load, or when nurses have no profes-sional aspirations – these are views of professional people viewed over the years. Indeed, the opposite is true, lifting children, large and small, on and off examination couches with and without plaster of paris casts means the work can be very heavy and physically demanding.

Out-patient services have been the referral centre of the hospital, the family doctor requests a child to be seen by a consultant or specialist doctor for their opinion – this is often the first contact a family has with the hospital and first impressions are lasting and important.

It should be remembered that babies and children are attending an out-patient clinic over periods of months – even years – in contrast to in-patient admissions. It is often the careful monitoring and management of children as out-patients while they are being cared for at home that helps to prevent expensive hospital admis-sions. Additionally, a serious accident or illness may necessitate an admission to hospital which may be the beginning of a longer-term problem requiring continuing follow-up at clinic before the child and family are finally discharged. It is at this point that children need to feel confident and happy within the hospital environment as this is often their first introduction to hospital – that place where they do nasty things to you! Therefore, it is important to view the hospital and the children's out-patient department especially through the eyes of a child to reduce anxieties and fears and to promote confidence and calm.

This should be part of the Children's Unit Philosophy of Care and should demon-strate that the children's out-patient department equally fulfils a clinical role in the child/family's care. The children's clinic provides the significant link for all families between hospital and home.

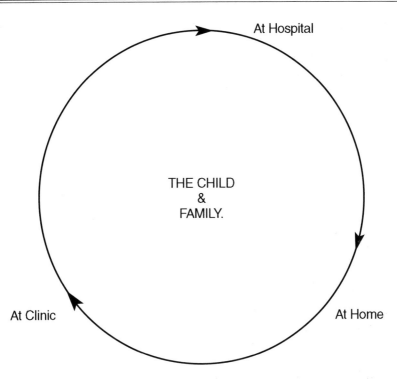

Fig. 4.1 The continuum of care – hospital – home. Source: Stower (1991).

THE FUTURE

It has been well documented that children should be nursed or cared for by their family at home with as many supportive services as possible: 'Children should only be admitted to hospital when the medical treatment they require cannot be given in other ways without real disadvantage'. (CHSC, 1959). Often during this process of a child being cared for at home, the care is co-ordinated and reviewed by nurses and physicians from the hospital, the Children's Clinic provides the venue and is central to all the decisions which are made.

Indeed, future trends will increase this vital service need and place even greater demands on the out-patient facility. As the continuance of care between hospital and home increases the need for a well-equipped family-centred department and a deep commitment to provide that vital link will become even more important.

NOTTINGHAM MODEL OF CHILD CARE

The unique relationship between child, family and hospital is one that warrants special attention. The Nottingham Model of Child Care includes the child in hospital, the significant role of the family and the special nurse or primary nurse.

This complex interaction of care members helps to bring about a change or an improvement in the child's problem or need, and to enable the child if physically possible to resume a near normal life activity as quickly as possible.

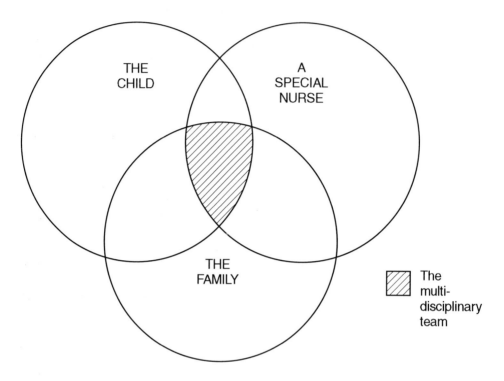

Fig. 4.2 Relationships built and developed with the concept of family-centred care.

The Nottingham Model of Child Care is based on a family-centred philosophy. This includes providing plans of care with children and their families, not children in isolation, and looking at the total needs of the child within the family context and other family members if appropriate. This means encouraging other family members to contribute to care of the child in hospital, to whatever degree they wish. This has obvious benefits for the child as they are more familiar with their parents caring for them than a stranger.

Philosophy of Care

Family-centred care is a salient feature of the Nottingham Model of Child Care. The children's clinic or out-patient service needs to be family-centred for it to be effective in meeting the needs of all the family at all times.

The staff of the Children's Clinic should establish from the outset the philosophy for the department and objectives for the year.

CHILDREN'S CLINIC

Philosophy and Aims (1991)

It is the philosophy of the children's out-patient department staff to adopt a pleasant, caring and professional attitude, making the visit of the child and family pleasant, relaxed and informative.

Aims for 1991

1. To improve play facilities for children by providing large play areas suitable to the age ranges of children and give a wider choice of toys to children from ethnic minority groups.
2. To encourage parent education with the use of videos and relevant accurate information leaflets written in English and ethnic languages.
3. To encourage regular liaison with support services and particularly with ward staff to provide a continuation of care to the child and family.
4. To provide improved facilities for the nursing mother.
5. To establish a Nursing Enuresis Clinic providing much needed support for these families.
6. To undertake a Family Satisfaction Survey and aim to use the information effectively and bring about change.
7. Encourage staff to participate in study days and the update of clinic knowledge.
8. To provide a safe environment adapted to the age and needs of the child and family.
9. To gain the confidence of children by wearing brightly coloured tabards and no uniform.
10. To develop the new department into a centre of clinical excellence for children and their families.
11. To be sensitive to the needs of the child and family when child abuse is suspected and being investigated in the department.

It is important for the staff to agree collectively on this issue, to have ownership and commitment to achieve a common goal. Indeed, when a new department is being developed, the philosophy will become the baseline and establish the culture which will develop.

Parents should be included and consulted in the care treatment and management of their children at all times.

Out-patient work can be seen as an extension of ward work. Encouraging staff from the wards to attend in clinic does have obvious benefits, as indeed does a child who needs admission in the future being prepared in the Children's Clinic and visiting the ward before admission. Introductions to staff at this stage make the ordeal a lot less frightening for the child and allow the staff an opportunity to meet the whole family.

The Children's Clinic should be used solely for children and their families whenever possible and in a department where this is not possible a designated area for children is preferable and the environment should be suitably decorated. Children playing noisily in an adult department may disturb the elderly client, and indeed they may disturb the child but in very different ways.

The Children's Clinic at the City Hospital in Nottingham is a national demonstration site sponsored by the Department of Health in 1990. It has as its focus the commitment to good practice in Children's Out-Patient Services. Nursing staff were involved in the planning stages, and throughout the development, to provide a voice for the child and family; and the families' input was obtained by carrying out a Family Satisfaction Survey.

Staffing and Skill-mix

In Nottingham the Children's Clinics are staffed by first-level nurses who hold the RSCN qualification and who are committed to caring for sick children and their families.

The question of skill-mix in out-patient departments has been discussed fully over the past two years, especially since the Value for Money Report, which questioned the skill-mix of out-patient staff. This report puts to the test the need for trained, experienced, credible nurses to care for children in the out-patient department.

The children's unit in Nottingham advocates that out-patient nurses need to:

1. Attend to the child's and family's immediate needs in clinic by a process of assessment, action and evaluation.
2. Provide support and help in the clinic setting and arrange for its continuation at home.
3. Provide guidance and advice on aspects of health care and undertake both a general and health education role. Preventive medicine is one way to help reduce expensive hospital admission.
4. Provide information, teach and counsel families with children who have chronic illness, such as asthma and cystic fibrosis – and they need a sound knowledge base to be able to do this.

This is not an exhaustive list, but staff need to be able to carry out routine screening such as taking blood pressures and urine tests and know the implications of the results, being able to interpret them and take the appropriate action. They need to undertake nursing duties, give detailed explanations of treatments and investigations and, as well as all of this, prepare children and their families for hospital admission thoroughly and with care. Therefore, this is a job for trained, experienced, credible nurses – not care assistants.

The staff provide a constant deluge of innovative ideas which are produced; such as attractive children's designed sheets and pillow cases for the examination couches and attractive fabrics for arm slings, strap-on sandals with teddy bears on for small children who have long leg plasters in situ, bravery badges and certificates, brightly coloured tabards for the nurses and not forgetting the day-trip outings and visits to the pantomime.

Innovations and motivations really do exist in out-patient departments.

In the new Children's Clinic the service available to families is of the highest standard and this can be immediately demonstrated in the large circular play park; curved walls and windows at low level enhance a bright department decorated in primary colours. High regard is given to play and stimulation. The play area is divided into sections dedicated to different age groups of children and play is well organised and planned carefully to cater for the changing needs of the clinic's clientele. It is a flexible arrangement and the children would not have it any other way. The play area extends through reinforced french windows into the garden area where outside play activities can be found, enabling children to play on the grass in fine weather. Because the department is at ground level, it is necessary to make this an important feature as children's units are often in large multi-storey buildings and have no outside facility to play. Play is encouraged and supervised by play leaders who hold the NNEB qualification.

There is a choice of waiting areas for families; bright red contour seating allows parents to sit in the play park area if they wish and a quiet area for the older child, teenager, mums and dads has also been provided. A television, video and computer games are available to keep the youngsters happy during the wait. Books and up-to-date magazines are provided for parents. This area is very popular and well used by these age groups; young people do prefer to wait in an area away from small children as their needs are naturally very different.

The decor in each of these areas is appropriate to the needs of the family member, although primary colours featured throughout provide a bright welcoming atmosphere. This includes the brightly colour-co-ordinated consulting rooms – there are six in total, each with a large number on the door, which children take great delight in counting as they walk down the corridor.

Two wall-mounted scenic boxes, hand-crafted and specially made by Arthos (The Arts in Hospital Trust (Arthos) Ltd) depict two scenes – one of Sherwood Forest and the second of Nottingham Castle, which add a sparkle of culture and creative play. For the department to be really successful the following top three favourite toys are recommended.

1. Coupee Car (The Little Tykes)
2. Home Corner Play House (Wendy House)
3. Activity Centre – interchangeable imaginative play shop. This changes each day to something different, e.g. optician, shoe shop, greengrocer, etc.

The reception area is purposefully designed with plenty of space to allow uncongested 'flow-through' of families. Frequently the whole extended family attend the clinic, so plenty of room is essential. The child-friendly reception desk is at low level so that children can have eye contact with the receptionist. The desk is so placed and curved to allow a panoramic view of the department, which is essential for security purposes.

A nursing room for families is provided so that they can sit in comfort to feed their babies and toddlers; a separate nappy changing facility is provided. A highchair, crib, bottle warmer and microwave are available for use. These rooms are available to both parents so that fathers can do their share of the work also. Facilities also exist for disabled visitors.

A buggy park allows families to park prams and buggies in an area that is visible. This prevents congestion in the department, therefore enhancing safety. To protect buggies a security system could be installed.

For safety reasons hot drinks are not for sale in the department but parents have access to hot drinks a short walking distance away. The WRVS provides a small range of 'healthy' snacks approved by the dietetic department. Families are a captive audience in the department, therefore sweets and cola are not available. Healthy eating starts here in hospital and promotion of a healthy diet has to be encouraged. Refreshments for children with certain illnesses such as diabetes are also provided.

Child Protection

Issues relating to child protection have often been neglected in the past. Facilities for this client group are often inadequate. Families attend hospital for examination and interviews and are kept waiting sitting on a busy ward corridor. It is obvious to all – other parents, staff and children – why they are there. These families feel anxious, uncomfortable and guilty, and their presence on a ward is unnecessary and inappropriate. Therefore designated facilities should be available for these families. An interview room in the Children's Clinic provides an ideal setting for this purpose. These families attending on child protection issues need to be attended to sensitively; a pleasantly decorated interview room is much better than a busy ward corridor. 'There is a need to treat parents with circumspection, sympathy and understanding. This will be better achieved in an appropriate environment' (NSPCC, 1976).

Department Base for Professionals

Additional accommodation in the Children's Clinic enables the whole multidisciplinary team to be based in the department for the child and family. This includes the specialist nurses such as diabetic, cystic fibrosis, asthma and family therapy sisters, social workers, dieticians, etc. The interview room also provides a room for visiting consultants, clinical psychologists, etc. Family-centred care means emphasising the importance of having as many care professionals based in the department as possible.

Children with special needs cared for in the community will have a special or primary nurse, who will be in attendance at clinic. Keeping all staff together is better for the families, who otherwise would have to locate each specialist in different parts of the hospital.

A seminar room provides a venue for meetings, case conferences, lectures and a meeting place for staff and visitors. The room is furnished in a comfortable manner and provides an ideal location for groups of young people to meet informally with their peers; for example, a group of teenage diabetics. This encourages discussions on health education and topical issues as well as enhancing independence of the individuals.

A New Focus in Children's Care

A new focus in children's nursing for the future will emphasise the importance of the Children's/Young Persons' Clinic. This issue needs to be addressed now. Nurse-led clinics, nurse practitioners' roles and unbooked, walk-in clinics are some of the innovations currently taking place in paediatric out-patient care.

The Value for Money Report mentioned earlier discusses some of these factors. If the question of skill-mix is an issue, nurses in out-patient departments must be seen to hold a credible role in the department. Nurse-led clinics will provide a new forum for nurses to develop their role and their autonomy. A nurse-led clinic is one in which the nurse, working in a specialist area, leads and co-ordinates the clinic independently. This does not exclude the child/family from seeing a doctor, but it does mean that there is not a need for the child/family to see a doctor at every visit. The nurse-led clinic can take on the responsibility of health education and promotion, teaching and educating children and parents in their illness/condition as well a reviewing and assessing their techniques for specific procedures. Often problems can be expertly dealt with by nurses. In Nottingham, nurse-led clinics are established or planned in the following areas:

● Plastic surgery dressings clinics
● Diabetic clinic
● Enuresis clinic
● Family therapy clinic
● Nebuliser clinic
● Cystic fibrosis clinic
● Asthma clinic
● Renal clinic

The important considerations regarding nurse-led clinics are that the nurse functions independently of the medical staff and works as an autonomous practitioner. However he/she will have the ability and provision to refer the child on to be seen by a doctor if necessary. Nurse-led clinics enable the nurse to pursue the role of nurse practitioner, one which will increase in the future with the expanded role of registered nurses and the reduction of hours for junior medical staff.

Both the nurse practitioner and nurse-led clinics have clearly designated criteria which are adhered to by strict protocols. This will promote quality and safety for the child/families and help to protect individual members of the nursing team.

Unbooked Walk-in Clinics

This clinic can be run at a specific time each day and is a quick referral system for GPs, health visitors/social workers. If these professionals have a problem and feel the assistance of a paediatrician would be of benefit, they can refer the same or following day. This system is of particular benefit if the hospital site does not have an Accident and Emergency Department. This clinic could cater for the immediate community providing an urgent, high-quality paediatric service.

The Benefits of a Quality Circle

Innovative practice has to start somewhere, and often it is getting started that is the most difficult. A Quality Circle can look at a problem or potential problem area and within it team members help to generate solutions. As a result new ideas and developments can be generated which will influence innovative practice. The nurse practitioner role, nurse-led and unbooked clinics are examples.

In-service education and customer training days have been developed in order to assist staff with identifying our clients' needs. It is generally accepted that the Children's Clinic is the shop window of the unit for the hospital, and therefore it is important to give the child/family a first impression of confidence in caring and then a firm belief that they are respected as individuals.

Another key innovation in paediatric out-patient practice is the significance of a Family Information Service. On a recent study tour it was noted that the service provided by the Canadians is impressive. At the Sick Children's Hospital, Toronto, the family information service is a key element in high-quality paediatric care. Information for families should start at a very basic level, with information written in an easily understood language. This may mean its being translated into a different ethnic language, which caters for both social and cultural backgrounds.

Information is constantly changing, so information needs to be regularly updated and reviewed. A Family Information Centre should be a resource available to families on all topics relating to health, living, illness and disease. Written information, audio tapes and videos can also be displayed for use.

Most of the innovations which have taken place in Nottingham were largely as a result of asking the families for their views. This was done by undertaking a family satisfaction survey. It is necessary to do this so that the views of children and their families can be obtained and used as a catalyst for change – for example, change from uniform to wearing own clothes. Families preferred the informal relaxed atmosphere. The nursing staff in the department were keen to eliminate barriers between themselves and the children; wearing their own clothes and brightly coloured tabards has proved to be a very successful attempt. Colour photographs of all the staff who work in the department, including medical staff and departmental pets, are mounted in a glass display cabinet so that families know the names of those attending them in clinic.

Providing an environment which is appropriate and complete to meet the changing needs of families isn't easy, especially as the clientele is constantly moving and changing. However, it is possible to achieve with thought and commitment. The proof can be seen without any doubt from the children when they enter the department. The expressions of pleasure and excitement tell a convincing story.

Family Care Assistants

A considerable benefit to establishing a family-centred philosophy of care at both ward and out-patient department level is the increasing developing role of the family care assistant. This role has been developed to care for the needs of the whole family in the hospital environment. The family care assistant spends time with parents on the ward, in the parents' unit and at clinic. A familiar welcoming face helps families to cope with the anxious times they encounter at hospital with their children. In clinic she/he will spend time with families chatting, arranging coffee mornings and encouraging integration of families with similar problems.

Innovative practice in out-patient departments is very much alive and kicking. It is not an area where times never need to move on, but a department which will play an ever-increasing part in the continuum of care, between hospital and home.

In the future the importance of heightening the profile of paediatric out-patient care and giving both the speciality and the staff who work there the kudos they deserve, must be recognised.

REFERENCES

Central Health Services Council (1959) *The Welfare of Children in Hospital: Report of The Committee* (Chairman Sir Harry Platt). London: HMSO.

NHS Management Executive (1990) *The Role of Nurses and other Non-Medical Staff in the Out-Patients Department.*

NSPCC Battered Child Research Team (1976) *At Risk*. London: Routledge & Kegan Paul.

Stower S (1991) The continuum of care. *International Journal of Health Care and Quality Assurance*, **4**(6).

5

Accidents in Childhood

Eileen Thomas

Accidents to children are commonly regarded as an unfortunate but almost necessary evil in the trial-and-error learning that leads to adulthood. However, this view that 'accidents will happen even in the best of households' (Dickens, 1968) reinforces the belief that there is only one kind of childhood accident, the type that results in little more than a bruised knee, wounded pride and a greater awareness of the adult world. The reality is, of course, that not only are accidents 'the most important epidemic in the western world today (Jackson and Wilkinson, 1976), but are also the commonest cause of death in children between the ages of 1 and 15 years (OPCS, 1991).

The following pages focus on the major causes of accidental injury in childhood, but most important, and the main purpose of this work, is that it demonstrates that, with anticipation, many accidents might be prevented.

CHILDHOOD ACCIDENTS - COUNTING THE COSTS

In epidemiological terms, mortality rates have long been used as the most important indicator of the significance of a condition or disease. Deaths, especially those in childhood with infectious aetiology, have shown the most dramatic reductions this century and are now thankfully rare events. Accidental injuries resulting in loss of life have also fallen over the past twenty years, especially during the past five years, from 865 in 1985 to 534 in 1991 (HMSO, 1992). As a result, in an average District Health Authority, there are likely, on average, to be around five accidental deaths a year (Jackson, 1988).

The death of a child under any circumstances is a cost far too high for any family or community to bear and is one from which some may never recover, such is their grief (Murray Parks, 1983). An overview of the main causes of these deaths will therefore provide an insight into a potential for prevention (Table 5.1).

In terms of mortality there are marked differences in causes between specific age groups. For the under-fives the most important causes of death occur in and around the home and are, in order, fires, drowning, inhalation and ingestion of food causing obstruction or suffocation, falls, mechanical suffocation, poisoning by medicines and other substances and scalds. For older children, road accidents become the most important cause of death, reflecting the increasing time spent away from the home. Throughout the whole age spectrum boys are far more likely than girls to die as the result of an accident (Table 5.2).

Table 5.1   Fatal accidents in the United Kingdom, 1987 – children under 15 years

Type of Accident	Number of Deaths	% of Total
Pedestrian (road)	260	31
Burns/fires	119	14
Vehicle occupants (road)	96	11
Pedal cyclists (road)	73	9
Drownings (home & elsewhere)	63	7
Choking on food	50	6
Falls (home & elsewhere)	40	5
Suffocation	34	4
Others*	107	13
Total	842	100

*Others include electrocution, falling objects and poisoning.
Source: OPCS (1991).

Table 5.2   Deaths from injury and poisoning by sex and age – 1988–90

Age Group	1988 Male	Female	1989 Male	Female	1990 Male	Female
Under 1 year	67	42	51	39	57	33
1–4 years	141	109	164	87	156	90
5–14 years	328	118	322	134	278	135
Total	536	269	537	260	491	258
Total Male and Female	805		797		749	

Source: OPCS (1991).

Accidents resulting in death are a harrowing but numerically small tip of the massive and obscure iceberg of morbidity. Nationally, Hospital Accident & Emergency Department attendances and in-patient data provide some measure of the great magnitude of the problem, but must still on the whole be regarded as estimates. Computerisation has been slow to develop in the majority of Accident & Emergency centres, many of which have relied on the labour-intensive manual recording of patient information until the recent introduction of the NHS internal market. One result is that varying methods of recording accident statistics have evolved in different areas with the result that information has been unreliable and not comparable. Moreover, even in the places where computerised information systems have been successfully established, hospital attendances and admissions are known to be subject to the influence of extraneous variables such as home distance from the unit and social class (Milner, Nicholl and Williams, 1988; Quick, 1991).

In 1976, in an endeavour to provide more accurate information on childhood accidents nationally, the Home Accident Surveillance System (HASS) was established by the Department of Trade and Industry for the recording of non-fatal accidents. HASS takes its statistics from attendances at twenty hospitals in England and Wales from those which operate a 24-hour service and have at least 10,000 new patients a year. During the 1980s organisations such as the Child Accident Prevention Trust (CAPT) and the Royal Society for the Prevention of Accidents added to the existing body of knowledge by conducting their own research in the field of childhood injuries. Some of this research included an enquiry into the financial costs of injuries in childhood which although encountering 'many difficulties in the collection and analysis of accident statistics' concluded that an estimate of £200 million was justified in terms of the hospital costs (Whalley, 1992).

This largely preventable and unacceptably high cost reflects that around one in six children will attend their local Accident and Emergency Department each year (CAPT, 1991a), a far greater number than those attending paediatric outpatient clinics (BPA, 1987). However, even these high numbers do not reflect the overall severity of a reason for attendance, which can span the whole range of the spectrum from a minor bruise to a major head injury (Hill, 1989; Walsh and Jarvis, 1992).

The growing evidence provided to government bodies, especially by CAPT, took the form of research studies, work programmes and audio-visual aids designed for a range of professional groups. During the late 1980s and until 1992 articles in medical journals and in the popular press increasingly focused on accidental injuries in childhood and their subsequent prevention. The enormity of the problem became unavoidable. In the spring of 1992 the Government produced a White Paper, 'The Health of the Nation', which included five target areas for prevention; accidents was one of the five.

ACCIDENT-PRONE OR CHANCE OF FATE: WHICH CHILDREN HAVE ACCIDENTS?

On a typical Saturday afternoon in an average District Accident and Emergency Department, several children are likely to be brought in by concerned parents and guardians. There will be children of different ages and backgrounds, but some will be represented in greater numbers than others; identifying these high-risk groups can help in the planning of preventative programmes. The two most vulnerable groups are:

- Boys: boys have more accidents than girls at all ages (CAPT, 1989).
- Children whose parents are in social class 5 are six times more likely to die or be injured than those with social class 1 parents (CAPT, 1991b).

From the age of about 1 year, boys are more likely than girls to sustain an injury as a result of an accident, outnumbering girls by a ratio of 3:1 (Alwash and McCarthy, 1987). A brief observation of young children at play offers an immediate insight into the contributory reasons for this difference, for male play is, even from a very early age, much more physical than that of a female child (Golding, 1986). This in part stems from the way that male children are treated even from the moment of birth in Western cultures, where female infants are talked to more and handled more gently than baby boys (Neubauer, 1979). These differences help to establish the stereotypical activity of boys, which leads to a heightening of adventurous and risk-taking behaviours (Rivara *et al.*, 1982).

The circumstances in which a child lives are known to have a profound effect on the likelihood of an accident occurring. Repeatedly, studies have shown a clear social class association between deprivation and childhood accidents (Brown and Davidson, 1978; Pearn, 1978; Constantinides, 1988). This relationship is one that extends across all age groups, but is especially marked in children and has created much debate regarding the causality. One view is that people with restricted incomes experience multiple concerns, which in themselves distract away from routine child care issues, towards the struggle for day-to-day survival (While, 1989). Another view is that poor housing alone is responsible for large numbers of injuries in children (CAPT, 1991c; Thomas, 1991).

The main contributors to high childhood accidental injury rates are almost certainly so closely intertwined that separating one from another will always be a complicated matter. However, one trend which can be observed without the need for complex interpretation lies in the geographical distribution of accidents. It is known from work such as the Black Report that the poorest in the community, those with the fewest resources at their disposal, will be those who experience the worst health (Black Report, 1980; Mitchell, 1984). Nationally, studies demonstrate that accidental injury in childhood is much more frequent in the north of England (Avery *et al.*, 1990) and that this north–south divide extends also to affluence and access to better housing (Eyles, 1987).

The principle of applying national indicators of deprivation to a local situation is not a new one and is an approach adopted by Brian Jarman (1984, 1989) as a means of identifying those areas where people live with the greatest disadvantage. The use of this kind of informative data can help to plan child accident programmes to focus on the areas of greatest need. Many systems which help to highlight relative deprivation are now in use; some use GP consultation rates as the measure (Balarajan, Yuen and Machin, 1992), but still the most commonly used, the Jarman 8 system, is based on census data. It uses factors which were considered by GPs in 1981 to be the most important indicators of social deprivation. The result is a 'score' for each electoral ward, made up of a weighted average from the following variables: pensioners living alone, children under 5 years of age, one-parent families, unskilled socio-economic groups, unemployed people, high population mobility and households headed by a person born in Pakistan or the New Commonwealth. Virtually every District Department of Public Health has a database of Jarman scores, which provides a map of deprivation and contributes to the service planning process. Scores for districts in England and Wales vary from −35 (extreme affluence) to +55 (extreme deprivation).

Within the Wessex Health Authority Region, Southampton and South West Health Authority holds the highest Jarman 8 score. However, compared to those districts in the north of the country or in London these are still comparatively low. Still, in local terms Jarman scores have been found to be valuable in the assessment of local deprivation, which is known to show a clear association with the incidence of childhood accidents (Agass *et al.*, 1990; McKee *et al.*, 1990). There is some debate regarding the ethical nature of targeting health promotional activity at just one group in society. The Department of Health shows no such doubts and urges a 33 per cent reduction in childhood injuries by 2005 (HMSO, 1992), and proposes that preventive action 'should relate to vulnerable groups' (ibid., p. 108).

AN ACCIDENT BY ANY OTHER NAME: WHAT KIND OF ACCIDENT DO CHILDREN HAVE?

Recently, there has been a rapid expansion in the use of technology to identify health service utilisation patterns (Hoare, 1992). There are still gaps in knowledge relating to the preceding circumstances which lead to an accidental event, and even much of this knowledge is a result of relatively small-scale studies. However, there are some facts which help in the planning of preventive programmes, and these are based on a number of studies or associations made over a number of years. It is known, for example, that the majority of accidents to children under 5 years of age, occur in the home, the place with the strongest associations with safety (Murdock and Eva, 1974). It is also known that many childhood injuries are a direct consequence of normal play behaviour, which can in turn be closely linked to a particular age or developmental phase (Kay, 1983; Thomas, 1989). Accidents that occur as part of the normal developmental progress of a child are most marked up to the age of 5, after which the more adventurous nature of the child results in road accidents in particular taking their toll (Greig, 1987).

Age-related accidents are most marked in children under 5 years, simply because, in order to become proficient in any skill, standing, walking and running, practice is a prerequisite. Such practice takes place without an awareness of the adult world, without knowledge of the hazards and without reading ability to understand necessary warnings. The parent or guardian is the agent for such knowledge but it is 'impossible to watch them 24 hours a day' (CAPT, 1991d). Despite the difficult role the parents and guardians have in the protection of their children there are some ways in which their job can be made more simple, and this lies in the identification of age group-specific risks as part of a health education programme.

Under 1 Year

The infant aged under 1 year is totally dependent on those adults, who also carry responsibility for his or her safety. New manipulative and gross motor skills appear with dramatic and unexpected speed and it is this very rapid escalation of ability that takes an adult by surprise. The occurrence of an accident is sometimes the first time that a child has been able to demonstrate a particular movement and the consequences are heart-rending. Parents attending Accident and Emergency Departments with their children frequently lament, 'I just did not know he/she could do it' (roll over, off the bed; pull the cup full of hot tea). Most accidents under 6 months of age occur as a result of falls and scalds. Innovations designed to assist development

have caused their own group of casualties. One of the clearest examples is the association of the 'Baby Walker' with burn and falls-related injuries, when the child propels
himself into danger and is unable to escape (Reider, Schwartz and Newman, 1986).

Some infants will begin to crawl at 6 months and child care books which give
definitive ages for a particular developmental skill to appear have contributed to a
false sense of parental security which lulls the adult into thinking their child is safe
from certain injuries for a period to come. These are just ranges and general parameters into which most children will fit, but not all do so neatly to a universal
plan. Some children do crawl at 6 months but others have walked at this age also.
In either case the child will usually develop along set lines and as he or she grows
stronger and more mobile, pulling up to standing becomes a prelude to walking
and access to a whole new range of dangers. The child who is able to reach and
pull articles down is subsequently at risk from falling objects and especially those containing hot liquids.

From 1 to 2

Many children are able to walk at 1 year. Even if this is not the case, most are mobile
by one means or another. The world is expanding very rapidly for the child of this age
and their curiosity is boundless, and certainly exceeding parental patience! From the
age of 1 year children remain at risk from the earlier causes but also, because of refine-
ments in motor skill, their ability to turn and open objects such as bottles becomes a
real possibility. Object permanency is gained around this age and parents find that out
of sight out of mind does not apply any more. The child in this age group will relent-
lessly pursue any object, hidden in the very most inaccessible place and sometimes in
the most dangerous manner.

2 to 3 Years

Very little is safe from the inquisitive 2 year old, who may understand the oft-used
word 'no' but will generally pay it little heed. The title 'terrible twos' is not awarded
lightly! Access to the garden increases at this age and so frequently to the contents of
the garage. Substances which were previously kept out of reach whet the appetite of
the young explorer. Generous to a fault, 2 and especially 3 year olds will often share
their poisonous booty with another little friend. A quiet 2 or 3 year old is often one
who is distracted by mischief; when there are two quiet children of this age it is a
virtual certainty.

4 to 5 Years

The 4 year old will have discovered the outside world and may seem very confident.
Natural imitators, they will copy older siblings and adults to the best of their
ability. When this involves activities outside the home the risks escalate. The
garden, if there is one, together with playgrounds are potentially painful areas for
children, particularly if they attempt to copy the more rehearsed skills of older

friends or brother and sisters. This is particularly true when bicycles and roads are involved, when inexperience, lack of strength and speed become important.

From 5 to 15

By the time a child has reached school age, pedestrian accidents resulting from collision with motor vehicles become a real and deadly possibility. Cycling accidents increase between the ages of 5 and 9 and remain a significant cause of injury until the young person leaves school.

SUFFER LITTLE CHILDREN: WHAT MAKES THEM HURT?

Road traffic accidents and burns and scalds claim the most young lives, but even when the injury is not fatal these causes result in the longest and most painful hospital in-patient periods (Sunderland, 1984). In one London study, 59 per cent of the children were scalded by hot water, tea or coffee. A further 8.2 per cent of burns were caused as a result of an adult giving the child a drink or bath that was too hot, as opposed to the child finding it for themselves, and a further 20.4 per cent of burns caused by a child playing with hot objects such as an iron (Consumer Safety Unit, 1983; Working Party, 1985). Information obtained from a five-year analysis of childhood accident data in Southampton has demonstrated that of the children who attended hospital with burns and scalds, 40 per cent resulted from spilt tea or coffee. Furthermore, 78 per cent of these attenders in this group were aged under 2 years (Southampton Community Health Service Unit, 1992).

Head injuries are another important reason for attendance at Accident and Emergency Departments, but many of these, although highly significant in numbers, will simply be minor bumps that shock the child and frighten the parent or guardian. Old wives' tales are still very prevalent in this sphere and all too often one hears parents say something like 'He cried immediately, so I didn't worry' or conversely, 'He didn't cry immediately, so I thought I had better take him to hospital'! Head injuries in children are usually a result of a fall, the higher the fall the greater the risk. In some cases the child may fall from a low height but impact with a sharp object which may cause considerable harm (Casey and Ludwig, 1986). Falls are, of course, a significant cause of hospital attendance in all age groups (Livesley and Atkinson, 1974).

Cuts and lacerations are always numerically important, but most frequently require little more than first aid and very rarely an in-patient admission.

Ingestion of Toxic Substances

In the Brent study (Agass et al., 1990), the second most common reason for attendance at hospital was for poisoning in childhood (the most common reason was given as falls). It was found that some 46 per cent of poisons were found by the children outside their normal storage place, such as in a handbag. In 1987, the

Proprietary Association of Great Britain conducted a study into the aetiology of childhood poisonings. The findings were that children under 2 years of age were the largest group and of these a little more than a half (54 per cent) were boys. In 75 per cent of cases the incident occurred in the child's home. More than half (59 per cent) involved medicinal products and more than one third (37 per cent) were household or garden substances. The child was alone in a room in half (52 per cent) of cases, another child was in the room in a further quarter cases (24 per cent), and an adult was present in 15 per cent of cases. In a subsequent audit of 600 homes, medicines were found in nearly all (97 per cent) where there were children under 5 years of age and the average number of products was 10 per home studied. Of these just 4 per cent were kept in locked cupboards (Proprietary Association, 1987). To a young child it seems as if most substances, especially those which are brightly coloured, are worth a taste.

Drownings

Drownings claimed the lives of 54 children in 1988 and it is estimated that for every fatal incident, there are at least two near drownings, which require admission to hospital (CAPT, 1990).

Bites

According to the Child Accident Prevention Trust, bites from domestic animals represent a real risk to children, especially those under 5 years of age. However, the publicity given to such events has recently heightened the awareness of the public, but in proportion to other injuries animal bites accounted for less than 1 per cent of the total number of child attendances in the Southampton data.

Accidents to children between the ages of 5 and 14 years are likely to occur as a result of most of the causes relevant to the under school age group. However, road traffic accidents, which occur as a result of pedestrians impacting with moving vehicles, claim more young lives than any other cause (DoT, 1989). The vast majority of these were as a result of the child running out in front of the vehicle and most of these occurred close to the child's home. One study examined the expectations of parents regarding a child's ability to cross a busy road. Many thought that it would be safe from around 5 years of age. In reality children are not capable of the kind of judgement which is necessary to estimate the speed of an approaching vehicle until they are well past their twelfth birthday (Constantinides and Walker, 1989).

Most parents will purchase a bicycle for their child when he is quite young, the child obtaining considerable benefit from practising balancing skills and gaining from the increased independence the new toy offers. However, bicycles can be a deadly means with which to acquire new skills. The United Kingdom is probably slower than most countries in getting to grips with a potentially lethal machine.

One study which examined bicycle injuries found that the mean age for consultation at Accident and Emergency Departments was just 9.4 years. Of the children studied, 70 per cent were boys, and of these only 2 per cent were wearing protective helmets. Over 80 per cent of the injuries occurred within half a mile of the child's home and were responsible for 49 per cent of skull injuries (Bull, 1988). Other studies verify these facts (Weiss, 1986; Selbst, Alexander and Ruddy, 1987; *Lancet*, 1988; Thompson, Rivara and Thomason, 1989; Halpern, 1990).

CHILDHOOD ACCIDENT PREVENTION: WHOSE RESPONSIBILITY?

Accident prevention in childhood has long been hampered by a lack of overall strategy and commitment at a high enough level to ensure its implementation and success. The White Paper, *Health of the Nation*, certainly gives the highest level of approval, but does not offer any additional resources to ensure its success. Preventive programmes are still dependent on the interest and goodwill of the many and varied professionals and volunteers who regard this work as a priority. It is also primarily dependent on parents having the financial and emotional resources to be able to anticipate an accident and take the necessary avoiding steps. These in turn are dependent to a certain extent on knowledge of the risks of childhood, and responsibility for imparting this knowledge must lie with individual professional groups. For the under-fives, the groups most likely to be able to perform this activity are health visitors, GPs and, increasingly, practice nurses. Volunteers working with young children and parents also have an opportunity to undertake this work but may need the support and encouragement of a professional to do so. For the over-fives, accident prevention needs to be considered an integral part of school activities and not just an odd subject for a rainy day during the last week of term. The heavy cost of injury and death is too high for such a low place on the curriculum.

One of the greatest opportunities for accident prevention work lies in the collective activities of primary care teams, working together towards the achievement of clear and specific health objectives. For children this would mean that each member of the team would agree the goal and contribute to its achievement. This involves each person working within the GP surgery or health centre, from the receptionist who suggests the health promotion session to parents and guardians visiting the surgery, to the health visitor who will provide the same advice as all the other members of the team to people in their own homes. The surgery would monitor its progress towards a reduction in childhood accident rates, and might even display accident numbers on its notice board. Such a collective approach involves the whole team in a concerted and focused manner. It is such an approach, integrating all professionals and others around one patient/client group, which will offer the best chance of changing the health of the young nation.

REFERENCES

Agass M, Mant D, Fuller A, Coulter A and Jones L (1990) Childhood accidents: a practice survey using General Practitioner's records and parental reports. *British Journal of General Practice*, **40**, 202–5.

Alwash R and McCarthy M (1987) How do child accidents happen? *Health Education Journal* **46**(4), 169–71.

Avery J W, Vaudin J N, Fletcher J L and Watson J M (1990) Geographical and social variations in mortality due to childhood accidents in England and Wales 1975–1984. *Public Health*, **104,** 171–82.

Balarajan R, Yuen P and Machin D (1992) Deprivation and general practitioner workload. *British Medical Journal*, **304,** 529–34.

British Paediatric Association (1987) *Surgeons and Casualty Surgeons in A. & E. Departments.* London: BPA.

Brown G W and Davidson S (1978) Social class, psychiatric disorder of mother and accidents to children. *Lancet*, **1,** 378–80.

Bull J (1988) Cyclists need helmets. *British Medical Journal*, **1,** 296.

CAPT (1989) *Basic Principles of Child Accident Prevention – a guide to action.* London.

CAPT (1990) *Child Safety Review*, **3,** London.

CAPT (1991a) *Preventing Accidents to Children: a training resource for health visitors.* London.

CAPT (1991b) *Approaches to Local Child Accident Prevention Projects.* London.

CAPT (1991c) *Safe as Houses.* London.

CAPT (1991d) *You Can't Watch Them 24 Hours a Day.* London.

Casey R and Ludwig S (1986) Morbidity following minor head trauma in children. *Pediatrics*, **78,** 497–502.

Constantinides P (1988) Safe at home? Children's accidents and inequality. *Radical Medicine.* Spring, 31–3.

Constantinides P and Walker G (1989) *Child Accidents: Inequality in a London Borough.* Research Report to N.E. Thames Health Authority.

Consumer Safety Unit (1983) *Domestic Thermal Injuries: a study of 1100 accidents admitted to specialised treatment centres.* London: DTI.

Department of Health and Social Security (The Black Report) *Inequalities in Health* (1980) London: HMSO, p. 329.

Department of Transport (1989) *Road Accidents in Great Britain.* London: HMSO.

Dickens C (1968) *David Copperfield.* In *Giants of Literature.* (Ed.) Lows L C. Milan: Arnoldo Mondadori Editore.

Eyles J (1987) *The Geography of the National Health.* London: Croom Helm.

Golding J (1986) In Butler N R and Golding J (Eds) *Accidents 'From Birth to Five'.* London: Pergammon Press.

Greig T (1987) The G.P.'s role in child accident prevention. *Practitioner*, **231,** 1612–16.

Halpern J (1990) Bicycle helmets for children. *Journal of Emergency Surgery*, **16,** 36–40.

Hill A (1989) Trends in paediatric medical admissions. *British Medical Journal*, **298,** 1479–83.

HMSO (1992) *The Health of the Nation: a strategy for health in England.* London.

Hoare J (1992) *Tidal Wave: New Technology Medicine and the NHS.* London: Kings Fund Centre.

Jackson R H (1988) The doctor's role in the prevention of accidents, *Archives of Diseases in Childhood*, **63,** 235–57.

Jackson R H and Wilkinson A W (1976) Why don't we prevent childhood accidents? *British Medical Journal*, **1,** 1258–62.

Jarman B (1984) Underprivileged areas. *British Medical Journal*, **289,** 1587–92.

Jarman B. In While, A (Ed) (1989) *Health in the Inner City.* London: Heinemann, pp. 95–115.

Kay E P (1983) A model for the development of priorities in health visiting with special respect to the prevention of accidents in childhood. MA (Ed) Dissertation. University of Southampton.

Lancet (1988) Editorial. When are cyclists going to wear helmets? *Lancet*, **1,** 159–60.

Livesley B and Atkinson L (1974) Repeated falls in the elderly. *Modern Geriatrics*, **11,** 458–67.

McKee C M, Gleadhill D N S and Watson J D (1990) Accident and emergency attendance rates by G.P. practice. *British Journal of General Practice*, **40,** 150–3.

Milner P, Nicholl J and Williams B (1988) Variation in demand for accident and emergency departments in England from 1974–85. *Journal of Epidemiology and Community Health*, **42,** 274–8.

Mitchell J (1984) *What is to be Done about Illness and Health?* Harmondsworth: Penguin.

Murdock K and Eva J (1974) Home accidents to children under 15 years: a survey. *British Medical Journal*, **3,** 103–6.

Murray Parks C (1983) *Bereavement*. Harmondsworth: Penguin.

Neubauer P (Ed.) (1979) *The Process of Child Development*. New York: Meridian.

OPCS (1991) *Mortality Statistics Cause 1990*. London: HMSO.

Pearn J (1978) Predisposing factors leading to child trauma. *Journal of Epidemiology and Community Health*, **32,** 190–3.

Proprietary Association of Great Britain (1987) *Accidental Poisoning in Childhood: a survey*. The Proprietary Association, July.

Quick A (1991) *Unequal Risks: accidents and social policy*. London: Socialist Health Association, p. 10.

Reider M J, Schwartz C and Newman J (1986) Patterns of Walker use and Walker injury. *Pediatrics*, **78,** 3.

Rivara F, Bergman A, LoGerfo J and Weiss N (1982) Epidemiology of childhood injuries 2: sex differences in injury rates. *American Journal of Diseases of Children*, **136,** 502–6.

Selbst S M, Alexander D and Ruddy R (1987) Bicycle-related injuries. *American Journal of Diseases of Children*, **141,** 140–4.

Southampton Community Health Services Unit (1992) *Department of Primary Care Development*. Special Projects Report.

Sunderland R (1984) Dying young in traffic. *Arc. Dis. Child.*, **59,** 754–7.

Thomas E P (1989) Accidents will Happen. *Nursing Times*, **85,** 26–9.

Thomas E P (1991) Unstable lodgings. *Nursing Times*, **87**(30), 42–4.

Thompson R, Rivara F and Thomason D (1989) A case controlled study of the effectiveness of bicycle helmets. *New England Journal of Medicine*, **320,** 1361–7.

Walsh S and Jarvis S N (1992) Measuring the frequency of 'severe' accidental injury in childhood. *Journal of Epidemiology and Community Health*, **46,** 26–32.

Weiss B (1986) Bicycle helmet use by children. *Paediatrics*, **1,** 159–60.

Whalley J (1992) When playtime's over. *Health Service Journal*, **102,** 5313, p. 22.

While A (Ed.) (1989) *Health in the Inner City*. London; Heinemann.

Working Party of the Child Accident Prevention Trust (1985) *Burns and Scald Accidents to Children*. London: Bedford Square Press.

6

Children with Disabilities

Chris Betts and Gill Meyer

In this chapter consideration will be given to the disabled child, his/her family and those who are closely involved in setting up support systems. Obviously, in such a short space it is not possible to look more than superficially at the issues involved, but it is hoped that this will lead the reader to examine some of them in greater depth.

One of the basic philosophical principles behind recent concepts of service delivery for disabled children is that each child, irrespective of race, colour, culture, sex, level of disability or the position of his/her family within their community, is worthy of respect, dignity and equality of access to services, opportunities and activities appropriate to his/her age. They should be respected and accorded dignity simply because they are human; entitled to equality of access because the society that does not offer this is failing to face its own inadequacies.

Unfortunately, discrimination within most modern societies against people of all ages with disabilities is so rife that it has to be regarded as the norm. Attempts to improve their lot through legislation have been of limited success, in some cases lacking even the political will to ensure effectiveness (witness the failure of Parliament to implement key sections of the Disabled Persons Act 1986, six years after its enactment). However, legislation spanning nearly 20 years, from the Chronically Sick and Disabled Persons Act 1970 to the Children Act 1989, *has* contributed to attitudinal change in society. Unfortunately there is still no Act, even on the horizon, to outlaw discrimination in the United Kingdom, and the environment which can turn even normally placid and compliant parents into aggressive fighters for their children's rights seems destined to continue for some years yet.

TERMINOLOGY

It is important to understand the terminology commonly used and to grasp the concepts and philosophies that are now preferred by children, parents and carers. These are forming the core of modern legislation and care practice.

Some alternative definitions for three key words are a useful starting point (World Health Organisation; Cooper, 1981, p. 15).

Impairment: 'A lack or loss of some physical or intellectual function. An intellectual impairment suggests the incomplete development (or loss) of mental abilities.'
Or 'A basic biological fault in a tissue or organ.'

Disability: 'The situation where someone is unable to do certain things because of their original impairment. A learning disability refers to a person's restricted or

reduced ability to learn as quickly or as readily as people without impairments.'
Or 'The limitation of function consequent upon impairment.'

Handicap: 'A person is handicapped when because of a disability he or she has fewer opportunities to take part in everyday life than the non-handicapped person. The real handicap may be other people's attitudes or prejudice.'
Or 'The resulting personal and social disadvantage.'

The word *retardation* is now rarely used in Britain, but would appear still to be widely used in the United States. It suggests a falling behind in norms of development, and has been assumed to imply a permanent reduction in intellectual function (Cooper, 1981, p. 16). It is also used by the World Health Organisation in the classification of people with mental handicaps by using IQ scores (Heddell, 1988, pp. 75, 84), i.e.

Mild retardation ....IQ 50–70
Moderate retardation..IQ 35–50
Severe retardation ....IQ 20–35
Profound retardation ....IQ < 20

Such definitions can be quite powerful, and may be used as tools in an attempt to define a child's ability or disability. Caution needs to be exercised, however, to avoid misusing these words as labels.

The use of terms such as 'child-centred' and 'holistic care' encourage providers of services to focus on the needs of the child. 'Normalisation' and 'age-appropriate care' convey the understanding that individual children are going to be offered normal, homely environments with social activities and recreation that matches their years. Dignity, enabling, consultation, information and the forming of partnerships in care are words that aim to convey support and understanding.

It should be remembered that the term 'disability' covers a very wide range of conditions, from impairment of vision or hearing, or limb deficiency, in a child who otherwise functions within normal parameters, through to profound and multiple handicaps.

THE IMPORTANCE OF APPROPRIATE ASSESSMENT

In order to identify the specific needs of a disabled child – and possibly his/her family also, for in such families it is difficult to separate the needs of one family member from the rest – it is necessary to carry out an assessment. The value, power and protection that a properly conducted assessment offers the child, his or her carers, or the professionals involved, should not be underestimated. The greater the sense of importance that is placed on an objective assessment, the more helpful it is likely to be in the enabling of opportunities to a child.

The professionals involved in assessing a child with disabilities need to be acquainted with the law, policy, service provision, social and personal relationships, and the various methods of information gathering and decision-making. The Children Act 1989 requires that, during the process of any assessment requested by a court, the feelings and wishes of the child are considered, as well as his/her physical, emotional and educational needs, and the likely effect of any change of circumstance. These principles should be acknowledged as good practice and applied to any assessment, whether or not ordered through court proceedings.

Various types of assessment may be employed:

● Health/medical/developmental.
● Care and care requirement.
● Educational.
● Psychological.
● Psychiatric.

A developmental assessment would focus on five key areas of a child's development (Woolfson, 1991, p. 11):

1. Gross motor development (limb/body control and balance).
2. Visual motor development (eye/hand co-ordination).
3. Language development (receptive/expressive language).
4. Social and emotional development (interaction/independence and self-help skills).
5. Intellectual development (ability to adapt and cope with new experiences).

Educational assessment highlights skills that have been achieved and those that have not yet been mastered, and those that need to be maintained and/or developed. These needs are identified clearly in the assessment, and subsequent 'Statement of Special Educational Needs', under the 1981 Education Act. One of the intentions of the Act, which was implemented in 1983, was to offer children with special educational needs the right to integration within the community. The Act also offers parents the right to participate in the assessment process, to submit material towards and comment on the draft Statement, and to appeal against the proposals (Heddell, 1988, p. 174).

Unfortunately, the Audit Commission Report of 1992 identified some serious deficiencies in the way in which children with special educational needs are provided for, among which were a lack of accountability by schools and local education authorities for progress made, or resources used, and lack of incentives for LEAs to implement the 1981 Act.

Statements sometimes identify provision in such general terms that they cannot guarantee a specific level of provision. Such vagueness is admitted by some authorities to be deliberate, since, faced with limited resources, the LEAs avoid open-ended commitments. Parents can find such statements very difficult to use, when endeavouring to ensure that their child's educational needs are met (Audit Commission, 1992).

While all assessments are becoming progressively more specialised, it can be seen that there is a common base from where each process starts. Most assessments have three functions:

1. To *describe* the child's problems/requirements.
2. To *make a judgement* about the nature of the problems.
3. To *make recommendations* regarding the form of intervention required to resolve or alleviate the problems (Grimshaw and Sumner, 1991).

In each case, accuracy and a succinct method are vital. Attention needs to be given to short-, medium- and longer-term goals, and an automatic review policy in order to evaluate progress.

Assessments may be carried out in a variety of ways. Some professionals use observation over a given period, requiring a team to submit judgements and recommendations at the end. Others may require one experienced individual to consider the needs of a child through the eyes of several colleagues, with whom he/she would then have close liaison to discuss the implications of the care or treatment that might be appropriate.

A useful approach to assessment is that of 'cross-planning' (Browder, 1991, p. 30), i.e. considering skills that are used across different areas or domains, e.g. motor, self-care and recreation skills. Because they are related to the activities of daily living they are called 'related' skills. It is essential, therefore, that no professional should conduct assessments in isolation from other disciplines.

THE DISABLED CHILD IN SOCIETY

An OPCS survey (Bone and Meltzer, 1989) showed that there are approximately 360,000 families in Great Britain with one or more children under the age of 16 years, who suffer from one or more disabilities. In the South-East of England alone there are 76,000 families where there is a disabled child being cared for at home. Statistics produced by Kushlick and Cox (1973, pp. 748–59) indicated that in Western Europe, in a population of 250,000, there could be 340–350 children under 18 years of age requiring mental handicap services alone.

The responsibility on each Health Authority, under the NHS and Community Care Act 1990, to assess the health needs of its population provides an opportunity to respond to the specific requirements of children with disabilities. In order to meet the needs of this dependent sector of society effectively, the costs of services to local and central government must not be underestimated. Extensive research has also illustrated the enormous costs incurred by carers (Drew, 1989).

MULTI-AGENCY INVOLVEMENT

It could be argued that in the field of disability more than any other, the importance of effective interdisciplinary co-operation is paramount. The havoc and distress caused by breakdowns in communication have costly implications – both in monetary and human terms.

The specialist input required by a profoundly multi-handicapped child requires not only constant review, but an on-going appreciation of the developing skills of the parents, who often become multi-skilled carers (Meyer, 1990). That is, they assume not only the multifaceted role that is parenthood, but also become nurse, dietitian, physiotherapist, teacher, etc.

Since needs change from time to time (sometimes from day to day), it is difficult, if not impossible, to include all those who might be involved with a family, when reviewing a child's situation. Clearly, there will be periods when one agency or professional has a high degree of input, which is gradually reduced as needs change. However, especially where the child has profound or multiple handicaps, it is sometimes startling just how many agencies or individuals are involved when the situation is analysed (see Figure 6.1). It is not difficult to imagine how easy it can be for families either to 'fall through the net', or be passed between authorities and departments, all of whom appear to have the protection of their budget as their top priority. Of course, there are many examples of good practice, where agencies work in close and effective collaboration, but unfortunately, many families find this ideal to be the exception rather than the rule.

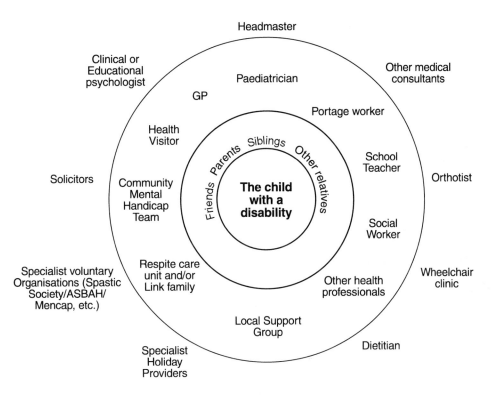

Fig. 6.1 Multi-agency involvement.

High demands are made on specialist support services, which require not only awareness of each other, but thoughtful and sensitive co-ordination between all areas. An effective and prompt communication network is essential for the well-being of the child and his/her family. The community mental handicap team is often a pivot for specialist help. A member of this team might be appointed as key worker, liaising with other professionals, gathering and disseminating information, so that the family is not inundated by a large number of well-intentioned people, each wanting to consider different aspects of the family's needs. However, such protection is viable and justified only so far, since one person cannot be a 'multi-specialist'.

In order to offer the child good care and treatment, services need to be flexible, local where possible, and able to accommodate children in appropriate environments according to their needs, and the associated needs of their parents.

The Children Act 1989 requires that where children are cared for in residential settings, they are reviewed on a regular basis. This ensures that the placement does not 'drift', and that short-, medium- and longer-term goals are regularly reviewed.

If professionals communicate effectively, and early, with the family and with each other, crisis management can be avoided. Forward planning helps parents to face problems before they become intractable. A clear respect of each other's boundaries and involvement avoids duplication of work and unnecessary defensiveness. More importantly, the child is likely to be offered a better service by those who work in a co-ordinated manner. Joint clinics, when properly thought through, can conserve resources and save time and frustration for families and professionals alike. A paediatrician, orthopaedic specialist and liaison nurse, for example, with access to a physiotherapist, orthotist and dietitian, would be an efficient and effective example of collaborative working.

RESPITE FROM CARE

In recent years, and most recently in response to the Children Act, many local Social Services Departments have developed their own short-term care units, or have recruited 'Link' or 'Befriending' families to offer parents occasional breaks from the care of a disabled child. This reflects the preferred approach of providing local care in the community. However, more parents now feel able to demand choice with regard to the services they are offered, rejecting vociferously the take it or leave it attitude which has characterised statutory provision for so long.

Choice is a complex ideal to strive towards, since it depends on all parties having sufficient information on all theoretical and actual options and entitlements, as well as local resources and the budgetary constraints of the statutory authorities. Additionally, a parent – or child – may not have developed sufficient skills to be able to cope with diverse choices.

Developments in community care are welcomed by all, but unfortunately an appropriate range of services is not uniformly available to all families. This is particularly noticeable when considering the respite care requirements of the parents of a profoundly multi-handicapped child who needs medical oversight or specialised nursing care; similarly, the disabled child with challenging behaviour. Carol Youngs, Director of 'Contact-A-Family', an umbrella organisation for several hundred specialist support groups, states that the greater the degree of disability, the less relevant the statutory respite care available to a parent.

In particular, few paediatric nurses would argue with the fact that an acute paediatric ward is not an appropriate environment for a handicapped child to be given respite care. Neither is a local authority hostel for children with a learning disability suitable for a child who also has complex physical problems.

If it is to benefit the family at all, the experience of respite care must be a positive one for the child, as well as offering the family the confidence to take a proper break. This means that they should be comfortable enough with their child's situation to go away – if that is what they want to do – secure in the knowledge that staff can meet their child's needs, and that, barring an emergency, they will not be called to collect the child because he/she has developed a rash or a temperature, or has had a series of fits.

Because of the shortfall in suitable statutory provision, a network of highly specialised support has developed within the charitable and voluntary sector for these unique groups in society. The growth in the number of children's hospices is but one example: also organisations offering domiciliary/palliative care, and other innovative support mechanisms, which in many areas would not be possible to arrange through local statutory provision. In the purchaser/provider environment created by the NHS and Community Care Act it is quite appropriate that authorities can purchase services which they could not cost-effectively provide within their own boundaries, for groups of children whose numbers within any one geographical area will only ever be very small. Difficulties remain, however, as provision is patchy, and some areas are much better served than others.

CARE WHICH ENABLES – OR REINFORCES DISABILITY?

There is a danger that the child with a chronic health problem or disability may be seen as a medical condition or a set of problems, instead of as a young individual who has personal preferences, and a positive capacity to contribute, albeit in a limited way. Consequently, he/she may be seen as being 'ill', as opposed to well, but having an on-going need for specialist support. This affects the way people speak to them, and the expectations that are held of them. This in turn influences the child's own self-image and expectations.

It is a natural instinct for parents to want to protect their vulnerable handicapped child. Even so, and in spite of a high level of respite care support, good social work input and medical supervision, an articulate father of a child with Rett Syndrome, a relatively rare genetic disorder which affects only girls, resulting in profound mental and physical disability, has said:

'Every parent aspires to protect their very young children from the harsher realities of life, and give them a tranquil yet stimulating childhood. Rett parents are not different, and yet they cannot protect their daughters, and so can only observe the sufferings of their child in anguish. A deep well of often unexpressed grief and anger is often sunk, and even with the most rational will in the world, one is left stranded with accompanying feelings of guilt, and loneliness.' (Field, 1990)

However, the desire to protect can sometimes become confused with wanting to maintain control, leading parents and professionals into a pattern of caring which reinforces the child's disability, instead of enabling him/her to achieve potential.

It might be useful to repeat here that people can impose handicaps on others by their attitudes and/or prejudices. This can be brought about through not under-standing fully what the difficulties are. If care is to be child-centred, it is essential that professionals not only listen, but that they really hear what the child or the parent is trying to say. Sometimes it is impossible to appreciate the problems until a direct part has been played in caring practically for someone who has special needs. There is an old Chinese proverb which says:

I hear and I forget
I see and I remember
I do and I understand

No one, neither parent, nor professional, has absolute control over a child, even though each input may be valuable. Each has individual accountabilities, making for a joint responsibility. This emphasises the importance of good teamwork, and the ability to see problems in the context of other needs that the child and his or her family might have.

Nevertheless great caution is required in the way that confidential information is used in the decision-making process. The National Children's Bureau's 'Who Cares?' and 'Who Says?' projects clearly document the opinions of young people on this subject, and how they consider themselves to be labelled and spoken for by professionals who are relative strangers, and are too often ill-informed (Page and Clark, 1975; Gardner, 1987). Direct involvement in the management needs that these children require reduces the likelihood of making incorrect assumptions.

DIRECT CARE

Positioning and Mobility

The importance of correct posture for the child with physical disabilities can hardly be overemphasised, for so many other things depend upon it – including lung function; the ability and opportunity to communicate meaningfully and learn; feeding – and therefore nutritional status; maintenance of mobility; renal function; and the opportunity to gain or maintain continence. To some extent then, every body system depends on appropriate positioning. Once this basic truth is grasped, the significance of appropriate seating, toilet and feeding aids becomes apparent.

All children learn through experience and rely on their carers to provide them with that experience. The responsibility, therefore, to make those experiences positive is obvious.

A wheelchair should be seen as a means of moving from one place to another, and never as a child's only seating during their waking hours. In the same way that anyone moves during the course of the day through multiple positions as different activities are undertaken, so should the physically disabled child be given the opportunity to experience a variety of positions, and therefore diversity of stimulation.

Regular standing is crucial, no matter what the level of disability. It aids blood flow, respiration, urinary drainage, digestion, the prevention of osteoporosis and flexion deformities, and encourages the development of the acetabulum. Far from being pointless if the child is not expected to walk, or not worth the bother because it may take the effort of two or more people to achieve a satisfactory position, it is usually rewarding for all concerned, the extra elevation and different perspective offered being enjoyed by the child, who is often better able to participate in activities or games. There is now a variety of different pieces of equipment which can offer good posture, according to each child's assessed need.

Weight bearing generally needs encouragement, even if the only practical application is standing transfers from chair to bed or to toilet, which may make all the difference in enabling the family to continue coping with the child's needs at home, without injury to themselves. Side-lying boards, toilet seats and alternative forms of seating should also be considered, but the equipment used must offer a good position – an outgrown chair is not just uncomfortable but actually harmful to the child, who is likely to develop deformities or exacerbate those already established (Thistlethwaite, 1989).

For children unable to make purposeful movements, or only of some parts of the body, passive movements of all joints need to be undertaken on a daily basis – and preferably at least twice a day. There is no question of this being seen as purely the province of the physiotherapist. To be of maximum value it must be taught to the principal carers as part of the child's essential routine. Many functional stretches which enhance more formal positive movements can be incorporated into other aspects of care, such as stretching adductors while changing nappies, or raising arms above the head, and rolling the knees from side to side as a routine when a child gets up after a rest period. This makes correct positioning easier and increases body awareness.

Feeding and Nutrition

Correct positioning is also essential to the establishment of a beneficial pattern of feeding and achieving a good nutritional status. This in turn increases the child's resistance to infection; improves skin condition, reducing the likelihood of developing pressure sores; and reduces mealtime stress, perhaps making it possible for meals to be taken with the rest of the family.

The role of the speech therapist in assessing the child's swallow, oral skills for eating and development of correct techniques is not always understood. Parents, nursing and care staff need to learn how to inhibit unwanted reflexes, such as tongue thrust, bite and hypersensitive gag reflexes, which are often misinterpreted as behavioural responses. These have to be overcome before more mature and safer feeding patterns can be established.

The increased use of videofluoroscopy to establish just what does happen to food and fluids introduced into the mouth has resulted in a better understanding of the need for adequate assessment. On some occasions the results are very alarming, demonstrating all too clearly why the child is so prone to chest infections! Mince – that much loved institutional answer to every child's 'need' for a meat meal – is actually one of the least suitable foods to offer a child with swallowing problems, the mixed texture being very difficult for them to deal with, and frequently resulting in inhalation.

One result of such revelations in recent years has been an increasing trend towards enteral feeding, whether by nasogastric tube, gastrostomy or jejunostomy. If oral feeding is shown to be unsafe – or unsuitable as the principal route of nutritional intake – and an enteral route is chosen, the child and the family are often released from what has become a daily battle to achieve a certain calorie intake. They may need reassurance at this point that they have not failed their child.

With the pressure off, oral feeding may be reintroduced at a later stage as a means of encouraging tongue movements and of introducing pleasurable tastes and textures rather than as the only way to maintain the child's diet.

Dietary reassessment for all children with disabilities, at intervals which reflect either changes in weight or condition, are crucial to the child's well-being. It is as important that a child does not become overweight as it is to maintain or gain weight in a child who is undernourished. The child who becomes obese compromises lung and renal function, and puts unnecessary demands on his or her own circulatory system, not to mention the carers' backs! The argument that 'food is the only thing he/she takes pleasure in' is a difficult one to counteract, but compromises can often be reached. Custards and sauces made with skimmed instead of full cream milk, low fat cheeses used when cooking and the use of ultra lean meats, together with the use of diet drinks, and replacing sugar with artificial sweeteners, are examples which need not take the pleasure out of eating.

Skill Development

The handicapped child painstakingly learns new skills at home and school, and unless he/she is given every opportunity and encouragement to keep practising those skills, there is a danger that they will be lost. Each new skill enhances a child's sense of self-worth, and frequently the ease of management.

It is a source of great pain to those who have watched over a child's slow acquisition of skills over a period of years, when that young person reaches 19 years old and risks losing them because an appropriate home environment cannot be found. Too often, a profoundly handicapped school leaver, who has learnt alternative means of communication such as Makaton, or simple eye pointing to make choices, cannot be cared for at home by parents whose own health may be at risk. Placed in long-term residential accommodation because there is no suitable alternative, they are faced with a situation where staff are not conversant with their communication skills, or simply do not have the time to allow choices to be made. Dignity is so closely tied up with the means to make wishes and feelings known, but sadly this is often sacrificed too.

Controlling Behaviour

The development of certain skills is achieved by some parents and professionals through behaviour modification. This is based on the idea that what we do is influenced by what happens immediately afterwards. If when we do something, what happens next is something pleasant, we will be likely to want to do it again. If it is unpleasant, we will be less likely to want to do it again.

Thus, the will, determination and developing skill of the parent and of involved professionals are crucial. However, good co-ordination, communication and support are necessary to ensure sustained improvement in the child's behaviour. It is important for the parents – and the child, too, where possible – to participate in the setting of goals and to understand the aims and rationale behind a programme that is set up. Such efforts are not always rewarded with success, however, and it is also important that parents do not perceive failure to achieve the goals set as personal failure on their part.

THE CHILD WITH A LIFE-THREATENING CONDITION

The families of many profoundly handicapped children, and those with degenerative conditions, live with the constant threat of critical ill health, which may be life-threatening. Parents lurch from one crisis to the next, desperately trying to maintain a positive outlook when they are exhausted, worried, financially hard-pressed and/or experiencing marital problems.

Working with these children, their parents and the professionals who give care, treatment and therapy brings a realisation of how very important today is to each child and the parents. If today is a good experience for the child, then he/she and everyone else will feel better about tomorrow; and so it is sometimes possible to help create or regenerate positivity in the most difficult circumstances.

However, it is not really that simple. Good working relationships are based on trust, openness, honesty, information sharing and mutual respect; but some professionals find it hard to be honest, if that means giving painful news. Others choose to give parents only a certain amount of information for fear of causing unnecessary anxiety. Such paternalism does not always help (Woolfson, 1991, p. 11).

On matters such as levels of specialist nursing or medical intervention – for example, whether or not it is appropriate to pass a nasogastric tube at a particular point in time – it is vital for the parents to be consulted frequently and in sufficient detail for them to feel involved and respected as responsible people. Health professionals – especially medical and nursing staff – still sometimes consider that they are helping parents by making decisions for them, forgetting or failing to acknowledge that by so doing, they are inadvertently undermining them. Informed consent goes hand in hand with this crucial issue, but can only be achieved by people who listen, are flexible, and are capable of consistently keeping the child and his/her needs as the centre of focus.

WHAT OF THE FUTURE

To consider the future in terms of care and support for the disabled child and his/her family, there are three influencing factors. These broadly are:

1. Legislative matters and government policies.
2. Social change: changing attitudes; the growth of support and pressure groups to work for further legislative or attitudinal change.
3. Advances in knowledge: e.g. in paediatric neurology and genetics; medical and surgical techniques; diagnostics, medication, and special diets.

These three forces are slowly having far-reaching and positive effects on the disabled child. As a result of policy, the numbers of children with disabilities living in institutional care – either children's homes or mental handicap hospitals – has reduced dramatically during the past fifteen years. Although foster care placements have grown in number, many more are needed if children with disabilities are to be offered the chance of family life.

Similarly, a dramatic increase in the numbers of 'Link Families' is needed to support families who want to continue to manage their disabled children within their own community. Resources, sadly, rarely follow the rhetoric of stated government intention.

Integration of disabled children into mainstream schools is currently being achieved in many areas, under the provisions of the 1981 Education Act. Although this is considered by some to be the ultimate goal for all children with disabilities, it is doubtful whether all children's needs could realistically be met in this way. This is a debate which will undoubtedly continue for some years yet; in the meantime some children who would clearly benefit from full integration are still being prevented from entering mainstream schools through a combination of lack of appropriate facilities or funding and lack of vision – or will. At the same time, some parents whose children's needs are not being met within mainstream education are having to fight through the courts for access to facilities such as speech therapy, which the child has formally been assessed as needing.

The Audit Commission Report (1992) has recommended changes to the state-menting process in order to increase the level of accountability of both schools and LEAs, specifying the obligations on each, and it is to be hoped that this will assist parents to identify whether their child's needs are being met appropriately within the system.

At the time of writing, an Education Bill is crawling through the parliamentary process. A chapter devoted to 'Pupils with Special Educational Needs' incorporates proposals set out in the consultation document 'Special Educational Needs; Access to the System' (Department of Education, 1992). This aims to improve access to assessment and statementing; to set time-limits within which these processes must be accomplished; to give parents the right to express a preference for a particular ordinary or special maintained school for their child; to require the LEA to meet the parents' preference after appropriate consultation, providing certain conditions are met; and to provide for extended rights of appeal. It remains to be seen how much of this reaches the statute book.

The Children Act 1989, together with documents and policies such as *The Welfare of Children in Hospital* (DoH, 1991a), and *The Patient's Charter* (DoH, 1991b), have the potential to make significant differences to the way in which care and treatment is delivered, and should begin to do so when nurses and others become fully acquainted with them and begin to use them as levers to influence change.

Social changes such as the increased expectations of working mothers, the con-tinuing rise of family breakdown and single-parent families, as well as the greater mobility of families and the recognition of the special needs of ethnic groups all contribute to the changing and developing pattern of the society in which these children grow up.

In 1987, the National Association of Health Authorities, The British Paediatric Association and The King's Fund set up a working party to 'provide guidelines for health authorities on the care of those groups of dying children for whom plans could be made' (Baum, Dominica and Woodward, 1990). As a consequence of this, and various other initiatives in different parts of the country, the whole profile of the terminally ill child has been raised.

Advances in medicine and developments in practice and care are happening at an increasing pace, apparently offering an opportunity for triumph for the child and his/her family; but in reality, according to a paediatric neurologist, Dr Edward Brett (1991, p. vii), 'Small profits and slow returns' describe the outcomes in many cases. 'The initial diagnostic exercise may have been brief or prolonged, but the diagnosis is not the end of the story, merely the start of another chapter.'

REFERENCES

Audit Commission (1992) *Getting in on the Act – Provision for Pupils with Special Educational Needs: The National Picture*. London: HMSO.

Baum J D, Dominica Sister Frances and Woodward Robert N (1990) *Listen. My Child Has a Lot of Living to Do. Caring for Children with Life Threatening Conditions*. Oxford: University Press, in association with The Institute of Child Health, Bristol.

Bone Margaret and Meltzer Howard (1989) *O.P.C.S. Surveys – Disability in Great Britain. Report No. 3: 'Prevalence of Disability Among Children'*. London: HMSO.

Brett Edward (Ed.) (1991) *Paediatric Neurology*. 2nd edition. Edinburgh: Churchill Livingstone.

Browder Diane M (1991) *Assessment of Individuals with Severe Disabilities. An Applied Behavior Approach to Life Skills Assessment*. 2nd Edition. Maryland: Paul H Brookes.

Cooper Brian (Ed.) (1981) *Assessing the Handicaps and Needs of Mentally Retarded Children*. New York: Academic Press.

Department of Education (1992) *Special Educational Needs: Access to the System*. London: HMSO.

Department of Health (1991a) *The Welfare of Children in Hospital*. London: HMSO.

Department of Health (1991b) *The Patient's Charter*. London: HMSO.

Drew Sarah (1989) *Disability Benefit – An income to support my needs*. London: The Spastic Society.

Field P (1990) Rett Syndrome. *Interlink (Cerebral Palsy Overseas)*. May.

Gardner R (1987) *Who Says? Care and Control in Care*. London: National Children's Bureau.

Grimshaw Roger and Sumner Maggie (1990) *What's Happening to Child Care Assessment? An Exploratory Study of New Approaches*. London: National Children's Bureau.

Heddell Fred (1988) *Children with Mental Handicaps*. Marlborough: Crowood Press.

Kushlick A and Cox G (1973) The epidemiology of mental subnormality. *Developmental Medicine & Child Neurology*.

Meyer Gill (1990) Listen to the parents. *Paediatric Nursing*. May.

Page R and Clarke G (1975) *Who Cares? Young People in Care Speak Out*. London: National Children's Bureau.

Thistlethwaite Belinda (1989) Apparatus and services. *Paediatric Nursing*. May.

Woolfson Richard (1991) *Children With Special Needs. A Guide for Parents and Carers*. London: Faber & Faber.

World Health Organisation, Cooper, 1981, p. 15.

FURTHER READING

Ainsworth-Smith Ian and Speck Peter (1982) *Letting Go: Caring for the Dying and Bereaved*. London: SPCK.

Carr Janet (1980) *Helping Your Handicapped Child: A Step-by-step Guide to Everyday Problems*. London: Penguin.

Davies Brian Meredith (1990) *Community Health and Social Services* 5th Edition. Sevenoaks: Hodder & Stoughton Educational.

Goodall C (1992) Preserving dignity for disabled people. *Nursing Standard*, 20 May.

Griffiths Margaret and Clegg Mary (1988) *Cerebral Palsy: Problems and Practice*, Human Horizons Series. London: Souvenir Press.

Jepson Marion E (1983) *Community Child Health*. Sevenoaks: Hodder & Stoughton Educational.

McCormack Andrina E (1985) *Coping with your Handicapped Child*. Edinburgh: Chambers.

McKendrick Olive (1991) *Assessment of Multihandicapped Visually Impaired Children: Discussion Paper from the Working Party on Services to Multihandicapped Visually Impaired Children and Young People*. London: Royal National Institute for the Blind.

Morris J (1991) *Pride against Prejudice: Transforming Attitudes to Disability*. London: The Women's Press.

Sines David and Bicknell Joan (1985) *Caring for Mentally Handicapped People in the Community*, Lippincott Nursing Series. London: Harper & Row.

Walsh Alison (Ed.) (1991) *Nothing Ventured: Disabled People Travel the World: A Rough Guide Special*. London: Harrap Columbus.

Wynne-Jones Pat (1985) *Children, Death and Bereavement*. London: Scripture Union.

7

Transcultural Aspects of
Paediatric Nursing

Jim Richardson

The idea of transcultural issues in nursing has been gaining popularity among British nurses as a topic worthy of study. This is clearly seen in the number of published papers and books on this subject which have appeared recently in the United Kingdom. The need for nurses to take a professional interest in the area of cultural factors is obvious now that it is accepted that the United Kingdom is a multicultural society. Most of us now regularly meet, both socially and professionally, people from 'cultures' other than our own. Even if this were not so, however, the areas of interest of transcultural nursing would be of great importance since, in the broadest sense, culture is central to *every* individual – nurse, client or patient. We should consider cultural issues in care planning if this care is to be truly person-centred and holistic.

Although, as will be shown, cultural issues are highly significant for children and families, little of the publishing activity in this area has been by or specifically for paediatric nurses. This is a surprising gap since pregnancy, childbirth and childrearing inevitably bring people into contact with the health services.

At this stage it will be useful to define just what is meant by the idea of 'culture'. This, in fact, is not altogether straightforward since culture is a large, complex and abstract concept. The word culture is also often used in many ways and in many contexts adding to the confusion. Culture is sometimes used to mean 'nationality' or 'ethnic group', or it can be used to describe the artistic or literary production of a group. Many workers from several different social sciences, such as sociology and anthropology, have attempted to clarify a definition of culture.

Perhaps one of the clearest and simplest definitions is offered by a medical anthropologist, G. J. Helman:

'culture can be seen as an inherited "lens", through which individuals perceive and understand the world that they inhabit, and learn how to live with it. Growing up within any society is a form of *en*culturation, whereby the individual slowly acquires the cultural "lens" of that society. Without such a shared perception of the world, both the cohesion and the continuity of any human group would be impossible.' (Helman, 1990 p. 3)

This definition emphasises the important features of culture: it is learned, so it is passed from generation to generation; it consists of shared views, beliefs, habits, values and customs, which form the basis for the rules that allow humans to live in and derive support from groups. Culture, therefore, allows people to identify a group to which they belong, although this can also be the basis for friction between groups.

There has been a tendency among nurses, and others, to see culture in terms of groups which appear exotically different from one's own. In fact, nothing could be further from the truth (Weller, 1991). Culture is integral to everyone and it could be argued that each of us belongs to several cultures. We belong to the culture of our parents, but that differs slightly from the culture we share with our age-group peers, e.g. the culture of youth. When we complete professional or vocational education we enter the culture of people who do the same job. Nursing has a strong and distinctive culture. Values, beliefs, habits and customs are transmitted through education to each succeeding generation of nurses (Ashworth and Morrison, 1989; Bradby, 1990). This is often to the despair of those who seek to bring about changes in this rather conservative culture/profession! The analogy of nursing as a culture can be used to demonstrate other features of this phenomenon. Although members of a defined culture share beliefs, values and customs to some extent, there is also a wide range of variation in the degree to which these features are shared. For example, one nurse may feel that it is politically important for nurses to campaign for better pay and working conditions even to the point of striking, believing that this will ultimately benefit users of the health services. Another nurse may feel that her patients are owed a duty which would preclude her ever participating in strike action. This illustrates the individuality within cultures which makes assumptions and generalisations about a person on the basis of his culture potentially unreliable. Identification of a person's cultural features is possible only by asking that person (Littlewood, 1988). Culture may impose some difficult obligations on its members so individuals exercise some degree of choice as to the degree to which they will adhere to these obligations. This can be seen as one of the reasons for the so-called 'generation gap' between parents and adolescent children who are beginning to exercise choice in the formation of their world-view and those actions based on this. This example also illustrates the fact that culture is not static – it is constantly shifting and slightly changing with time in response to the environment to which the culture is exposed. If the environment changes rapidly, then cultural norms can be expected to change also. This can be seen in the case of the emigrant who suddenly finds himself in a completely alien environment; this person may then experience *culture shock*, which has been defined by Brink and Saunders (1976) as the situation when an abrupt transition, with many major and minor differences in lifestyle, is made from a familiar to an alien environment. A South-East Asian refugee in the United States described the feeling as 'being like a goat in a herd of cows' (Rairdan and Higgs, 1992). Any nurse who has spent time working abroad will recognise this description! This is a feature of the discomfort experienced by, for example, families from the Indian Subcontinent when they arrive in Britain. Sometimes these families will require the help of the health services and will be shocked and bewildered not simply by the ill health necessitating this contact but also by the alien norms of this new culture surrounding them.

The process of coming to terms with and adapting to a new culture is termed *acculturation*. People do not, however, simply abandon their old culture and adopt a new one, 'It is . . . the creation of a new culture which has mixed the values of the original and adopted cultures and is producing something quite distinct from both' (Parfitt, 1988). This phenomenon can be observed among those immigrant families who appear to have completely assimilated the majority culture's norms but who react unexpectedly when they experience a crisis (Hartog and Hartog, 1983). An example of this might be seen in the situation in which a South Asian family's teenage daughter wishes to eschew the tradition of arranged marriage and select her own partner. This may cause enormous conflict within the family and may be the sort of situation in which a paediatric nurse may find herself at a loss. This points to an important feature of culture in that the most deeply-held and cherished cultural values are embodied in rituals marking important life events such as birth, marriage and death (Dobson, 1991). These rituals serve as *rites of passage* marking a change in the situation and status of the individuals involved. The fact that many of these rituals centre on childbirth, childrearing and coming of age emphasises the importance of paediatric nurses developing an understanding of culture's rôle in the lives of their patients/ clients and their families. Gaining an appreciation and understanding of cultural issues is, of course, rather more easily said than done. A wry North American Indian proverb runs, 'Never judge a person until you have walked a mile in his moccasins.'

Much of the activity in nurse education concerning this topic has centred on isolated exposés of the cultural features of the major cultural minorities represented in the United Kingdom (Stokes, 1991). This is naturally important and relevant, but long 'shopping lists' of facts, though initially interesting, can be difficult to absorb and will ultimately become tedious without a better understanding of the basic concepts of culture. Would it perhaps be more constructive to concentrate less on culture-specific information and more on ideas shared by people from many different cultures but interpreted and expressed in different ways (Tuck and Harris, 1988; Lynam, 1992)? Consider for a moment some of the rituals following childbirth, particularly if the baby is unwell. A Christian family may wish to have the baby christened, a Hindu family might wish to write the mantra 'Om' on the baby's tongue with honey (Henley, 1982a), while a Muslim family may wish that a male relative whisper the Islamic call to prayer into the baby's ear (Henley, 1982b) and perhaps attach an amulet round the baby's neck or wrist. All of these very different rituals might be seen to have a common purpose: (1) to welcome the baby into the human community, and (2) to offer some ritual protection to the baby and ensure his well-being. The motivation for these ceremonies is therefore shared but expressed in different ways.

Perhaps one of the most useful things a nurse can do in striving to understand cultural issues is to explore his/her own culture (Melia, 1987; McCall, 1991). Our own culture is so much part of ourselves that many of our beliefs and values are virtually subconscious so that actions based on cultural orientation are almost reflex-produced, without thought or analysis. We are all, therefore, to a greater or lesser extent *ethnocentric*, we have absorbed the values of our culture, hold these important, are often willing to defend them, and measure other peoples' cultural values against them (Thiedermann, 1986). It is then a short step to judging others' cultural norms negatively against our own, which we consider the best and most appropriate. It is important to stress that these value-judgements are often subconscious and unintentional – but no less damaging for that. An example of this might be seen in the attitude of many British nurses who feel, rather patronisingly, that the rôle of women in traditional Islamic families is 'wrong', judged against their own benchmark of women's rights, and may go so far as to try to persuade Muslim women to adopt British norms of self-determination and choice – this though with little insight into the rôles or dynamics of the Muslim family and society. This might be seen as counterproductive in the caring relationship, and potentially offensive. Another danger of unthinking ethnocentrism is that it requires only a short step before such thinking becomes the repellent phenomenon of *racism*, defined by Mares *et al.* (1985) as beliefs based on cultural prejudices and actions based on these beliefs – treating someone in an unfair way because of his or her membership of a particular cultural group. This may lead even to difficulty in gaining access to health care (Health Visitors Association, 1989). Of course, this attitude is usually not based on factual knowledge. It is not an easy task to begin unravelling our own cultural beliefs and our ethnocentrism, but success in this venture is richly rewarded in a deeper understanding of our own responses and those with whom we have a professional relationship (Anderson, 1990).

We have a duty to our patients/clients to consider that they might not share our perspectives or interpretation of events. The importance of this to paediatric nurses is immense because since children are developmentally immature and culture is learned, children are in the process of assimilating their own cultural norms and may be deeply confused and anxious if these norms are breached by a well-meaning but ignorant nurse. Since culturally determined issues are often subconscious, simply accepted as reality, and children often have difficulty in expressing their views whether through immature language skills or because English is not their first language, effort is demanded of the nurse in clarifying these questions. Partnership between the nurse and the child's parents in providing care is imperative. Put very simply, cultural norms form part of the child's everyday routine. Paediatric nurses are well aware of the serious effect on any child of disrupting his routine. We must, therefore, be sufficiently flexible to adapt to different practices.

Culture is usually expressed in behaviour seen as customs or habits. These customs are visible expressions of a shared philosophy and as such are usually held to be important. These customs usually have a rational basis in terms of being a response to the environment in which the culture was originally formed. Often, as cultures and living environments change, the original response behaviours become 'fossilised' and retain no useful purpose other than as a badge of belonging to a group. Certain cultural and religious groups have dietary laws which prohibit the eating of certain foods, such as pork and shellfish. These groups tend to have their origin in environments which have hot climates. Under these conditions such foods spoiled rapidly and might have caused food poisoning. It can be seen that such 'public health laws' lose their relevance in the context of modern Britain but retain importance as markers of commitment to belonging to a group who share this habit of avoiding such foods. Some of these practices may strike the ethnocentric British person as strange, but one Jewish adolescent patient in a children's ward described the thought of eating pork as seeming to her like the thought of eating snake might appear to me!

Some of the customs and beliefs which contribute to culture can be illustrated by considering ordinary, everyday questions.

RELIGION

Religion is closely interwoven with culture and is similarly a large and difficult-to-define idea (Smart, 1989). The Concise Oxford Dictionary defines religion thus: 'a particular system of faith and worship, human recognition of a superhuman controlling power, effect of such recognition on conduct and mental attitude' (Sykes, 1982). Religions function in many ways as social codes, laying down rules for behaviour. They also allow people to feel a sense of belonging to a group from which they derive support and comfort. As with culture in general, religion finds expression in rituals which adherents recognise as affirmations of their religious faith. Religion also provides through faith, explanations for otherwise inexplicable and frightening events, such as serious illness. Religion also offers comfort to beleaguered people through specific guidance and through prayer. Nurses must recognise these functions in the people they care for even though they may not always understand what is happening. Space and time must be created to respect the privacy required for ritual or prayer (Sampson, 1982). I vividly remember caring for a 4-year-old boy from a devoutly religious community in London, who required emergency surgery. The entire children's ward was threatened with upset by the child's family's very vocal prayer and distress. A wise and sensitive ward sister, however, quickly organised a private area for the family and the company of a nurse who could calm as well as answer queries and concerns, and above all tolerate this ritual behaviour. A manifest respect for such behaviour, determined by culture and/or religion, is essential and fosters a feeling of acceptance in such families in trouble. This lays the foundation for an equal and respectful relationship between families and paediatric nurses.

Religious and cultural traditions are often intertwined and it is often difficult to tease these apart. An example of this is the ritual genital mutilation, the so-called 'female circumcision', practised by certain Muslim communities (McLean and Graham, 1981). In fact, Muslim thinkers and leaders strenuously oppose this practice. Performing this mutilation is now punishable by law in this country and may be the cause of a dilemma for health care workers. The practice is enormously damaging physically and psychologically, but at the same time a girl who has not endured this may suffer difficulties in being thus different from her female siblings, relatives and friends. For some communities this custom is felt to be necessary to ensure that virginity is protected until marriage. The girl who has not been so mutilated may be seen as 'unclean' and unmarriageable – a terrible fate in such traditional communities. This issue starkly illustrates the dilemma of defining one culture's norms as 'right' against those of another as 'wrong'.

FOOD

Food is vitally important to all of us. We need food for growth and strength; food satisfies hunger – one of our most basic drives. Food provides satisfaction and enjoyment. We offer food to those we love as a tangible expression of our affection and regard. It is not surprising, therefore, that food and eating are an important part of culture. We learn our tastes and preferences for food as children when provided with the food that our culture defines as important. Food is also central in many of our cultural rituals; special dishes are prepared for festivals such as the Christian Easter and the Hindu Diwali. Since food is generally held to be important in establishing and promoting health, it follows that food is usually held to be important when someone suffers ill health. Again, this is a feature common to all cultures, but each interprets and expresses its attitude towards food in its own distinctive way.

In many cultures food is seen as having either 'hot' or 'cold' properties, which have nothing to do with their actual temperature but rather with their effects on the body (Karseras and Hopkins, 1987). An explanation of this can be seen in the Chinese concepts of yin and yang. Yin is the cold, wet and dark principle, while yang represents the hot, dry and light: all of life including health depends on these two principles being in harmony, in balance. This is known as the *humoral theory of health*. Some vital body organs are seen as intrinsically yang and some as yin, so disturbances in their function are seen as disturbances in the yin–yang balance. Since foods can also be classified as yin or yang in character their consumption may alleviate or worsen bodily balance disturbances. For a yang disorder a yin food may be taken almost as a medicine. Some vestiges of this sort of belief might be seen in the British belief of, 'feed a cold and starve a fever', or in the practice of taking hot drinks for a cold. There is great variability between cultures in the classification of foods and health disorders into yin and yang, hot or cold. The only way to obtain reliable information about this is to ask the family concerned. This system of belief may be very significant for the health care worker when, for example, pregnancy is seen as a hot disorder so hot foods are avoided, placing the pregnant woman at potential risk of dietary insufficiencies. If a health care worker's advice runs contrary to a person's nutritional beliefs and customs he may quite simply ignore this advice and fail to comply. Personally acceptable solutions thus have to be negotiated in order to secure benefit for the person concerned. It is obvious that families will often use this system of treatment by food alongside orthodox treatment. It may be alarming for a parent to find that a nurse offers his child a food which he believes to be capable of worsening his condition. During health assessment it is important not only to establish the child's normal dietary pattern but also to find out which foods the child's parents would like to be offered.

Given the importance of food it is logical that many cultures define foods which are not suitable for consumption, which may be unclean or polluting, and also the means by which acceptable foods are prepared for eating. These rules can be complex, and while it is important that the nurse has access to sources of information on this subject to provide guidelines, authoritative and reliable information is only to be had from the people themselves. This is particularly important for paediatric nurses as a child will often be unable to explain what foods he should or should not eat, whether this is because of a cultural prohibition or because he has diabetes mellitus. It is deeply offensive and alarming for parents to find that their child has been offered and perhaps eaten a food which they find distasteful. It is part of the paediatric nurse's established rôle to monitor the dietary intake of the children in her care and it is a relatively simple matter to take cultural factors into account in this assessment.

Many cultural and religious traditions include the habit of periodic fasting as a religious obligation or as a sort of 'cleansing'. By and large, children, pregnant or breastfeeding women are not expected to fast but nurses should be aware that fasting may be an added pressure for anxious, tired parents, for example, during the Muslim festival of Ramadan or the Jewish Yom Kippur holiday (Berkovits, 1988). Cultural groups often have strongly defined practices in infant and child feeding which may be felt to be undesirable by health care personnel of the dominant culture. Many Asian women who very much want to breastfeed their babies nevertheless do not wish to give the baby the colostrum, fearing that it is weak or even potentially harmful (Taylor, 1985). Nurses, aware of the nutritional and immunological benefit of colostrum, may attempt to promote giving it to the baby thus causing confusion and possibly conflict. A tactful and sensitive offering of information will allow the mother, and her female relatives, to make an informed choice in the matter. This choice must be respected and facilities for formula feeding arranged until the mother is producing breastmilk. It is significant that in such important matters older women in the family may be instrumental in decision-making. In the extended family these matriarchs may be pivotal in defining and defending cultural norms, and their experience and wisdom are respected within the family and their decisions deferred to (Beare, 1983; Friedemann, 1991). This makes it constructive to include these family members in discussions about health and treatment. This also highlights the fact the various cultures define gender rôles and expectations very differently; this applies also to children and we may often detect very different expectations within families of boys and girls.

DRESS

The mode of dress used by a person is an immediate signal of his cultural orientation. This can be illustrated by the wide range of national costumes seen in the world. Some of these are for everyday use, others are reserved for festive and ceremonial use. Interestingly, when the use of a specific costume is declining, it is generally older women who are last to abandon wearing it; again, women can be seen to have a role in preserving cultural norms and habits. The style of dress is generally related to the climatic conditions of the place from which the culture originated. Clothes also meet the needs for modesty required by a culture. Many cultures feel that it is important that women dress modestly, covering their limbs and hair. Even small children develop modesty and should be assisted in a manner sensitive to this; unnecessary exposure should be avoided and the attentions of a same-sex nurse are helpful.

Jewellery and other adornments often have specific meanings and should not, in general, be tampered with by nurses. If it is accepted that these objects may have a similar meaning to the wearer or his family as a wedding ring does in native British society, then it is natural to make efforts to maintain their use safely for their wearer. For some time the use of *surma*, a black eye cosmetic, on South Asian children has caused some concern since this may contain high levels of lead and may lead to poisoning. Since the use of this cosmetic has significance to parents, attempts to change habits and encourage the use of a similar, safe product must be made in a culturally sensitive way. This method, combined with the involvement of health care workers from the South Asian community who have an understanding of the cultural basis of the custom, is proving successful in Derbyshire (Smart and Madan, 1990).

HYGIENE

Good hygiene is essential for comfort and health and is also crucial for a person's social acceptability. Cleanliness has a physical aspect but also, for many, an abstract, ritual meaning. Many will want to wash prior to prayer, seeking both physical and spiritual cleanliness. Not all cultures, however, agree on how best to get clean. The British may like a good, hot bath, while the Finns would prefer a sauna. Many Asian people prefer to wash in running water so that the dirt is borne away with the water flow. This is another area where cultural and spiritual requirements may be modified by personal preference and standards. Many cultures have specific hygiene, purification customs for preparing the body after death (Neuberger, 1987; Green and Green, 1992). These cultures may also have very clear ideas of bodily pollution and how to avoid this in these circumstances. Personal grooming is also often dictated by tradition and habit. It is well known that adult male Sikhs generally do not shave but often less well known that Muslim children may, as newborns, have their hair shaved off completely.

LANGUAGE

Language tells us many things about a person, the language spoken, the dialect, the accent and again, as ethnocentric beings, we compare the speech we hear with our own and make judgements. Children naturally acquire language as they develop, so again, child health nurses have an advantage in that they work with patients who have widely varying language ability. Non-verbal communication and cues are an integral part of all communication but we note and act on these often at a subliminal level. Bringing these to consciousness is an important step in becoming a skilled communicator, particularly with children. Through language we give directions, information and comfort – not to understand the speech of those around us is a bewildering, possibly even frightening, experience (Haigh, 1988). It can be particularly terrifying for a child if he does not understand or communicate. Parents often act as 'interpreters' for small children who are just beginning to speak and in the same way should be similarly encouraged if the child's mother tongue is not English. Should the parents not speak English it is important to use all alternative communication facilities ranging from interpreters to picture boards (Watson, 1985; Hayward *et al.*, 1991). It is not advisable to use an older child in the family as an interpreter since he may be frightened and not understand what is happening. This habit, which is still unfortunately widespread, can only be condoned in an emergency until alternative arrangements are made. Many minority communities have interpreter services which a health authority can negotiate to use. The potential for misunderstanding is great when there is a language barrier. Many strategies will reduce this risk: speaking directly, slowly and clearly to a person, keeping sentences short, avoiding complicated words and jargon, keeping information offered to the minimum and repeating as necessary are all helpful. These are all methods which paediatric nurses are skilled in using, placing them at a distinct advantage. It is important though that if these strategies are used, a patronising manner is not communicated.

All of the issues discussed briefly above point to the importance of culture in people's lives and how vital it is that this aspect is taken into account when health care is planned or offered. This will help to ensure harmony and co-operation between health care worker and client/patient. If the nurse does not make an attempt to see a person's situation from his point of view, there is a risk that her explanations and solutions do not match his and the opportunity for collaboration and success in the caring encounter is lost. The patient/client or his parents may quite simply choose to disregard the nurse's advice if this is in conflict with their beliefs (Kleinman et al., 1978). Advice must therefore take such beliefs into account. The nurse must try to see her client's world-view.

The very everyday nature of the examples used above to illustrate aspects of culture and how they affect people point out how important this issue is for nurses. This does not simply mean the industrious learning of long lists of details about each specific culture; this would be an enormous task and would ultimately carry the risk of inflexibility – people once identified as belonging to a cultural group might be *stereotyped* with all the things so laboriously learned. This is neither a helpful nor a reliable approach (Mason, 1990). How much better if the nurse addresses those common themes of culture which bind us all but which we know vary to a greater or lesser extent between groups. The nurse will then have an insight into the sorts of areas in which people might have particular needs or preferences. These are the issues which may be significant to *any* individual or family – explanations of health and ill-health, preferred sources of health care and advice (orthodox or folk), religious rituals, diet, dress and modesty, hygiene, family structure and decision-making strategies.

Paediatric nurses are increasingly intent on 'plugging into' family resources in order to empower, to initiate and promote positive coping and health behaviours. This then is dependent on a healthy, egalitarian, co-operative relationship between the child, the family and the nurse. Such a relationship cannot flourish unless there is broad mutual understanding of the aims, hopes and fears on the one hand, and customs, beliefs, values and priorities on the other hand, of all those involved.

Transcultural nursing theory can provide us with important information about cultural groups but given the individual and personal nature of culture this can only be the 'broad brushstrokes'. For the fine detail of a picture of the family we must ask the family members themselves (Baxter, 1988). This process of *negotiation* of information is essential. As nurses we already complete assessments of the needs of our patients and their families, but how often do these assessments include information on the family's cultural background? Many systems of cultural assessment have been devised by nurses and social scientists, and these can give valuable cues for direction in cultural discovery and in the organisation of information but most are probably too complex for routine use (Tripp-Reimer et al., 1984; Giger and Davidhizar, 1990). The simplest and most practical means of gathering information on a family's cultural beliefs and customs probably lies in a simple expansion of the range of information sought on routine health assessment. It has been demonstrated that cultural issues touch all the everyday concerns of life, so it is not unreasonable to include in an assessment interview and in observation related data when establishing a child's and his family's normal everyday routine. For example, the Roper–Logan–Tierney model's Activities of Daily Living should comprehensively cover the important cultural issues in the health care context (Roper et al., 1981). A heightened awareness of cultural questions will allow the nurse, for example, when seeking information on a child's nutritional habits not simply to enquire about his eating habits and likes and dislikes, but also to find out specific dietary prohibitions. Similarly, we usually ask about a family's conception of a health problem, but rarely proceed to find out what their opinion is of what made the problem occur, what treatment they feel is necessary and how it will affect the whole family.

It is thus obvious how important an appreciation of cultural ideas is for paediatric nurses who are striving to care for a child in collaboration with his family who are his principal care givers. Working together in this way is an imperative not simply on philosophical or humanitarian grounds but also ethically. The United Kingdom Central Council for Nursing, Midwifery and Health Visiting, in its recently updated Code of Conduct states,

'As a registered nurse, midwife or health visitor you are personally accountable for your practice and, in the exercise of your professional accountability, must recognize and respect the uniqueness and dignity of each patient and client, and respond to their need for care, irrespective of their ethnic origin, religious beliefs, personal attributes, the nature of their health problems or any other factor.' (UKCC, 1992)

Investigation of cultural issues helps also to ensure the success of our nursing efforts and allows us access to a rich appreciation of people in all their diversity.

Cultural consideration is one more step towards provision of care which is truly child and family centred. Children have culture too!

REFERENCES

Anderson J M (1990) Health care across cultures. *Nursing Outlook*, **38**(3), 78–82.

Ashworth P and Morrison P (1989) Some ambiguities of the student's rôle in undergraduate nurse training. *Journal of Advanced Nursing*, **14**, 1009–15.

Baxter C (1988) Culture shock. *Nursing Times*, 13 Jan, 36–8.

Beare J (1983) Parenthood in other cultures. *Nursing* (Second series) 19, 563–4.

Berkovits B (1988) *A Guide to Jewish Practice for Nurses and Medical Staff* (Beth Din leaflet No. 9). London. Court of the Chief Rabbi.

Bradby M (1990) Status passage into nursing: another view of the process of socialisation into nursing. *Journal of Advanced Nursing*, **14**, 1220–5.

Brink P J and Saunders J M (1976) *Cultural Shock: theoretical and applied*. In Brink P J (Ed.) *Transcultural Nursing: a book of readings*. Englewood Cliffs, NJ: Prentice Hall.

Dobson S M (1991) *Transcultural Nursing*. London. Scutari Press.

Friedemann M-L (1991) *Exploring Culture and Family Caring Patterns with the Framework of Systemic Organisation*. In Chinn P L (Ed.) *Anthology on Caring*. New York: National League for Nursing Press.

Giger J N and Davidhizar R (1990) Transcultural nursing assessment: a method for advanced nursing practice. *International Nursing Review*, **37**(1), 199–202.

Green J and Green M (1992) *Dealing with Death: practices and procedures*. London: Chapman & Hall.

Haigh H (1988) 'OK?' – Communication across the language barrier. *NATN News*, Apr/May, 11–15.

Hartog J and Hartog E A (1983) Cultural aspects of health and illness behavior in hospitals. *The Western Journal of Medicine*, December, 910–16.

Hayward P J, Woo M and Kangesu E (1991) One solution to the linguistic problems faced by health visitors. *Health Visitor*, June, 185–7.

Health Visitors Association Racial Issues Working Party (1989) *Entitled to be Healthy: health visiting and school nursing in a multiracial society*. London: HVA.

Helman G J (1990) *Culture, Health and Illness*. 2nd edition. London: Butterworth-Heinemann.

Henley A (1982a) *Caring for Hindus and their Families: religious aspects of care*. London: Department of Health and Social Security/King Edward Hospital Fund for London/ National Extension College.

Henley A (1982b) *Caring for Muslims and their Families: religious aspects of care*. London: Department of Health and Social Security/King Edward Hospital Fund for London/ National Extension College.

Karseras P and Hopkins E (1987) *British Asians – health in the community*. London: Wiley.

Kleinman A, Eisenberg L and Good B (1978) Culture, illness and care: clinical lessons from anthropologic and cross-cultural research. *Annals of Internal Medicine*, **88**, 251–8.

Littlewood J (1988) The patient's world. *Nursing Times*, 20 Jan, 29–30.

Lynam M J (1992) Towards the goal of providing culturally sensitive care: principles upon which to build nursing curricula. *Journal of Advanced Nursing*, **17**, 149–57.

Mares P, Henley A and Baxter C (1985) *Health Care in Multiracial Britain*. Cambridge: National Extension College/Health Education Council.

Mason C (1990) Women as mothers in Northern Ireland and Jamaica: a critique of the transcultural nursing movement. *International Journal of Nursing Studies*, **27**(4), 367–74.

McCall J (1991) Ethnic minorities. *Surgical Nurse*, **4**(4), 20–3.

McLean S and Graham S E (1981) *Female Circumcision, Excision and Infibulation*. London: Minority Rights Group.

Melia K (1987) Balance of power. *Nursing Times*, 24 June, 42–4.

Neuberger J (1987) *Caring for Dying People of Different Faiths*. Lisa Sainsbury Foundation Series. London: Austen Cornish.

Parfitt B A (1988) Cultural assessment in the intensive care unit. *Intensive Care Nursing*, **4**, 124–7.

Rairdan B and Higgs Z R (1992) When your patient is a Hmong refugee. *American Journal of Nursing*, March, 52–5.

Roper N, Logan W W and Tierney A J (1981) *Learning to Use the Nursing Process*. Edinburgh: Churchill Livingstone.

Sampson A C M (1982) *The Neglected Ethic: cultural and religious factors in the care of patients*. Maidenhead: McGraw-Hill.

Smart A and Madan N (1990) Surma: a cause for concern. *Health Visitor*, November, 379–80.

Smart N (1989) *The World's Religions: old traditions and modern transformations*. Cambridge: Cambridge University Press.

Stokes G (1991) A transcultural nurse is about. *Senior Nurse*, **11**(1), 40–2.

Sykes J B (Ed.) (1982) *The Concise Oxford Dictionary of Current English*. Oxford: Oxford University Press.

Taylor M M (1985) *Transcultural Aspects of Breastfeeding – USA*. New York: La Leche League International Lactation Consultant Series.

Thiedermann S B (1986) Ethnocentrism: a barrier to effective health care. *Nurse Practitioner*, **11**(8), 52–9.

Tripp-Reimer T, Brink P J and Saunders J M (1984) Cultural assessment: content and process. *Nursing Outlook*, **32**(2), 78–82.

Tuck I and Harris L H (1988) Teaching students transcultural concepts. *Nurse Educator*, **13**(3), 36–9.

United Kingdom Central Council for Nursing, Midwifery and Health Visiting (1992) *Code of Professional of Conduct*. London: UKCC.

Watson P (1985) Towers of Babel? *Nursing Times*, 3 Dec, 40–1.

Weller B (1991) Nursing in a multicultural world. *Nursing Standard*, 17 April, 31–2.

8

Primary Nursing in a General Paediatric Medical Ward

Breda Gahan and Margaret Rogers

'Children suffer from passing through too many pairs of hands. For the child's own welfare a method of nursing which gives him a sense of security through being nursed by a familiar person ...'

Platt, 1959, para. 38

This chapter explores the development of primary nursing in one paediatric setting. It is a description of what has actually happened: preparing for the change, the skills that are developed, and the improved quality and continuity of care, and ultimately how some families have been empowered by this type of nursing, by the use of negotiation skills within a partnership in care (Casey, 1988). The importance of evaluating any changes in nursing practice will be emphasised throughout the text, and evaluation methods will be described. Finally, some common questions and concerns about primary nursing will be answered.

To set the scene, primary nursing will be defined as a system of organising nursing care and developing nursing practice. The difference in this type of nursing and other forms of nursing will also be highlighted.

Primary nursing is about responsibility and nurse/patient (family) relationships. It is the giving and acceptance of responsibility, with the accompanying authority. The primary nurse is given the authority, by the ward sister, to make decisions about nursing care for her own caseload of patients throughout their hospital stay. When this happens, she experiences a gradual increase in her level of autonomy as her clinical skills and her knowledge develop. She learns to evaluate her own practice and share her experiences and knowledge with her peers. The ward sister, as the clinical specialist and leader, encourages this sharing and evaluation, so creating collaborative practice among her team. These attributes are inherent in the philosophy of primary nursing. Good team work is not lost, but is enhanced. The result is comprehensive, high quality care for the child and family, smooth, direct communication channels, and continuity of care. All trained nurses are accountable for their practice. Primary nursing, with its focused responsibility, means that nurses 'feel' accountable, and recognise the positive attributes of being an accountable practitioner.

The major difference between primary nursing and other forms of nursing, is that in primary nursing, responsibility is focused not shared, and the primary nurse can begin to work in a more professional way. Being accountable to individual families for their care 'is the mark of individualising care' (Pearson, 1988). When other forms of nursing are adopted or developed, the organisation may be seen in isolation from the need to develop nursing practice. For example, if team nursing is implemented as an organisational concept alone, the team leader may focus on the supervision of the team and task completion, rather than the clinical development of herself and the team. Responsibility and accountability will remain unclear, and collaborative practice will be difficult. As Manthey states, 'Shared responsibility equals no responsibility' (Manthey, 1992). Primary nursing cannot be implemented successfully without the development of individual nurses, whereas team nursing may be 'working' without such preparation.

IMPLEMENTATION

The ward concerned is a general medical ward for children aged 0–2 years. With 24-hour admissions from the casualty department and booked admissions, the workload can be unpredictable and the dependency of the children variable. The reasons for change were identified and explored before it was agreed by the team that primary nursing was the way forward (Gahan, 1991). This was then followed by in-depth planning and preparation which proved to be essential for the successful implementation and development of primary nursing. Once implemented, the planned changes were monitored closely and evaluated, and objectives agreed accordingly. It was essential during preparation to create an atmosphere and culture on the ward that were conducive to both the philosophical and organisational aspects of primary nursing. Before primary nursing can begin, the traditional role of the ward sister must change. This helped to facilitate and support individual trained nurses in preparation for primary nursing and development of their role within primary nursing.

Although the ward sister is the manager of the ward, the controlling emphasis of this role needs to be reduced. This meant more emphasis being directed towards the supportive, teaching and facilitative aspects of the role. As well as devolving power and autonomy for patient care to primary nurses, the ward sister encouraged nurses to think laterally; to examine and develop their self-awareness, and their own individual skills in relation to nursing practice and patient care. By knowing themselves well and being encouraged to deal with their own weaknesses, they were better able to nurse patients and support their colleagues.

The ward sister is the key person responsible for the way the ward functions, for the overall standards of care and the tone and climate of the ward (Pembrey, 1980). These roles were especially important through the development and transition phase of primary nursing, and were reflected in the way nurses practise, relate to each other and communicate with the families and the multi-disciplinary team. It was essential for all members of the nursing team to be fully involved in the whole process of preparation and change.

Meetings were held every 1 to 2 weeks and provided a forum for staff education, discussion, feedback and reflection. The process of change began by nurses examining existing practice, how care is delivered at present, what and why they needed to change. All nurses took on the responsibility for educating themselves and their colleagues about primary nursing. For example, getting into small groups to review the available literature, and then sharing this information with the rest of the team at these meetings. Notes kept from these meetings were used to inform all nurses, and proved to be valuable for future evaluation. Once confident and articulate about primary nursing, the process of disseminating the information to the rest of the multi-disciplinary team began. The nursing team need to convince others of the benefits of the change (Wright, 1990).

The point of implementation was reached when the nursing team were knowledge-able and articulate about primary nursing, and when each nurse understood and anticipated her change in role, as far as was possible. The benefits of planned change during the preparation gave nurses the confidence to approach the final change to primary nursing and to deal with the early challenges. Because the preparation was thorough, the team was cohesive. A final consideration was that staffing levels were at an optimum to enter the transition phase of primary nursing.

CONTINUITY OF CARE AND SKILLS DEVELOPED

The level of continuity provided in primary nursing has not only benefited the child and family, but also facilitated nurses to develop their skills to a much higher level. Each nurse is individually assessed and appraised by the ward sister to assume the primary and associate nurse roles, and the duty rota plays an important part in plan-ning for continuity of care. This is part of the ward sister's management role, and requires more skill than just 'covering the ward'.

Assessment Skills

Assessment skills are enhanced because the primary nurse is a trained nurse, cares for the child and family on a continual basis, and gets to know the family more thor-oughly and in a shorter length of time. These skills have also been developed through clinical practice, by linking theoretical knowledge with the practical care. Because the primary nurse is responsible for that child's total nursing care, she ensures that her clinical knowledge of the child's condition is detailed and thorough. Knowing the child and family well, she is in a much better position to assess the child's progress and response to treatment, and can do so more promptly. The relationship she has with the child and family also assists her to assess the whole family unit, especially in terms of psychological and social aspects of care. The primary nurse can also offer her families a greater level of confidentiality, where some information may not need to be shared with the whole ward team.

Assertiveness

The increased knowledge that nurses have of their families has given them the confi-dence to be appropriately assertive, and act as the family's advocate within the multi-disciplinary team, if and when this is necessary. These assertiveness skills are complemented by supportive behaviour offered to associate nurses, health care assis-tants and students. This ensures continuity of care in her absence, that her care plan is followed carefully, and that the evaluation of that care is continuous. The primary nurse has an essential role in facilitating the associate nurse to develop the skills essential to become a primary nurse. She achieves this by acting as a role model and by teaching at the bedside.

Teaching

Primary nurses on the ward have felt a greater responsibility for teaching both nurses and families. They want to ensure that their associate nurses have an in-depth knowledge of the child's illness and how this affects their nursing intervention. The teaching at the bedside increases, and formal teaching sessions tend to reduce in number. Case presentation is used to share and evaluate the total care given to particular families. This encourages nurses to identify what nursing care and management a family needs. It also reassures student nurses, who sometimes have the misconception that they might not get as varied experience if they look after fewer patient 'types'. Students can sit and learn how nurses assess, plan and evaluate the care for particular patients, in relation to the medical diagnosis and treatments. This is opposed to being 'taught' about different conditions and nursing care in isolation.

The primary and key associate nurse, who is also a trained nurse, act as link nurses for one or two students throughout their placement. This allows for more support and supervision in the clinical area. Students have valued the opportunity of this type of learning, and often identify that they are developing their management skills, and experiencing an increased level of responsibility. Two student nurses commented:

'as a student it has helped me to learn to take a greater responsibility for the care I am giving and to take a more active role.'

'I gained valuable management experience, the chance to contribute my ideas and point of view when planning care and see it acted on if it was appropriate, the opportunity to learn when planning care with a senior member of staff ... the feeling of being supported and the chance to work alongside trained staff.'

This type of preparation and experience will be of great value for the Project 2000 student leading to registration.

Documentation

Nursing documentation has improved in primary nursing, because one person, the primary nurse, has responsibility for the nursing record. Although the primary nurse is ultimately responsible, the process of assessing, planning, implementing and evaluating care is a collaborative activity, with her associate nurses. The primary nurse and her associate nurses sit down regularly to discuss the nursing care of their patients, and update the care plans. Therefore, when a primary or key associate nurse is not on duty, it will be easier for another nurse who does not know the family as well to look at the care plan and know exactly what care is planned and the needs of the child.

The documentation also reflects the involvement of family members in the planning and evaluation of care, and that negotiation of care is taking place. To achieve a partnership with the family it has been essential to document that discussion has taken place between nurses and family about the family participation in care, and that this is reviewed on a daily basis. Paediatric nurses may have felt content that they do a lot for families, by allowing parents to be resident and 'do all care'. Family involvement in care is often recorded in the following way: 'Mum doing care' or 'Parents involved in care' (Rogers, 1990). This may be without clarification of what 'care' or 'all care' is, and with no indication that negotiation has taken place, or that families have even been asked. In other words, nurses have assumed what role families would like to play.

Handovers

There has been a noticeable change in the length and content of information given at the general report sessions at midday. These sessions have changed, because only information that the whole ward team need to know is exchanged, so the information is prioritised. It does take some time for nurses to develop the confidence required, and often students find this difficult. But when it is realised that more detailed information is gained about their own patients at the bedside, and that the care plan is up-to-date and specific, confidence is gained. The benefits include the reduction in time of lengthy report sessions and the overstrenuous note-taking, as well as an increased level of confidentiality for the family. Others have found this confidence of great value in primary nursing (Cole, 1991). The need not to share all of the information about a family, if this is not essential, is reassuring when considering social and emotional problems. Maintaining these changes is difficult. The experience of the primary, associate and student nurses is variable over time. The reassuring aspects of traditional communications – 'tell everybody everything and there is a chance it won't be forgotten' – is easy to slip back into for the less experienced nurse.

The common theme, when considering the skills that have been developed, is continuity. Continuity of carers is essential in primary nursing for delivering high quality care. It can be alarming how many different nurses can be involved in the care of a hospitalised child in other systems of organising care. Assessing this number for individual patients is a worthwhile exercise to demonstrate that continuity of care needs to be improved. If 20, 30 or more nurses have been allocated to care for a family during their hospital stay, it is hardly surprising that care plans are not kept up-to-date, communication is fragmented and families are sometimes confused about what is being expected of them. If in addition to this no one trained nurse is taking responsibility for teaching or supporting the family, a very confused picture emerges. However, continuity of carers, without matching the skills of the nurse with the needs of the family, will not equal quality. The allocation of patients to primary nurses is based on the experience and skill of the nurse, the workload and the needs of the family. None of these things can be taken in isolation, and reallocation may be required.

WHAT PRIMARY NURSING MEANS TO FAMILIES

When nursing changes its culture so dramatically it can be expected that families will also change the way they behave and respond. Traditional nursing will receive traditional feedback from families, that is, if families are asked to evaluate the care they have received at all. 'Everyone has been wonderful', or 'the nurses work so hard' will be common responses, and the occasional complaint may arise from some families who may risk being labelled 'a difficult family'. The relationships and trust that have developed between nurses and families in primary nursing have encouraged honesty and openness. The primary nurse opens herself up to scrutiny, and the families will feel more comfortable about giving constructive as well as favourable feedback.

The feedback from families has been a key motivating factor for primary and associate nurses, and 'the difficult family' becomes a rarity. Families have been able to articulate how primary nursing has helped them to feel totally involved in the care of their child, and in control, even if they are unable to remain in hospital all the time. It has taken some time for all families to identify the particular benefits of primary nursing, although from the very early stages responses were enthusiastic and favourable. If a family is experiencing their first hospital admission, they think that this type of practice is the 'norm' for paediatric hospital care, and find it difficult when they are moved to wards and hospitals that are not practising primary nursing. Those families who have had previous hospital experiences have been able to identify the differences very clearly. Families have also valued the opportunity to give feedback about other experiences during their hospital stay, for example, about the facilities available for resident parents. As primary nursing has developed, so families have become more articulate and definitive about what they value in primary nursing. The following two parent statements show that these families have been involved in the negotiation of care and have experienced a partnership with the nurses:

'For the first time in a "hospital situation" I felt *included and not patronised* and felt the nurses valued our contribution as we did theirs.'

'I feel that the primary nursing approach treats patients and parents as co-workers in the process of nursing care, not just passive recipients.'

One mother wanted to write a great deal about her experience with primary nursing on this ward, and clearly demonstrates how she felt empowered in the care of her child:

'the difference in this to other forms of nursing is that the most important person of all is the child, no offence to other forms of nursing, but in my experience of what I've seen, I much prefer primary nursing, for their skills and knowing that the two main nurses looking after him are professionals in every sense ... I still feel involved, and not pushed out, and not feel just like a visitor after a while, that's been one of the most important things to me regarding this type of nursing. I feel involved, I can't stress how much the difference to me ... helps me to be more able to cope with him when he gets home.'

EVALUATION

Evaluation is critical for any change in nursing practice. It is no longer acceptable for nurses to say 'I know it's better' or 'it definitely works' without some sound evaluation. This evaluation can take many forms, from making notes at meetings through the development of primary nursing, to the use of formal evaluation tools. A combination of different types of evaluation is most valuable, as results are then being validated against each other. It is particularly important to evaluate primary nursing in the hospital paediatric setting, as relatively few paediatric wards have developed this practice and shared their experiences.

An action research process (Winter, 1989) was identified as being appropriate for the development and evaluation of primary nursing on this ward. Others have found this process valuable for developing nursing practice and implementing change (Webb, 1990). The action research process follows a spiral, with continuous planning, action, observation and reflection, which begins with the analysis of practice leading to changes in practice. It is itself a collaborative activity which complements primary nursing; the whole ward team decides which areas to evaluate in depth, and what data to collect. The following methods were used:

Before and after Evaluations

Documentation Audit

At The Hospitals for Sick Children a standard 'Nursing Documentation' was written, and an audit tool developed. An audit was carried out across the two hospitals in 1990, and two sample documents were evaluated on each ward. On this ward a larger sample of documents was evaluated as one before-primary-nursing measure, and re-evaluated a year later following the introduction of primary nursing. The most obvious improvement in the documentation at this time was the increased recording of communications with community staff and the more detailed discharge planning. More recent audits have identified an increase in the recording of family involvement, and negotiation of care.

Nurse/Patient Allocation

The number of different nurses allocated to individual families was assessed both before and one year after the introduction of primary nursing. An allocation book was kept, where on each shift the allocated nurse's name was written next to the patient's name. The total numbers were cumulative; one child who was hospitalised for 2 months had over 40 different nurses allocated. It is not difficult to see how this number could be achieved during this time, with possibly three changes of student nurses and the use of agency staff. The after-primary-nursing assessment demonstrated that there was a consistent reduction in the total number of nurses allocated, by ten or more in some cases. In addition to this a core group of nurses led by the primary nurse cared for the child throughout his stay, and for short-stay patients (fewer than 5 days) the primary and key associate nurse were always allocated for some of the shifts (see Rogers and Gahan, 1992).

Participant Observation

The 'action researcher' spent periods of time working on the ward. Before the implementation of primary nursing this helped to identify areas that could be changed, and the readiness of the team to go ahead. After the implementation she returned and worked as an associate nurse and helped to evaluate the changes that had taken place. Having not worked in a primary nursing setting before, it was a learning experience, and gave the opportunity to consolidate her theoretical knowledge of primary nursing with the practice. It was easy to identify the different 'feel' of the ward and to observe the obvious ease that parents felt in reading the nursing documents and charts. To experience the different type of communications, to see primary and associate nurses together at the bedside, and individual nurses involving the family in the care planning – these observations were then shared with the ward team at their meetings and confirmed that change was actually happening.

Ongoing Evaluations

Notes from Meetings

The meetings continue as a forum for discussing nursing practice, and notes continue to be recorded. The notes taken during the preparation and implementation demonstrate the importance of careful planning. It meant that at each meeting the previous meeting could be quickly reviewed, so issues were not 'over'-explored. It was a way to identify the strong interests or concerns of the whole ward team, and facilitated the writing of the ward objectives to be achieved. It has also meant that all nurses could feel that their own interests or concerns would be dealt with and shared with those who were not present at a particular meeting.

Feedback from Families

Each family is given an information and feedback sheet. On one side of this sheet the names of the primary nurse, the key associate nurse and other nurses involved in their care are written; also the names of medical staff and the times of their visits to the ward. On the reverse side is a request for the family to write or inform the nurses of their perceptions of the care they have received. Some families are very keen and interested to do this, and return the sheets before discharge or post them from home. A large percentage of families do not speak or cannot write English, and a key objective for the future is to obtain information from these families. Although the personal and non-verbal feedback individual nurses are receiving is very favourable, this needs to be confirmed by verbal communication. This is the most valuable and rewarding data for the nursing team to have, showing that their efforts and achievements are fully recognised by the families themselves.

Feedback from the Multi-disciplinary Team

Throughout the development of primary nursing medical staff and others have been asked for their perceptions of primary nursing. After one year a letter was sent to senior medical staff asking for some feedback. Although mostly favourable, a few of the registrars still expressed their liking for the ward sister to do the 'ward round', and were somewhat irritated by not being able to walk around the ward in a systematic way. Generally there was recognition from the medical staff that the primary and associate nurses had an in-depth knowledge of their families. One consultant wrote: 'The way in which they [primary/associate nurses] report on their patients is impressive, accurate, and informative.' Other comments mentioned how doctors had experienced, over the years, many changes in nursing, but no real change in nursing practice had ever been identified by them, until the introduction of primary nursing.

Feedback from Student Nurses

The majority of students have enjoyed and made favourable comments about primary nursing. Junior students often adapt to primary nursing more readily, as they have not experienced as much socialisation into traditional nursing. Occasionally, senior students will voice their dislike of primary nursing as they can only look forward to the 'being in charge' role of the newly qualified staff nurse, and there is the need for 'management' experience. An audit of the learning environment carried out by the school of nursing identified that the needs of the student were being met most appropriately in this form of nursing.

Feedback from Community Staff

From the time primary nursing is implemented the type of conversation that takes place between a primary nursing ward and the community staff changes. No longer is the sister or 'nurse in charge' assuming the role of community liaison; nor are messages left for other members of the team to contact a health visitor, when they may know very little about the family. One of the first primary nurses who was an experienced staff nurse said, 'I can remember coming on a late shift and having a list of health visitors to try and contact.'

Discharge planning begins with the admission assessment, and the community staff are contacted at the earliest opportunity. This communication tends to be ongoing rather than a one-off phone call. If the health visitor calls to see how a patient is, the student nurse, who knows the family well, may be perfectly able to up-date her, if the primary or key associate is not on duty. One health visitor wrote: 'I felt valued because of the time and trouble that you took to inform me and keep me up-to-date . . . I felt very involved receiving and sharing information with you.'

Case Presentation and Peer Review

As well as being a method of teaching, case presentation offers the opportunity for a rudimentary form of peer review. The term 'peer review' can sound threatening; the idea of work colleagues carrying out appraisal and discussion about each other's practice is very new for paediatric nurses and is not widely used in nursing. However, when practising primary nursing, interpersonal problems are addressed in an open, mature manner. If problems do arise they become obvious and need to be dealt with. If not, they can have detrimental effects on staff morale and on patient care. For example, if a nurse fails to carry out the prescribed care on the care plan, or changes an agreed and negotiated plan of care unnecessarily, this situation needs to be dealt with promptly. It may be easier for that nurse to complain to a colleague. But nurses are encouraged to approach the nurse involved directly and sort the problem out in a mature way, so preventing the back-biting or the 'sweeping under the carpet' that occurs in the superficial 'harmonious team'. Case presentation is carried out by the primary and her associate nurses. One of their primary patients is selected, and the total care that the patient has received is presented to the nursing team. Each nurse presents a different aspect of the care, looking at the nursing needs of the child and family in relation to the hospital admission, treatments and discharge. This allows nurses to develop their presentation skills, as well as learning from each other's experience. It also encourages nurses to highlight the nursing care in relation to the medical care, rather than the medical diagnosis and treatments being the focus.

At the end of each presentation, questions and discussion are encouraged. Other trained staff may offer suggestions for aspects of care that could have been carried out in a different manner. This advice is offered in a supportive way rather than as a criticism. The ward sister's role is to ensure that this forum is 'safe', and that the freedom to discuss and challenge is seen in a positive rather than a negative light. This has also been helped by the sister giving presentations and encouraging staff to appraise her own practice and performance. She can also identify for herself areas in her own practice that could have been improved.

Staff Appraisal

It is inappropriate to have rigid criteria about who can and who cannot be a primary and associate nurse, especially if primary nursing is to be widely implemented. The ability to assume these roles is very individual; all nurses will develop at a different pace. Each nurse is assessed and appraised before becoming and while practising in the primary and associate nurse role. Informal and formal assessment and appraisal are carried out by the ward sister. As part of the informal appraisal each nurse carries out a self-appraisal where she is encouraged to examine her own practice and performance in detail. Nurses also outline what they have contributed to the ward and how they are developing professionally. Following this informal appraisal, plans are agreed and written, related to future development, support and educational needs of the individual nurse.

The individually assessed criteria for taking on the role of the primary nurse will include: that she can demonstrate an ability to contribute actively to assessment, care planning and evaluation of care; that she has an understanding of the responsibilities of a primary nurse, and that this has been demonstrated in the associate nurse role, by liaising regularly, and by carrying out the prescribed care to a high standard in the primary nurse's absence; that she has, through her practice, shown a sound clinical knowledge base, and applies research to her practice, and developed good communication skills, including the negotiation of care with families; that she has a good knowledge of the ward and hospital resources available to support the nurse, patient and family; finally, that she has the potential to use reflective practice to further her own and her associate nurse's development.

Using a structured evaluation process and an outside researcher or change agent is an undoubted advantage, but it is not essential to the development of primary nursing. Continuing the regular meetings, setting achievable objectives, sharing experiences and case presentation can all be achieved within the restraints of a busy ward. However, support and commitment from management are essential; nurse managers, tutors and clinical nurse specialists should be expected to offer pro-active support for any ward wanting to implement primary nursing.

CHALLENGES OF IMPLEMENTING PRIMARY NURSING

There is no doubt that implementing primary nursing in the acute paediatric hospital setting is an immense challenge. To maintain primary nursing, even in areas where it is well established, will continue to pose challenges, as nurses continue to be trained and socialised in a traditional way. When primary nurses move on to widen their clinical experience, the ward sister has to repeat the process of developing new staff into a primary nursing system. It will be some time before new staff will have the knowledge and experience to fit into a primary nursing system without this extensive input from the ward sister. The tradition and culture of medical staff need to change in response to the practice of primary nursing, and this will take a long time in some settings. The greatest challenges will be apparent through the transition phase of implementing primary nursing. Primary nursing will be given the blame for anything that goes wrong or does not work. A piece of information not delivered, a drug omission or even a busy, stressful day will all be the fault of primary nursing. As the duty rota is adapted and changed in response to offering continuity of carers, nurses may begin to worry about their requests being met. Finally, it may not be long before criticisms from peers start to feed through the grapevine; 'They can't be doing primary nursing, they're so busy', 'I've been to that ward and it doesn't look any different to me', could well be the 'canteen gossip' that is overheard.

How do the ward teams deal with this? The level of confidence and the preparation will give individual nurses the ability to ignore such comments and argue rationally with those who question primary nursing directly. A level of determination will be required, and although at first great effort will be made not to criticise other nurses' practice, eventually patience may be lost and nurses practising in primary nursing wards may just state that it is better. Although willing to share and teach from their experiences, the barriers against primary nursing may be very strong, and based on a lack of knowledge rather than any great understanding.

Primary nursing by its very nature is making a strong statement about achieving high quality care and professional practice. It is not surprising that other wards do feel threatened and feel that their own practice is being criticised. Determination to succeed will be needed by wards who experience these problems.

EIGHTEEN COMMON QUESTIONS AND CONCERNS ANSWERED

1. Do you need more nurses?
No. Whatever system of nursing is used the workload will remain the same. Primary nursing is not about increasing the workload, it is about individualising the care. Time can actually be saved by reducing repetitive routines and complex communication channels.

2. Who allocates patients to primary nurses?
It is not usually one nurse's decision. Many things need to be taken into consideration. The primary nurse must be able, in terms of workload and skill, to take on a

particular patient. Occasionally the ward sister or most senior nurse on duty may need to make or override decisions in terms of workload and nursing skill, but this would be unusual.

3. How many primary patients does a primary nurse have?
The number of patients will depend on the clinical setting and the dependency and needs of the family. For example, in an intensive care setting a primary nurse would only have one primary patient, in a general paediatric ward an average may be four or five primary patients.

4. Do primary nurses have to give all the care?
No. Primary nursing is often confused with the wrong definition of 'total patient care'. 'Total patient care' means that one nurse is responsible for the nursing care for a particular family for the length of that allocation. Primary nursing means that the primary nurse is responsible for the nursing care for the length of the admission. For both these definitions the nurse needs to give enough direct care to be able to assess, plan and evaluate the care. The literal meaning of 'TOTAL patient care' would only be possible if there was one nurse for each patient, and if each nurse had all the skills required.

5. What happens when the primary nurse or associate nurse is not on duty?
The term 'key' associate has been used to ensure that a second trained nurse is involved in the care of all families. Other associate nurses will also work with the primary nurse and her patients. These could be senior students, agency nurses, other primary nurses or the ward sister. It would be exceptional if one of these nurses were not on duty and unable to be allocated to care for a particular family.

6. Is primary nursing more stressful?
Primary nursing is not necessarily more stressful, but the potential for stress needs to be recognised. If the collaborative practice described is achieved, clinical support is very strong. The ward sister is the key person to assess the stress levels of her staff and intervene whenever indicated.

7. Do nurses get too involved?
Primary and associate nurses have a closer relationship with their patients families, so they are more involved. This means that they are more effective in the care they deliver. However, boundaries need to be identified, and a level of objectivity is essential if a therapeutic relationship is to be achieved. If nurses get too involved they will lose their objectivity; this will compromise the care and so can be dangerous. Nurses who have not been prepared for this type of relationship will be taking a greater risk of becoming too involved. However, there may be a small percentage of nurses who relish this type of involvement whichever system of nursing is being used.

8. What about difficult families?
Families may become labelled as 'difficult' because they are particularly demanding, or because they have 'complained'. Often these families have experienced the fragmented care and conflicting communication that primary nursing reduces. For the truly 'difficult' family, whatever that is, careful allocation is needed.

9. What if you don't like the family or they don't like you?
This is not a prominent problem within primary nursing, although it is a common concern. Having more than one trained nurse involved in the care of the family will help if the primary nurse feels that she is not achieving a very good rapport. If a sound decision is made to reallocate a primary nurse, this does not mean the primary nurse has failed in her role. The primary nurse may feel able to say to the family herself: 'We don't seem to be getting on, I think you should have another nurse as your primary nurse.' If the family request a change in allocation, this poses a more difficult problem, and will need a great deal of exploration and discussion locally. This is now an issue for all nurses, with the publication of the Patient's Charter (Department of Health, 1991).

10. Don't families become too dependent on the primary nurse?
If this happens the primary nurse has failed in her role. Only the nurse can perpetuate this type of dependency. If the primary nurse has fully involved her associates and works in a collaborative way, this will not happen. The family will have full confidence in the primary nurse's absence in the same way that families do when the ward sister is absent on a well-run traditional ward. If the nurse in question 7 meets the family in question 10, there could be a problem, but this could happen in any nursing system.

11. Where do night staff and part-time staff fit in?
To fulfil the role of primary nurse, enough direct care needs to be given to assess, plan, implement and evaluate that care. Clearly this will be difficult for some night staff and part-time staff, but not all. What is important is that all staff are involved in the preparation and implementation of primary nursing, and can identify and experience the benefits for themselves, and are valued for their contribution.

12. Isn't primary nursing the same as team nursing in practice?
No, not if primary nursing is actually being practised. There may be some grey areas where teams have been used to achieve primary nursing, but any simple evaluation will be able to identify what is really happening.

13. What grade should a primary nurse be?
Primary nursing is not about one grade or one level of experienced nurse. It is about developing nurses in the primary nursing role, from a recently qualified and prepared primary nurse who takes her first primary patient through to a primary nurse who is highly skilled and experienced.

14. How do you convince the doctors?
By demonstrating through your practice the benefits of primary nursing, by informing them and involving them in the preparation and evaluation of primary nursing. By not losing the co-ordination of the ward, or saying: 'We're going to do primary nursing whether you like it or not, and it's up to you to find and communicate with the primary nurses.'

15. Who can be a primary nurse?
Each individual trained nurse is assessed and appraised to take on the role of the primary and associate nurse by the ward sister. For a traditionally trained nurse it could

take 3–6 months for her to take her first primary patient. For a Project 2000 nurse it could take up to a year post-registration.

16. Do you still need a nurse in charge?
Yes. Clinical leadership, co-ordination, general management decision-making, guidance and support are essential on a shift-to-shift basis. This is the ward sister's role, and the senior primary nurse's in her absence.

17. How do you plan the duty rota?
The major change to planning the duty rota is that the demands of the ward are reflected more acutely, with careful, short-term planning. Whichever system is used attempts are made for the primary nurse to work opposite her associates.

18. I think we already do it?
If you only think you are doing it, you probably aren't. If primary nursing is understood and you are doing it there would be no doubt.

CONCLUSION

The final question that needs to be answered is, why change? The answer is that, if we want to achieve family-centred, holistic, individualised care, and want to practise as professional practitioners in partnership with our families, we need to move in this direction. Recently 'The Patient's Charter' (DoH, 1991) specifies that every patient will have a qualified named nurse responsible for their care. Primary nursing offers the most clearly defined form of named nursing at the present time. The potential that primary nursing can offer paediatric nursing is both exciting and achievable. It offers the opportunity to genuinely realise the philosophical theories which underpin modern paediatric nursing.

REFERENCES

Casey A (1988) A partnership with child and family. *Senior Nurse*, **8**(4) April.
Cole S (1991) Developing trust. *Paediatric Nursing*, **3**(5), June.
Department of Health (1991) *The Patient's Charter – a summary*. London: HMSO.
Gahan B (1991) Implementing primary nursing. *Paediatric Nursing*, **3**(9), November.
Pearson A (1988) *Primary Nursing – Nursing in the Burford and Oxford Nursing Development Unit*. London: Chapman and Hall.
Pembrey S (1980) *Ward Sister – Key to Nursing*. London: RCN.
Platt H (1959) *The Welfare of Children in Hospital*. Ministry of Health. London: HMSO.
Manthey M (1992) *The Practice of Primary Nursing*. London: King's Fund Centre.
Rogers M (1990) *Audit of the Nursing Documentation at The Hospitals for Sick Children – London*. Unpublished report.
Rogers M and Gahan B (1992) Improving the continuity of care. *Paediatric Nursing*, **4**(1), February.
Webb C (1990) Partners in research. *Nursing Times*, **86**(32), 8 August.
Winter R (1989) *Learning from Experience*. Brighton: Falmer Press.
Wright S (1990) *My Patient, My Nurse*. London: Scutari Press.

FURTHER READING

Gahan B (1991) Changing roles. *Paediatric Nursing,* **3**(10), December.
Ersser S and Tutton E (1991) *Primary Nursing in Perspective*. London: Scutari Press.
Wright S (1989) *Changing Nursing Practice*. London: Edward Arnold.

9

The Child in Accident and Emergency: A Philosophy of Care

Roberta Burton

INTRODUCTION

Charles Dickens' Mr Micawber says: 'accidents *will* happen in the best regulated families'! Staff working in Paediatric Accident and Emergency Departments know how true this is.

In a survey undertaken by the British Paediatric Association and the British Association of Paediatric Surgeons in 1987, it was found that children comprised one quarter of all patients attending A & E Departments annually. The reason for this is threefold: (1) children are immature and their lack of experience makes them vulnerable to accidents; (2) their immune systems are not fully developed and they are more susceptible to illnesses; the onset can be sudden and their condition can deteriorate rapidly, much more so than in adults; (3) their insatiable curiosity about the world, combined with their limitless energy, drive them to explore, to examine and to probe. They often inadvertently put themselves in danger of injury or accident.

Once an accident has occurred, the child will probably be brought to the A & E Department. This in itself can be a deeply frightening and traumatic experience. It can be their first introduction to the hospital environment. Everything about it is strange and terrifying – the atmosphere, the smells, the uniforms, the noise, and even other patients, can take on nightmare proportions. Their security is threatened. They will cling to their mother or father with unreasoning determination because in familiarity there is security. Even an abused child will cling to her/his abuser rather than trust the safe stranger who wants to help. Add to this the physical reason for the attendance, and it will be easy to understand the child's vulnerability and fear.

Wordsworth has said, 'the child is father of the man'. If children are not treated with great sensitivity and awareness of their needs, a visit to A & E may leave psychological scars which will be with them for a long time, if not for life; for this reason a Paediatric A & E Department must be very special. Every aspect of our care must be seen through the eyes of a child. Communication and environment must be child-oriented. *Time* must be child-oriented, for it takes much longer to establish a rapport with a child than with an adult; relationships need to be built up slowly – trust is not automatic, but must be sought for and won. Both medical and nursing staff need to develop skills in communicating with a child; they must never be talked down to or ignored. Nurses need to include them in their conversation, perhaps by taking an interest in what they are wearing or maybe discerning their interests from what they are wearing. It is often helpful not to hover over the child, but to come down to his level. Gaining a child's trust and confidence is one of the most rewarding aspects of a nurse's work and a very great privilege. Nurses who work with small children need to develop the ability to meet the inarticulated needs and to recognise that a silent, withdrawn child is actually shouting as loud as the screaming, struggling one. Nursing children in A & E is demanding and exacting, but it is also exciting and challenging. Every day we experience sadness and happiness, tears and laughter, humour and pathos. It can be an Alice in Wonderland situation (with shades of the Mad Hatter's tea party at times) but it can also be immensely satisfying and professionally rewarding.

A PHILOSOPHY OF CARE – THE PHYSICAL PERSPECTIVE

The physical conditions that children will present with are as varied and as numerous as pebbles on a beach. They range from fairly minor accidents to major trauma. Illness, too, will vary from the simple head cold to serious illnesses such as meningitis and septicaemia. Sadly, too often, leukaemia and malignant tumours are 'picked up' in the department. Abdominal pain can be an acute surgical condition such as appendicitis, intussusception, or may be due to severe constipation. In one 24-hour period, 108 children were seen in the A & E Department of the Royal Belfast Hospital for Sick Children. They were classified as follows:

Medical	33
Surgical	16
Accidents	20
Emergencies	3
Other	36

In spite of the variety of conditions, it is important to develop a standardised, systematic approach to nursing care, based on a nursing model. This will vary from hospital to hospital. Many departments have found difficulty in using a ward-based model in an A & E situation, and have evolved their own model on which their care is based.

The planning of care begins at the triage desk when a trained nurse interviews the parents and the child, identifies the problem, records the necessary data, assesses the priority of urgency and plans the individualised patient care. Parents have expressed their appreciation of being interviewed by a nurse immediately on arrival rather than by a receptionist. It is reassuring for them, and is an identifiable source of communication while they are waiting. The triage nurse has an important role in establishing a rapport with the child and in gaining his confidence before he is seen by a doctor. Triage is an opportunity for the nurse to listen and observe, and to assess the child and his parents, both physically and emotionally. Once the child's turn to be seen arrives, he is shown into a cubicle or room, which again will be full of unfamiliar equipment and seem very alien to him. Trust gained can be very quickly lost at this time. The child should be encouraged, if at all possible, to remain on his parent's knee, within the safety of his/her arms. The nurse must talk to him and his parents and involve the parent/s in his preparation for examination. Children will cling fiercely to their clothes; they see them as their last link with familiarity and normality: at this stage, it is much more reassuring if the parent rather than the nurse undresses the child. Take time to hold a small baby. Talk quietly and reassuringly to him. Physical procedures and treatments may be unpleasant; many are. Children all seem to have an inborn fear of 'the needle'. They need to be constantly reassured about every procedure and shown equipment before it is used. Many children fear something as simple as a thermometer, but, if they are encouraged to touch and examine it, they will more readily accept what is being done. Perhaps 'Teddy' or 'Tiny Tears' could have their temperature checked too!

Painful procedures should be explained with honesty, but played down if possible: 'This is going to hurt a little, but it will be over very soon.' Promises of bravery badges are a great incentive to tolerate procedures. In this day of hi-tech toys and expensive playthings, it is lovely to see the joy and pride with which these badges are worn. There should be no place in the nurse's vocabulary for jocular remarks such as 'I think we will have to cut his ear/leg/finger off.' The nurse may understand, the parents may understand, but to the child, this will only confirm his worst fears.

At all times, nurses must be sensitively aware of the danger of child abuse. They must listen and observe – not only physical observations but also the attitude of the parent or carer. Excessive display of parental anxiety may be an indication of child abuse. A delay in seeking help for an injury may be suspicious. The story of how the injury happened may be inconsistent with the actual injury. A parent who comes to A & E many times saying, 'she is always crying' or 'always vomiting', when no physical reason can be found, may be crying for help and saying: 'If someone does not help me, I will injure my child …' Nurses working in A & E need to develop a 'listening' ear, always sympathetic and never judgemental.

Many parents come to A & E Departments with their sick children rather than go to their GP. In a recent survey carried out in the A & E Department of the Royal Belfast Hospital for Sick Children, it was found that 45 per cent presented with medical problems such as tonsillitis, otitis media, upper respiratory tract infections, etc. It is tempting for the A & E nurse to question the validity of their visit to the Department.

In Pearson and Vaughan's (1986) *Models for Nursing Practice*, we read: 'all patients should have the freedom to identify their own needs and to decide on how these needs are to be met'. Parents are using A & E as a source of primary health care. In a study carried out in the Accident and Emergency Department of the Royal Belfast Hospital for Sick Children (Burton, 1989) comparisons were made between the parents' perceptions of the urgency of their child's condition and the nurse's assessment of the urgency of the child's condition. Fifty-two incidences were studied and results showed that 30 per cent of parents' perceptions agreed with the nursing assessment, 65 per cent underestimated the urgency, and only 5 per cent overestimated the urgency.

A PHILOSOPHY OF CARE – THE ENVIRONMENTAL PERSPECTIVE

The Standing Committee on Accidents in Childhood recommended in 1967 that 'the aim of our patient care should be to provide the best medical attention with the minimal emotional upset to the child. Children should be shielded from all unpleasant sights and sounds such as severely injured, noisy or drunken people.'

Many hospitals are now recognising the need for a separate waiting area in A & E for children; others, while recognising the need, are severely limited by lack of funds and/or lack of space. In the Royal Belfast Hospital for Sick Children, this problem does not exist. The A & E Department is an integral part of the Children's Hospital. It is there for all children under the age of 13 years. It provides a permanent 24-hour take-in service. It is the only A & E Department in Northern Ireland devoted exclusively to paediatric care. The waiting area serves several Outpatient Departments as well as A & E. An old photograph of the Department's waiting room in 1933 shows a dark, dismal picture of regimentally placed, rigid seats. There is no sign of toys or posters. The mothers look depressed, the children even more so! Today in 1993, the structure of the waiting area remains the same. However, work is due to begin on a new Department, in mid-summer 1995, but apart from this, by 1933 standards, it would still be unrecognisable. The walls are now painted a light colour, murals adorn the walls, seating is so arranged that a central play area is available. In this area there is a Wendy House, a toy telephone kiosk and many other toys. They are made of strong, durable plastic in bright, primary colours. They are easily washed. More important than this, they have been chosen for safety. There is a blackboard and chalk at toddler level, and scrap paper and crayons are available for diminutive Picassos! Very often the whole family will come to A & E with the sick child, and staff are dealing with bored, healthy children as well as the patient. Bored children can become noisy and demanding, distressing to others who are waiting. The provision of safe toys can help alleviate this problem. The little patients themselves feel less threatened in this environment. Occasionally, the sick child will make a sudden recovery when he sees the toys – to the great embarrassment of the mother or father! Children learn through play and perhaps the less boisterous will prefer to crayon pictures of how they perceive the hospital environment.

Chairs should be strong, wipeable and comfortable, as parents may be nursing a heavy, fretful baby or toddler. A hungry baby will soon make his hunger known, so the A & E Department should have a supply of pre-packed feeds and teats. Disposable cups and feeding beakers should also be available. Somewhere for a mother to breastfeed in privacy is a necessity, as well as somewhere to change a soiled nappy. Disposable nappies and barrier cream should also be available.

Video recorders have been installed in many Paediatric Departments. They are used, not only as a means of entertainment but as a valuable educational medium giving information on immunisation, for example. It is inevitable that the clinical examination area will contain many things which frighten the child such as auriscopes, instruments, syringes and needles. It is better that these things are kept on covered trays or in cupboards. Bright friezes (at child level) will help to capture a child's attention.

Things that rattle or move or make other interesting noises will often distract a child from what is going on, and also give a valuable indication of his developmental progress. 'Teddy' can often share the examination couch with the young patient. He, too, can be bandaged, have steristrips, have his heart listened to and his blood pressure recorded. The only difference is 'Teddy' will suffer no emotional deprivation if mishandled, but the child may. The total environmental aspect of the A & E care is important in maintaining the welfare of our patients and has an invaluable part to play in the holistic and family-centred ethos of our caring.

A PHILOSOPHY OF CARE – THE PSYCHOLOGICAL PERSPECTIVE

The nurse working in A & E must always adopt a sympathetic approach to the care of a sick child and his family. Parents very often come only for reassurance and advice, and the nurse must recognise this. Talking is the most obvious form of communication. Listening is a less obvious one but is an important vehicle of communication. It is important to include the child in the conversation, learn what his name is, and what he is usually called. Show an interest in the child, admiring babies and perhaps talking about current toys and television programmes. While talking, the nurse should also be listening and observing. Touch is important too – a worried and distraught mother will appreciate having an arm put around her by the nurse. Bereaved parents will not condemn a nurse because her tears mingle with theirs. The days of the 'stiff upper lip' are gone forever. Children only know and understand what they have already experienced in life. They may have no previous experience of a hospital visit or they may have had a traumatic experience. They are afraid of the unknown, uncertain about what is going to happen to them; they fear further physical pain and they may feel out of control in the situation in which they find themselves. More than anything, they fear separation from their parent/s; this should be avoided at all costs. Parents should be encouraged to remain with their child at all times and be involved in their care.

The child coming into A & E as the result of an accident may already be experiencing severe pain. Practical measures (such as immobilisation of the limb by splinting, topical anaesthesia and analgesia) should be taken and reassurance given. All these measures will help him to come to terms with his predicament. The expectation that a child will not cry is unrealistic when in A & E. Every child is different – some are unbelievably good, while others react in a violent and vociferous manner. Each of them needs a nurse who is patient and understanding and who has gained the trust and confidence of both parent and child.

Anxious parents too may be transmitting their fears to their child, adding to his distress. They may be blaming themselves for the accident and be experiencing feelings of guilt. The nurse has an important role to play in reassurance in this situation. Parents should be encouraged not to blame themselves, and to do all they can during the present crisis to calm and comfort their child.

In April 1990, a joint Working Party of the Royal College of Nursing A & E Forum and the Society of Paediatric Nursing published *Nursing Children in the Accident and*

Emergency Department. It contains comprehensive guidelines for the care of a child in A & E. They list the following pointers to help the nurse to establish a good rapport with the child. They are:

● Make a very gentle approach.
● Use a soft tone of voice.
● Talk with a toddler's parents first, then involve the child.
● Get down to the child's level, towering above him will only frighten him.
● Address the child by his usual name, frequently different from the one on the card.
● Discuss something personal to the child, perhaps a toy that he has with him.
● Elicit the child's help in all activities, ask the child to point out his buttons.
● Continue to involve the child's parents in the conversation.
● Take time to wait for replies.
● Never force an issue.
● Be thoughtful, be honest.

RECEPTION AND DOCUMENTATION

Usually on arrival at the hospital, most parents and their children will call at the reception desk, unless they arrive by ambulance or are emergencies. Here, details are taken of their name, address, date of birth, general practitioner and school (if applicable). They are then given their record card which they immediately present to the nurse at the triage desk. Clerical staff, too, must play their part in the well-being of a child and his parents; as they are often the first people to greet the patients, they need to develop personal communication skills and to speak with courtesy and interest.

The triage nurse interviews the child and his parents to add to the demographic data such details as:

1. Immunisation status.
2. If the child has a referral letter from his/her general practitioner.
3. The history of present accident or illness.

All the time, as she is speaking to the parents, she is observing and assessing, enabling her to conceive an individualised plan of care for this child. Preliminary observations and investigations can be carried out at this point, such as temperature, pulse, blood pressure, central nervous system observations, urine collection and testing. Injured limbs can be immobilised by splinting or the use of slings, lacerations covered with sterile dressings. The most important aspect of the triage nurse's responsibility is the gauging of priority of urgency. The nurse will communicate her observations and findings to her colleagues. The individual care plan will follow an established plan:

● Identification of the problem.
● Planning of care.
● Action taken.
● Evaluation.

The nurse will also see how many previous visits the child has had, whether the child's age matches his developmental age, his sleeping and eating patterns and his behaviour. Many people who come simply for reassurance and advice are already more relaxed at this stage. It is important that the triage nurse can be seen by those in the waiting area. He/she is the reassuring link during the waiting time.

The NAWCH Quality Review document (1989) recommended that Accident and Emergency Departments should keep a separate register for children aged 0–16. Children's cards should be filed separately from adults and can be a different colour. It should be possible to distinguish the cards of children of special interests, i.e. with medical or social problems, from other children. This is an important part of strategies for child protection. If information is collected on children who come into the A & E Department following accidents, it can be used to plan services for the prevention of accidents.

Many A & E records are now computerised and more are in the process of becoming computerised. This facilitates easy retrieval and quantification of attendances at A & E. Some departments keep no separate records of paediatric attendances. It is impossible to quantify the workload that children represent and so requests for funding cannot be backed by statistical evidence of need.

A PHILOSOPHY OF CARE – THE PERSPECTIVE OF OUTCOME

After a child has been seen in A & E, there are three possible outcomes:

1. Discharge home
2. Transfer to another hospital
3. Admission

Discharge Home

This is the most usual and desired outcome of any child's visit to the hospital. The NAWCH Charter (1984) states very clearly: 'Children shall be admitted to Hospital only if the care they require cannot be equally provided at home or on a day basis.' If discharge home is to be successful, it is imperative that they understand all the advice and instructions that have been given to them. Printed leaflets, with clear advice, are given to parents when a child is discharged home, e.g. (1) head injury advice, (2) care of plaster of paris, (3) control of pyrexia, and (4) management of diarrhoea and vomiting. They are always assured that staff are willing to answer telephone enquiries if they are worried, and that they may return to the Department at any time. Leaflets will need to be printed in languages other than English. Liaison between hospital staff and community is essential. The general practitioner, district nurse or health visitor may be involved in after-discharge care. The health visitor plays an important role in the totality of care. He/she usually calls to discuss discharges needing follow-up, any problems relevant to the previous 24 hours, and any other problems which may have arisen.

Staff in many A & E Departments have recognised the need for and are producing booklets, mainly for children, but giving advice to parents. A good example of this innovation is *Harry goes to Hospital*, produced by the staff of the A & E Department of the Royal Belfast Hospital for Sick Children, written in rhyming couplets and amusingly illustrated. This booklet is the first in a series called *The Adventures of the Belfast Gang*. An example of the advice given to Harry, who is in a short leg plaster of paris is:

Exercise your toes each day
Backwards ... forwards ... every way,
Even if it's rather sore
Gently try to move them more!

Transfer to Another Hospital

The situation may arise when a child requires transfer to another hospital for one of several reasons:

● The hospital may have no vacant beds.
● The child may require specialised care, e.g. isolation of infectious disease.
● If the A & E Department is in a general hospital, there may be no paediatric beds on the same site.

A joint statement from the British Paediatric Association and the British Association of Paediatric Surgeons (1987) says:

'A/E Departments where children are seen, and Children's Departments, should be on the same hospital site. Hospital and District Planning should take account of this. This is important not only because of the numbers attending, but because of the rapidity with which illness progresses in this age group! When transfer must take place, it should be planned carefully to ensure the maximum welfare of the child, both physically and emotionally.'

The staff must ensure:

● Full explanations are given for the reason for transfer.
● Assurance to the child that 'mummy and daddy can go too'.
● His/her condition should be stable before departure.
● Good communication between the two hospitals concerned.
● A nurse and/or doctor to accompany the child if necessary.
● Ambulance personnel should be made aware of any special needs the child has.
● Full details of illness and treatments including x-rays and blood tests to be sent.

Admission

Inevitably, some children will have to be admitted to the wards. This can cause them much distress. Old fears, temporarily allayed, will surface again, the fear of the unknown, separation from parents. They feel immensely vulnerable, tears will begin to flow again. Distress can be lessened if a 'named' nurse is responsible for their care from when they come into the A & E Department, right until the time they are handed over to the ward staff. This nurse will already have established a relationship with the child and should be involved in the preparation of the child for admission. She can explain, perhaps with the help of pictures, what the ward will be like and why the child has come in; she can promise the child that his/her parents will be allowed to stay. She will be responsible for seeing that the appropriate documentation is complete, for personally conveying what is already known about the child, his condition and his treatment, to the ward staff. While the parents are supporting their child, they may have many questions they want to ask, such as 'Am I allowed to visit my child at any time?' The manner in which the child and his parents are greeted by the ward staff will have a bearing on how quickly they settle down. It is important that busy ward staff do not give the impression that the child's admission is an imposition they could well do without!

A favourite toy or teddy can be 'admitted' too. Older children generally react to the news that they need admission with more panache and self-control, but they will need reassurance also, even if their fears are less vociferously articulated.

A PHILOSOPHY OF CARE – A PERSPECTIVE OF THE 'ULTIMATE' SADNESS

Edna St Vincent Millay said, 'childhood is the kingdom where nobody dies'. Sadly, nurses working in A & E Departments know this is not true. Edna Millay might well have said, 'childhood is the kingdom where children die too easily' for three children die every day in the United Kingdom as the result of road traffic accidents alone. Inevitably, the nurse will have to cope with sudden death while working in A & E. The unnecessary death of a child is always a tragedy. How can staff ease the pain of bereavement or offer comfort to a distraught grieving parent or grandparent? Not an easy question to answer. When a severely injured child is brought into A & E and dies, or when a dead baby is carried in, a victim of Sudden Infant Death Syndrome, one nurse is assigned to stay with the parents at all times. It is the responsibility of this nurse to keep the parents informed of what is happening, to help them contact family and friends, to make arrangements for other siblings to be looked after, to make arrangements for them to contact their minister or priest. The nurse must remain with the doctor when news of the child's death is confirmed. Words are inadequate vehicles of sympathy, but an arm placed around someone's shoulder can often speak louder than words. People will not always remember what the nurse or doctor said, but they will often remember that 'the nurse and the doctor cried too'.

Essentially, every A & E Department should have a bereavement or counselling room where parents can begin the grieving process in privacy – somewhere removed from the clinical area and waiting room. Parents are encouraged to hold their little one and to remain with the child as long as they want to. They may wish to be alone at this stage. How much nicer it is for them to look on their baby's face for the last time without being surrounded by all the paraphernalia of resuscitation. This provision for privacy is a Department of Health (1991) standard: 'Parents are given the privacy to grieve alone in a quiet room set aside for this purpose, with the body of their child if they so wish ...'

A & E nurses must be prepared to listen again and again to accounts of the baby's or child's last hours. Very often parents will cry, 'Is it my fault, nurse?' They should be encouraged to 'give sorrow words', as Shakespeare said. If properly handled, the grieving process and the healing process can become intertwined and indistinguishable until it would be difficult to say where one ended and the other began. A relative or friend can be given written instructions about the removal of the body, the funeral arrangements and the post-mortem. Parents may want to come back and talk to staff who were on duty at the time, and should be assured that this is perfectly acceptable. Nurses themselves need support, especially nurses in training. They should expect and receive counselling from their more senior and experienced colleagues. As one post-registration student said, 'I just wanted the baby to waken up. I steeled myself not to cry.' Death is the ultimate sadness for staff in A & E. A philosophy of care will have its foundations firm in the practicalities which come from familiarity and experience. Upon this foundation, which gives confidence, they can build with gentleness, with love and with a sensitive understanding of the enormity of a parent's loss.

A PHILOSOPHY OF CARE – THE RESEARCH PERSPECTIVE

Research is the buzz-word in nursing theory and practice today. It permeates every aspect of our thinking, influencing and altering cherished theories and traditions. It excites and challenges, stimulates and stirs us to question and evaluate whatever we are doing in a systematic and thorough way. Research no longer belongs to the academic isolationists, it has moved into the realm of reality and belongs to the practical as well as the theoretical skills. Research awareness should be fostered in Paediatric A & E Departments and research skills identified and developed.

'The objectives of scientific research are to answer questions, to discover or re-use facts or theories or to solve problems. Scientific research is every nurse's business' (Nottar, 1974). 'Every nurse' applies to the nurse working in A & E and he/she must be committed to research-based practice, not necessarily in carrying out research, but reading research and learning to apply it to his/her own practice. This will encourage A & E nurses to identify problems and to seek ways of solving them through research for the ultimate benefit of their patients. In Darling and Rogers' (1986) words, 'the corollary of accountability is a questioning approach'.

The word 'quality' has been introduced into the A & E situation over the past few years (see chapter one). Quality is defined as a 'degree of excellence of a thing' (Oxford English Dictionary). Paediatric A & E Departments are setting their own standards and auditing their practice. The Accident & Emergency Nursing Monitor is a quality assurance nursing audit designed for use in A & E Units. The Accident & Emergency Monitor provides a series of master checklists of observable, quality-related criteria, by which nurses can assess the quality of care. This document contains a Junior Supplement.

Many Paediatric Accident & Emergency Departments are designing their own quality tools, e.g. Parents' Satisfaction Questionnaires, and producing Plans of Action in response to identified deficiencies. Increasingly, parents are becoming more and more involved in the planning of their child's care and are perceived as being partners in caring. A cardinal principle of hospital services for children is complete ease of access to the child by his/her parents. This is *not* a luxury. It is now generally accepted that the care and comfort of parents for a child is *fundamental* to the care and treatment of children in hospital (DoH, 1991).

A PHILOSOPHY OF CARE – A STAFFING PERSPECTIVE

The standard of care given to the patient is to a great extent dependent on the staff available to deliver the care. The RCN, in its policy document 'Nursing the Child in A & E', recognises the need for specialist staff. It recommends that each A & E Department should attempt to recruit at least one RSCN to its staff. Ideally, a department should be staffed over the 24-hour period by an RSCN, but this is not always feasible. The RCN recommend quantifying the workload and its spread across the day. In a recent survey carried out over a 3-month period in a Paediatric A & E Department, the following figures emerged:

Time of Attendance: (New patients)
2 per cent of children attended between the hours of midnight and 6.00 a.m.
18 per cent of children attended between the hours of 6.00 a.m. and noon.
50 per cent of children attended between the hours of noon and 6.00 p.m.
30 per cent of children attended between the hours of 6.00 p.m. and midnight.

The afternoon and early evening was the busiest period of the day. In many hospitals a twilight shift (8 p.m. to midnight) has been introduced enabling nurses with young children to bring their knowledge and experience to the clinical area. Many other disciplines are involved in the staffing of a paediatric A & E:

1. The health visitor, who already has a contact with the family, has a valuable follow-up role to play. Her advice on accident prevention and safety will often be listened to when people are in their own home and not in the alien environment of a hospital.
2. The play specialist who encourages and supervises play.
3. The social worker works closely with the A & E team and is always available to give advice and check records where staff are concerned about the welfare or safety of a child. Social workers are contactable over a 24-hour period.
4. The dietitian may be called to give dietary advice, e.g. if a child who is complaining of abdominal pain is found to be severely constipated.

There are many other disciplines involved in the care of the child in A & E. The RCN Document (1990) makes the following recommendations for nurses working in A & E Departments. They need to develop specialist knowledge of:

1. The recognition of the alteration in physiology and the response of a child to illness or injury.
2. The psychological effects of injury, sickness and hospitalisation.
3. The support of the parents, siblings and other family members.
4. The care of the family immediately following sudden infant death and child death.
5. The recognition of child abuse and the procedures to follow.
6. The knowledge to provide advice and health education to families.

The Children Act 1989

On 14 October 1991, The Children Act 1989 became law. Designed to protect the interests of all children, the Act represents the most fundamental reform this century of legislation affecting children. It reflects the way we, as a society, want to see our children brought up and protected (DoH, 1991).

A number of important principles are embodied in the Children Act:

● The welfare of the child is the paramount consideration in court proceedings.
● Wherever possible, children should be brought up and cared for within their own families.
● Children should be safe and protected by effective intervention if they are in danger but this should be open to challenge by parents, in the courts.
● When dealing with children, courts should ensure that delay is avoided and may only make an order if to do so, is better for the child than making no order at all.
● Children should be kept informed about what happens to them and should participate when decisions are made about their future.

These are just a few points from the Children Act which are significant for nurses working in A & E Departments. The RCN and The Department of Health have produced a booklet, 'What every Nurse, Health Visitor and Midwife needs to know about the Children Act'. It explains the implications for District Health Authorities, NHS Trusts and Family Health Service Authorities, and answers many questions A & E nurses are asking, e.g. 'What are its implications for practitioners?' The Children Act defines a child in need. The Royal College of Nursing reminds us that, 'any nurses who come into contact with children may be the first people to alert others, in particular Paediatric nurses, nurses working in Accident & Emergency Departments, Psychiatric Nurses, Mental Handicap and Practice Nurses, who will need to have an agreed practice protocol' (RCN, 1992).

The Royal College of Nursing make the following recommendations:

THE CHILDREN ACT 1989
What you can do

● Find out who is the lead officer for the Children Act in your Unit and also for the Social Services department and contact them for local information, plans and procedures.
● Contact voluntary organisations to establish their approach to the Act.
● Discuss the Children Act with colleagues, particularly in a multi-disciplinary area, inviting knowledgeable speakers.
● Raise issues related to the Children Act and health care with those who plan services for children and their families.
● Develop links with appropriate key workers in social services and education departments.
● Ensure that there is access to legal advice where necessary.

CONCLUSION

'Injury has been the cause of human suffering through the ages, but in this modern era of sophisticated technology and high speed transport, it has assumed epidemic proportions. The brunt of this onslaught has fallen on the young in our society and, unfortunately, society has not catered sufficiently for the needs of children afflicted by degrees of physical damage, accidental or otherwise' (Alpar and Owen, 1988).

The A & E Departments are seeing the results of the dangerous environment that children live in today. As well as bringing the child to A & E following an accident, many parents are choosing A & E as a source of primary health care for their child. We are often tempted to judge the legitimacy of their visit to the Department. Pearson and Vaughan (1986) state that all patients should have the freedom to identify their own needs and to decide on how these needs are to be met. Nurses working in A & E are professionally obliged to meet their expectations and to give the best possible service to the children in their care. Childhood should be a treasured and wonderful time, jealously protected before 'shades of the prison house begin to close upon the growing boy' (Wordsworth).

This chapter has looked at the physical, environmental and psychological implications for the children in our care. Under this umbrella, we have looked at documentation, staffing, quality and research. The following are the major points which emerged:

- Children should be recognised as unique, developing individuals. Their inherent characteristics make them susceptible to accidental injury. Their immune systems are immature. They can become *very* ill, *very* quickly.
- There should be a separate area for children, away from the sights and sounds of sick, injured or drunken adults.
- Clinical and treatment areas must be child-oriented, bright and cheerful.
- At least one RSCN should be on duty at all times over the 24-hour period.
- A chart giving paediatric drug doses in emergencies, according to the weight of the child, should be displayed in the resuscitation room.
- A paediatric consultant with special interest in A & E should be supervising the work and children's services.
- There should be written guidelines for staff about the prioritisation of children according to urgency.
- Parents should be able to stay with their children at all times.
- Parents should be given written instructions about the care of their child at home, e.g.
    Head injury advice
    Care of wounds
    Plaster of paris
    Treatment of diarrhoea and vomiting.
- Special room should be available where distressed or bereaved parents can be alone or talk with staff and where they can grieve in private.
- Staff need special guidelines on procedure to follow when a baby dies of Sudden Infant Death Syndrome.
- Staff need to be aware of the procedure for dealing with children who have been abused.
- A liaison health visitor should be attached to the Department.
- A liaison social worker should be attached to the Department.
- Each Department should have a paediatric register or computer system which allows comprehensive monitoring of all paediatric attenders.

● There should be somewhere for parents to feed children and change nappies.
● There should be books and toys for children of all ages.
● There should be toilets available which can be used by small children.
(NAWCH (1989) Quality Review of Services to Children).

The checklist is designed for staff working in A & E departments. The complete checklist can be read in the Quality Review.

'Children are not just mini-adults; they are more vulnerable than adults and less aware of the dangers lurking in the modern environment. They are more dependent physically and emotionally, upon their families and indeed, must never be considered apart from them.' (Appley, 1988)

The whole ethos of our philosophy of care seeks to protect the physical and emotional welfare of the children who come under our care. It helps to have an inborn love of children and to develop selective deafness! Every day is a challenge.

Children react in so many different ways to their trauma; some with minor injuries are inordinately distressed; some with major trauma are incredibly brave. What could be more appropriate than to let a little child have the last word? When a delightful little 7-year-old boy was told his arm was broken, his immediate reaction was, 'Oh dear, and I was having such good fun!'

REFERENCES

Alpar E K and Owen R (1988) *Paediatric Trauma.* Tunbridge Wells: Castle House Publications.
Appley Graham (1988) Foreword, in ibid.
British Paediatric Association and British Association of Paediatric Surgeons (1987) *A Joint Statement on Children's Attendances at A & E Departments.* London: British Paediatric Association.
Burton R (1989) Shifting horizons – parents' perceptions of a paediatric A & E department. *Paediatric Nursing,* **1**(8), 19–20.
Darling J and Rogers J (1986) *Research for Practising Nurses.* Basingstoke: Macmillan.
Department of Health (1991) *Guidelines for the Welfare of Children and Young People in Hospital.* London: HMSO.
Department of Health (1991) *The Children Act 1989: An Introductory Guide for the NHS.* London: HMSO
Dickens Charles *David Copperfield.* In *Oxford Dictionary of Quotations.* Oxford: Oxford University Press.
Millay, Edna St Vincent. 'Childhood is the Kingdom'. In *Oxford Dictionary of Quotations.* Oxford: Oxford University Press.
National Association for the Welfare of Children in Hospital (1984) *Charter.* London.
National Association for the Welfare of Children in Hospital (1989) *Quality Review of Services to Children.* London: NAWCH.
Nottar L E (1974) *Essentials of Nursing Research.* New York: Springer.
Pearson A and Vaughan B (1986) *Models for Nursing Practice.* London: Heinemann.
Royal College of Nursing A&E Forum, Society of Paediatric Nursing (1990) *Nursing Children in the Accident & Emergency Departments.* London: RCN.
Royal College of Nursing and Department of Health (1992) *What Every Nurse, Health Visitor and Midwife Needs to know about the Children Act.* Manchester: HMSO.
Wordsworth William. 'My heart leaps up'. In *Oxford Dictionary of Quotations.* Oxford: Oxford University Press.
Wordsworth William. 'Ode, Intimations to Immortality'. In *Oxford Dictionary of Quotations.* Oxford: Oxford University Press.

FURTHER READING

Department of Health (1991) *Guidelines for the Welfare of Children and Young People in Hospital*, London: HMSO.

Royal College of Nursing A&E Forum, Society of Paediatric Nursing (1990) *Nursing Children in the Accident and Emergency Department*, London: RCN.

Royal College of Nursing and Department of Health (1992) *What Every Nurse, Health Visitor and Midwife Needs to Know about the Children Act.* Manchester: HMSO.

10

Paediatric Pain Management – An Imprecise Science

Noelle Llewellyn

Pain is often considered to be an integral part of the process of living. Only a limited number of people, for example those with tuberculoid leprosy or congenital insensitivity to pain, do not 'feel' pain in the way the majority of the population do. The process of becoming a patient, particularly a patient who requires surgery, frequently leads to an increase in the incidence of pain, yet the individuals concerned demonstrate high levels of satisfaction with the service they have received, perhaps indicating that they too perceive pain to be an irrefutable fact (Royal College of Surgeons and College of Anaesthetists, 1990). However, despite its universality, the problem of pain has been virtually ignored. More recently both popular (Rigge, 1990; Boelen, 1990; Doyle, 1991) and professional literature (Royal College of Surgeons and College of Anaesthetists, 1990) have begun to raise awareness of the problem of pain. The aim must surely be to bring about positive changes in the patients' experience. The need to improve pain management interventions is equally as pressing for the paediatric patient, as for the adult. This chapter will explore the vital role of the nurse in the assessment of the child in pain, and will also discuss some of the pain management interventions which may be utilised within the clinical area. For ease of reading the nurse is referred to as she, and the child as he.

THE COMPLEXITY OF THE PAEDIATRIC PAIN EXPERIENCE

McCaffery defined pain as 'whatever the patient says it is and exists wherever he says it does' (cited in Sofaer, 1984). Extensive research has been carried out to establish what factors influence the individuals' perception of pain and thereby contribute to their personal pain experience. Consideration of these contributing factors may be helpful to the nurse in her endeavours to assess pain accurately.

Age

The contentious issue of the influence of age on the pain experience has provoked much discussion. It is suggested that even embryos appear to have an aversive response to noxious stimuli; nevertheless many professionals still disagree about the age at which infants perceive pain (Gauntlett, 1987; Barr, 1990; McGrath, 1990). A reason for this controversy may be the subjective nature of the experience of pain, as describing the experience to others relies on communication skills which the young child may not yet have developed. Piaget (1930, cited in Hurley and Whelan, 1988) extensively described the ways in which children of different ages respond to and perceive pain. As with all aspects of paediatric nursing a working knowledge of the implications of the child's level of cognitive development and how to tailor nursing approaches accordingly may be a critical factor in the success or failure of the therapeutic relationship.

Gender

Despite attempts at sexual equality, there is still evidence to suggest that the socialisation of male children in Western society encourages boys to conform to stereotypical male roles, thereby reinforcing acceptable 'male' behaviour (Haralambos and Holborn, 1990). Certainly, it appears that society tolerates greater freedom of expression from females while encouraging a male child to be a 'big brave boy'.

Culture

The influence of culture on the perception of pain has been extensively documented, Zborowski (1952, cited in Walding, 1991) suggested that the further an individual was from the immigrant generation the less culturally-specific his behaviour became, a dilution of culturally-specific responses by the multi-cultural society in which the individual lived. However, Lambert et al. (1960, cited in Seers, 1988) propose that actual or perceived competition between different cultural groups may artificially maintain and reinforce cultural idiosyncrasies.

Significant Others

The reaction of the family to the child in pain will very rapidly teach the child how to behave in a manner which the family finds acceptable. If the child is given minimal comfort, and largely ignored when in pain, and is acknowledged or praised when no longer exhibiting distress, the child will learn to suppress and control himself when in pain, as he will learn that demonstrative behaviour affords him little if any solace and comfort.

Temperament

The general nature or characteristic mood of an individual is referred to as their temperament. Wallace (1989) suggests that identification of the child's temperament may enable the nurse to decrease anxiety, by creatively modifying the medical demands made of the child in such a way as to allow them to 'fit' with the child's perception of what is right and acceptable. Wallace suggests that children who are more overt in their demonstration of pain receive more analgesia than children who internalise their distress. Perhaps nurses feel more comfortable administering analgesics to children who are 'obviously' in pain; however, applying this criterion blindly may result in children who are overt demonstrators being over-medicated, and children who are covert demonstrators being under-medicated.

Even this very brief consideration of the factors which may affect a child's perception of his pain clearly demonstrates the confusion and conflict of information which may result when one aspect is considered in isolation. To identify an individual's perception of his own pain, an individualised holistic assessment, which is current in time, place, experience and cognitive abilities, is necessary.

PAIN ASSESSMENT

Pain assessment is often perceived to be the use of a validated assessment tool to quantify the individual's level of comfort or discomfort. However, to facilitate the effective use of a selected pain assessment tool, pain assessment should be integrated into the holistic admission assessment of the child and his family. Not only will this approach identify factors which may be crucial to effective pain management, but it will also identify pain as a priority issue, and the child and family may be reassured that a pro-active approach is being taken rather than the nursing staff simply reacting if and, more probably, when pain does occur. This acknowledgement of the existence or possible existence of pain may be the first step in effective management.

An ability to communicate effectively is one of the core skills of a nurse. Paediatric nurses interact not only with patients with a wide range of developmental abilities, but also with their families, who may be anxious, frightened or angry, or indeed experiencing a whole variety of emotions, which may influence their usual skills and behaviour. The nurse must encourage the development of a therapeutic relationship, so that goals can be mutually identified and appropriate strategies devised to achieve these goals.

The assessment interview and discussion should be calm and uninterrupted if at all possible. The child and family should be given an opportunity to become familiar with their surroundings and to feel comfortable with the staff, so that they do not perceive the interview to be an 'interrogation'. If the child appears shy, it may be helpful to talk to the parents or primary care-giver initially and to include them gently in the conversation. The use of puppets or toys as an intermediary may also be less threatening to the child. The assessment should be dynamic, but the nurse may use a framework, which can be modified to the individual needs of the child and family.

THE ASSESSMENT FRAMEWORK

Pain Words

As with many other behaviours, the child and the family may have developed their own 'pain language' (McCaffery and Beebe, 1989; Whaley and Wong, 1989; 1990). Instead of a pain they may have a 'baddie', 'boo boo', 'nasty' or a 'hurt'. Although words which may be associated with pain are commonly used, some families may use expressions which have no relevance or connection to pain to an individual outside the family unit. Identification of these words will facilitate communication, and also serve to emphasise the importance of the role of the child and family in the effective management of pain. If the child is admitted with a 'painful condition', it may be helpful to ask him to describe how the pain feels. Often one-word descriptions are woefully inadequate and a much clearer insight into the intensity, quality and subjective effect of the pain can be gained by listening to the child's description. If the child is unable to encompass how the pain feels using his verbal skills, he may be encouraged to 'draw' his pain (Ross and Ross, 1988). The important factor is the quality of the information which the child is enabled to disseminate to those who have primary responsibility for managing his pain, and not the medium by which this is achieved.

Pain History

Establishing the words a child and his family use to describe pain will also provide insight into the types of pain the child has previously experienced and his understanding of pain. These experiences can be used as a core of knowledge for the child and family to build upon. The child may be prepared for potentially painful procedures by comparing his previous experience to the planned procedure. Indeed, children often develop this strategy independently by asking questions which begin 'Will it be like...?' Fear of the unknown can increase the child's perception of pain and therefore using their previous experiences to increase their knowledge can increase their 'power over pain'.

Pain Behaviours

The behaviour which the child manifests when he is in pain is an integral part of the pain history. For example, what behavioural cues have the parents observed which they consider to be 'pain indicators'? It is important to establish whether there are two sets of behaviours, one for pain of a sudden onset, and one for pain of a more chronic nature. Being sensitive to the child's pain behaviours may enable the nursing staff to detect pain more readily and therefore intervene more effectively.

Pain Management Strategy

Many families develop a pain management strategy, which may include both pharmacological and non-pharmacological methods of relieving pain. Some families may have developed a strategy, but may be unaware that they have done so. The nurse should establish which analgesic the child is most commonly given, and whether there is a 'ritual' to the administration of the medicine, such as a certain spoon or drink to 'wash it down with'. Many parents make use of the more sophisticated non-pharmacological methods of pain relief, such as massage therapy, aromatherapy, relaxation and guided imagery. Providing there is no medical contra-indication to these interventions being used, the parents should be encouraged and facilitated to maintain their contribution to the child's pain management if they wish to do so. The child may also have a 'transitional object', a woolly, baby, bunnie or blanket, which is essential to them when they are distressed (Darbyshire, 1985). If this is established on admission, then anguish for the child and nursing staff can be avoided by ensuring the transitional object is available at all times. The parents may use a specific song, story or even video cassette to soothe their child, and this again is relatively easy to continue during hospitalisation, although many parents may feel inhibited by the strange environment and may therefore require con-siderable encouragement. In a situation where many parents feel powerless and inadequate, valuing their established methods of dealing with their child in pain may improve their sense of well-being, and it can also provide a valuable opportunity for education to enable them to modify their management if and when this is appropriate. It may be possible to integrate the home and hospital pain management strategies, thereby acknowledging the value of the parents' contribution while provid-ing a degree of continuity for the child.

Roles and Expectations

Many parents experience a crisis of confidence when their child is admitted to hospital. They do not feel that they have the necessary skills and abilities to care for him. Others feel that it is imperative to maintain their parenting role in the new situation and to develop their skills and abilities to accommodate the new and different needs of their sick child. The parents' and child's perceived role in the management of pain can have important implications when the selection of an appropriate management technique is being considered. A child who wants to be made better by others, with little or no involvement himself, may be an unsuitable candidate for a regime, such as patient-controlled analgesia which involves a high degree of co-operation from the patient. Parents who expect a more traditional form of pain management may express considerable anxieties about some of the less commonly used analgesic techniques. Some parents may have anxieties about being present during potentially painful procedures and may fear their own reactions, they may feel that their presence will do little to comfort their child, and therefore may not wish to be involved. If the parents voice these opinions, the nurse then has the opportunity to discuss their role and to help them decide on a plan which will address the needs of the child while also acknowledging their concerns. If the child and family expect that the analgesic technique used will result in the complete absence of pain, they are likely to be disappointed. It is perhaps more honest and realistic to discuss pain management as a 'little hurt', that, although they may realise it is there, will not stop them doing what they want to do (within the confines of their condition). For the younger child this is obviously a difficult concept to grasp, and the parents and nursing staff may have to rely quite heavily on the child's behavioural cues for an indication of their level of comfort. For the older child it may be appropriate to draw a comparison with a headache or toothache, how at first, although they know it is not 'right' they do not think it is 'bad enough' to need a painkiller, and if it gets worse it is they who decide to ask their parent for some medicine. In the hospital setting the child will again be the one who decides how much pain is 'too much', but they should not be led to expect no pain at all.

PAIN ASSESSMENT TOOLS

The subjectivity of the pain experience makes accurate pain assessment a difficult task to carry out. Unlike body temperature which can be measured directly and objectively by using a thermometer, pain is measured indirectly, using tools which have been created to evaluate the amount of pain experienced by focusing on certain aspects of pain.

Many assessment tools are available, each with its own characteristic strengths and weaknesses. They can be broadly divided into three categories; subjective or self-report tools, behavioural tools and physiological assessment. These three components are most commonly felt to comprise the experience of pain.

Subjective or Self-report Tools

For many years it was felt that children were unable to quantify such an abstract concept as pain (Beyer and Wells, 1989). Now a variety of assessment tools are available to enable the child to identify varying levels of 'hurt'. Self-report tools provide information not only on the amount of pain, but may also help the child to describe the location, quality and individual characteristics of the sensation (Beyer *et al.*, 1990), and may also be used to evaluate the efficacy of the analgesic intervention. It is important to recognise that although self-report tools are sensitive to changes in pain level, they are still considered to be an estimate of pain, rather than an absolute measure (Ross and Ross, 1988). They require a level of cognitive and communication skills which may preclude their use in certain groups of paediatric patients, such as the neonate, the educationally-challenged child or the child who has a limited command of the English language. Accurate use of a self-report tool may also be prejudiced by the child's concerns about the consequence of stating that the pain has worsened. This is especially true if the analgesic regime which is prescribed has a high degree of unacceptability to the child.

Selection of an appropriate self-report tool from the wide range available should be determined with regard to the child's cognitive and developmental abilities. The child should perceive the tool to be an aid to the effective management of their pain, and not another stressor. It is also important that the nursing staff are familiar with the chosen tool, to enable them to fulfil their role as educator and facilitator.

Behavioural Tools

Estimating levels of pain from the observation of behaviours is considered by many to have several advantages over self-report tools for the paediatric patient (McGrath *et al.*, 1985a; Ross and Ross, 1988). The verbal and cognitive skills of the individual child are irrelevant, and the scale is unobtrusive and requires no co-operation from the child. It is also suggested that the observation of behaviour is more objective than relying on subjective self-report tools which may be influenced by factors associated with pain, rather than the actual level of pain. However, many behavioural responses, with the possible exceptions of pain cries and facial expression in infants, are not unique to the experience of pain, and distinguishing between pain and distress can be very difficult. Tools which observe a variety of behaviours are more likely to give pain assessment rather than simply an assessment of distress. There can be little doubt, however, that the information obtained by using a behavioural tool is far less sensitive to subtle changes in the nature, quality and intensity of pain levels, which may be identified by a self-report tool when used effectively.

Physiological Assessment

Although a physiological response to a painful stimulus may be considered a part of the total pain experience, the value of physiological monitoring as a means of estimating 'pain levels' does have several limitations. The child in acute pain will experience a global, non-specific physiological arousal, such as increased cardiac and respiratory rate, and elevation of blood pressure. Other conditions, both physical and psychological, may well lead to the same global, non-specific arousal state (Ross and Ross, 1988). If the pain is allowed to persist, the autonomic response becomes modified by a process of adaptation, and the physiological signs will return to near normal. Therefore, if physical signs are taken as the only indicator of the child's pain level, it would be natural to presume that this return to normality is an indication of no pain. It is also suggested that physiological measures are less susceptible to children's control, and therefore are more objective than self-report or behavioural methods of assessment (Gedaly-Duff, 1989). There can be little doubt, however, that although physical responses are not as susceptible to voluntary control as self-report or indeed behavioural factors, the response may be altered or magnified by other factors, such as fear, anxiety and expectancy. Physiological measures also fail to give a true indication of the child's perception of his pain (Beyer and Wells, 1989). Some more complex physiological methods of assessing pain exist, but they are not appropriate for use within the clinical area, or would be considered ethically unacceptable for the child (McGrath et al., 1985b). Recording of vital signs may be of value in providing a more complete picture of the child's condition, but should not be relied on as the sole means of assessing their level of pain.

Further reading about the individual tools available is recommended and a reading list is included at the end of this chapter.

PHARMACOLOGICAL PAIN MANAGEMENT

Conventional pain management for children has invariably consisted of either the intermittent intramuscular injection of narcotics, oral or rectally administered paracetamol, or nothing whatsoever. An analgesic technique should be effective; it should reduce pain efficiently, achieve this relatively quickly and be acceptable, both to the child, his family and the nursing staff. If these three criteria are fulfilled then the vicious circle of pain, which involves not only anticipation and fear of pain, but also, in many cases, of the analgesia technique prescribed, will be avoided.

Increasing use is being made of peri-operative analgesia techniques. Nerve blocks and wound infiltration may provide adequate immediate post-operative analgesia and may reduce the child's overall analgesic requirements. Although the nurse caring for the child is not directly involved in these techniques she should understand the principles of the procedure to enable her to answer any questions the child or his family may have, and also to enable her to monitor the child appropriately.

There are many different analgesics available, both narcotic and non-narcotic, and these can be administered to the child via a variety of routes, namely oral, rectal, sublingual, extradural, intravenous, subcutaneous and, of course, intramuscular.

The crucial factors in achieving effective analgesia are the selection of the appropriate drug, via an appropriate route, and then the administration of the drug so that a steady plasma level is achieved. Administration of analgesics on a regular round the clock basis will result in a steady plasma level and therefore more effective pain control, as a preventive or pro-active approach is used. Analgesics administered on an 'as required' (PRN) basis often leads to requests for analgesics only when pain is being experienced. Peaks and troughs in the plasma level of the drug result from this reactive approach to pain management, and pain control is frequently inadequate.

Although the final decision on the choice of analgesic used may rest with the medical staff, the nurse has a responsibility to act as the advocate for the child and family, and, wherever possible, to include them in the decision-making process.

Many of the more commonly used analgesia techniques are discussed in other paediatric nursing texts (Tackett and Hunberger, 1981; Marlow and Redding, 1988; Whaley and Wong, 1989). Some of the less commonly used methods, specifically extradural (epidural) analgesia, patient-controlled analgesia and nurse-controlled analgesia will now be discussed.

Extradural (Epidural) Analgesia

Extradurally administered analgesia and/or anaesthesia has been most commonly used for adult pain management, particularly for the obstetric patient, but also for post-operative pain management (Rosen and Calio, 1990). It is a method of targeting analgesia to the appropriate spinal nerves affected by the proposed procedure, thereby preventing the conveyance of information from peripheral pain receptors to the central nervous system and also potentially from the central nervous system to the skeletal and autonomic nervous systems. The drugs used act within the spinal cord itself, on the nerve roots outside the dura mater, within the cerebrospinal fluid and also systemically. The advantages of this technique are that it provides a means of maintaining a constant level of analgesia without excessive sedation, and in this way the child is able to co-operate with post-operative regimes such as chest physiotherapy without fear of pain or drowsiness affecting their ability or willingness to participate (Bragg, 1989).

The technique can be used successfully for pain management following abdominal surgery, thoracic surgery and orthopaedic surgery of the lower limbs. Narcotics or local anaesthetics, or a combination of the two, may be used to achieve effective pain relief.

Wherever possible the proposed technique should be discussed with the child and family pre-operatively to enable them to make an informed decision about its use. Many children and their families express anxieties about the use of extradural analgesia, which are largely due to incomplete or erroneous information. If their misconceptions are addressed and they still express anxieties about its use, then another analgesic technique should be used if at all possible.

Common Extradural Analgesia Questions

When will the catheter be put in?

Many children are concerned that they will be awake when the catheter is inserted. Generally the catheter is inserted pre-operatively, when the child is under general anaesthesia. In this way the technique can be used to provide intra-operative analgesia, and the accurate placement of the catheter can be checked by the child's physiological response to the surgery.

Does the catheter go into the spinal cord itself?

The catheter lies outside the dura mater and the drugs diffuse across the membrane into the subarachnoid space and from there exert their action in the spinal cord and within the cerebrospinal fluid. There is no direct communication between the catheter and the substance of the spinal cord.

Will the child be able to feel and move his legs normally?

Many adults experience a profound sensory and motor block following extradural analgesia, and despite explanations that all will return to normal when the technique is discontinued they often find this distressing and frightening. The use of a continuous infusion of a combination of local anaesthetic and narcotic for children rarely results in a sensory block, though occasionally older children may complain of a slight 'pins and needles' sensation, which may be resolved by a fractional reduction in the rate of the infusion. Motor block does not appear to be a side-effect which is commonly seen in children, and indeed the children are encouraged to be as mobile as their surgical condition will allow.

Are there any other side-effects?

All analgesia manifests desirable and less desirable effects to some extent. If the child and his family are unaware of these effects, they cannot make an informed choice about the use of the analgesic technique. It is important that any side-effects are explained to the child and their family in a way that will not increase their anxiety. The potential side-effects may include:

Drowsiness, as a direct effect of the narcotics or as a result of the relief of pain and reduced perception of external stimuli.

Respiratory depression, due to the effect of the narcotic on the respiratory centres in the medulla which therefore have a reduced response to carbon dioxide. The respiratory pattern is typically slow and sighing (Park and Fulton, 1991). Although this potentially lethal side-effect is a very rare occurrence, the nurse must be constantly vigilant. Hourly recordings of respiratory rate and sedation scale should be maintained for the duration of the infusion and for 6 hours following its discontinuation, to facilitate immediate intervention should this occur. A reversal dose of intravenous Naloxone should be available at all times.

Nausea and vomiting, due to the action of the narcotic on the vomiting centre situated in the medulla and brain stem. This effect is worsened by vestibular stimulation, therefore nausea and vomiting may be more troublesome in the mobile patient. Narcotics can also cause contraction of the smooth muscle throughout the gastrointestinal tract, which leads to delayed gastric emptying and prolonged transit time. Intravenous Metoclopramide or intramuscular Prochlorperazine may be helpful in alleviating feelings of nausea and vomiting.

Itching. Although allergic responses to narcotics are rare, they can cause histamine release when administered systemically, which results in vasodilation, pruritus and erythema. When narcotics are administered, centrally itching can occur to a lesser extent; the precise reason for this response is unclear, as the receptors involved are still to be identified. A non-reversal dose of intravenous Naloxone or Chlorpheniramine may give some relief.

Urinary retention. The action by which this occurs in unclear and may be a result of the narcotic or of the local anaesthetic. A non-reversal dose of intravenous Naloxone may be of help if retention is as a result of the action of the narcotic. If this is not effective, an indwelling urinary catheter should be placed in situ for the duration of the extradural infusion.

Will the child have to lie flat while the extradural infusion is running?

Although adult patients occasionally experience hypotension as a result of sympathetic fibre blockage producing vasodilation of the lower limbs, and therefore are encouraged to remain flat in bed for the duration of the infusion, children do not appear to manifest this side-effect. Attempts to keep a child flat in bed if he does not wish it are largely fruitless and therefore the child may adopt any position he feels comfortable in. Sitting out and having cuddles with his parents, providing care is taken with movement to avoid inadvertent dislodging of the extradural catheter, should be actively encouraged, providing his condition allows this.

When and how will the extradural catheter be removed?

The extradural infusion will be discontinued when the child is demonstrating a reduced need for analgesia as his condition improves, and when a suitable alternative method of analgesia can be employed. The removal of the catheter is simply a matter of removing the adhesive dressing which has retained the catheter in the correct position, the action of removing the dressing exerts gentle traction on the actual catheter which results in its simultaneous removal. As only 4–6 cm of catheter is left in the extradural space, the catheter is usually removed with relative ease. Rarely, resistance is felt and the child should then be encouraged to flex his spine while traction is maintained. This invariably results in the removal of the catheter. After removal the catheter should be carefully checked to ensure that it is complete.

The nurse caring for the child receiving extradural analgesia must be aware of the specific care this technique requires, and should also have the necessary skills and knowledge to answer any questions which the child and his family may have and also to intervene should any adverse effects occur. The core elements of care are:

- Hourly respiratory rate and sedation scale.
- Record volume of fluid infused hourly.
- Check extradural lines and connections hourly.
- Nurse the child on a sheepskin.
- Change the child's position two-hourly to maintain skin integrity.
- Check the catheter insertion site two-hourly.
- Assess level of comfort hourly.
- Intervene appropriately if side-effects occur.
- Maintain child and family contact.

Patient-controlled Analgesia

Patient-controlled analgesia (PCA) is a way of enabling the patient to titrate the amount of narcotic analgesia he receives according to his level of comfort or discomfort. In this way plasma levels of the drug are maintained within a therapeutic range, with minimal side-effects (Bucknell and Sikorski, 1989). The most commonly used route of administration is the intravenous route, although the subcutaneous and extradural routes have been utilised successfully. The PCA infusion pump is simply a sophisticated infusion pump which allows a range of programming. This can include:

- A variable rate continuous infusion.
- Administration of supplemental bolus doses, on demand from the patient by using some type of handset, usually either electronic or pneumatic.
- A variable time duration lockout period, during which no further bolus doses will be delivered, regardless of patient demands.

Although these devices have been available for adult pain management since the late 1960s/early 1970s, it is only relatively recently that they have been used for paediatric pain management. The confusion which surrounds the concept of the paediatric pain experience may have led health care professionals to assume that children would be unable to cope with such an active role in their pain management strategy. There can be little doubt that this technique is not suitable for all children, and the following criteria must be fulfilled before the technique is implemented:

- The child must have the physical ability to use the handset.
- They must understand the relationship between using the handset and receiving medication.
- They must trust that the infusion pump has been programmed appropriately.
- They should understand that the expectation is alleviation of pain, and not complete absence of pain.

● They must demonstrate a willingness and desire to be actively involved in their pain management strategy.

In practice the minimum age at which children are able to use PCA effectively is between 5 and 6 years. However, it is imperative that an individual assessment is carried out for each child, so that their willingness and ability to co-operate is established and any questions that they or their family have may be answered. If the child is unable or unwilling to use the PCA infusion pump, then another analgesic technique should be used.

Common Patient-controlled Analgesia Questions

Will the pump give the right amount?

Many parents and children feel concerned that the infusion pump will give an inappropriate amount of analgesia, either too much or not enough. The pump is programmed according to the drug used and the child's weight, and therefore the dose is primarily calculated to ensure that it is a 'safe amount'. Reprogramming can be carried out at any time during the infusion if it appears to be necessary.

Will there be nurses around?

The presence of a sophisticated infusion device may lead some parents to believe that the level of nursing involvement with their child may be diminished. The nursing care required by children receiving this type of analgesic regime is no less than with any other type of analgesic method. It could perhaps be argued that because the nurses are not frequently checking and administering analgesia, they consequently have more time to spend 'caring' for the child.

Will the child use the handset like a toy?

When first confronted with the PCA infusion pump, some children demonstrate an understandable curiosity about it and the way in which it works. If they are given an opportunity to explore the pump and to learn about it through 'play' before they require it therapeutically, the 'novelty' of it is worked through and with support and reinforcement it is then used appropriately in the therapeutic setting. Children who may benefit from PCA who have a chronic or non-surgical acute pain, invariably value using the pump not because of its 'novelty value', but because it actually makes their pain better, therefore their use of the infusion pump is rarely inappropriate. Of course, these children may require more support and reinforcement in the early stages of using PCA.

How will you know if you have programmed the pump properly?

The child and their family should be forewarned that the PCA infusion pump is programmed for the non-existent 'average child'. How the individual child concerned will respond to their pain and to the use of PCA is an unknown quantity. Therefore, the programming should be checked at least twice daily, so that any changes which appear necessary can be made. The child should be reminded to press the handset every time he feels he needs some painkiller, although he will not receive a bolus on each occasion because of the lockout interval. The discrepancy between demands (using the handset) and good demands (using the handset and receiving a bolus of analgesic) will be a valuable indicator as to how appropriately the pump has been programmed. A large discrepancy between demands and good demands indicates that the child is still in pain, and therefore still demanding analgesia, or that they have not grasped the concept of PCA, and are therefore at that time not able to co-operate with the regime. Use of a background infusion to complement bolus administration is not usual for adult patients (McLintock and Hodsman, 1987); however, children often claim to have better quality analgesia when a background infusion is used. Individual programming will depend on the drug being adminis-tered, the choice of PCA infusion pump and the specific needs of the child.

What if something is going to happen that may cause the child pain?

Administration of a bolus of analgesic before potentially painful procedures such as dressing changes, movement or physiotherapy, may enable the child to co-operate with the procedure without undue distress. He should be reminded that the analgesic takes about 10 minutes to have its effect, and therefore the bolus should be adminis-tered 10–15 minutes before the proposed activity.

Will the child give himself bolus doses because he likes the feeling he gets?

The ill-founded concerns about addiction which frequently accompany the use of narcotic analgesics may also be expressed when the drug is administered via a PCA infusion device. The psychological benefit for the child of being in some control of the administration of pain relief may lead parents to worry about their child using the system inappropriately. There is no evidence to suggest that children become psychologically dependent on narcotics after their therapeutic use. The use of a PCA infusion device does have a limiting effect on the child's abilities because of the need to maintain venous access and to 'be careful' of the pump. For these reasons children appear very keen to abandon the PCA technique as soon as they no longer have a perceived need for it. Premature discontinuation, due to feeling well as a result of the narcotic, is a much more likely scenario than prolonged non-therapeutic usage.

Because this pump is going to be used, does it mean that the pain is going to be really bad?

The relative rarity of the use of PCA in children may lead some children and their families to presume that because the pump is being offered for use, there is an expec-tation that the child will experience extreme pain. The child and his family should be reassured that no one, not even the child himself, knows how severe the pain will be, but that by having the PCA infusion device available and educating the child in its use, the child should not experience extreme pain because he will be able to administer analgesics before that stage is reached. It is much simpler to discontinue PCA if the child does not require it, rather than attempt to explain the concept to a child who is in pain and therefore requires it.

Are there any side-effects?

The potential side-effects of narcotic administration apply equally to narcotics administered via a PCA infusion device. Although it is suggested that PCA may result in fewer side-effects, it is erroneous to presume that this means no side-effects. Side-effects may include:

● Excessive sedation.
● Respiratory depression.
● Nausea and vomiting.
● Itching.

These effects are explained in detail in the section on extradural analgesia.

When will PCA be stopped?

Discontinuing narcotic analgesics may give rise to concerns about the 'correct' length of time the drug is required. Individual requirements differ, and use of PCA facilitates the child to stop the narcotics when it is appropriate for him, rather than when the health care professionals presume it is the right time. The transition from narcotic analgesics to a non-narcotic regime may be facilitated by introducing the non-narcotic regime while PCA is still available. The child is then reassured that the 'strong medicine' is still available if he needs it, but that if the other medicine keeps him comfortable then he need not use the PCA.

   As with the child receiving extradural analgesia the nurse caring for the child using PCA must be aware of the specific care this technique requires, and should also have the necessary skills and knowledge to answer any questions which the child and his family may have and to intervene should any adverse effects occur. The core elements of care are:

● Hourly respiratory rate and sedation scale.
● Record volume of fluid infused hourly.
● Record amount of analgesia administered hourly.
● Check intravenous lines hourly.
● Check the intravenous infusion site hourly.
● Assess level of comfort hourly.
● Encourage the child in his use of PCA.
● Intervene appropriately if side-effects occur.
● Maintain child and family contact.

Nurse-controlled Analgesia

Several groups of children are unable to utilise the advantages of the PCA infusion device, for example, the very young, the physically challenged and the child who is educationally challenged. These children may benefit from the use of the PCA infusion device with a somewhat different programming. The aim is to achieve more or less adequate analgesia with a higher dose continuous background infusion, but with supplemental bolus doses available for administration before potentially painful procedures or if the child appears less comfortable, and other interventions do not give him comfort. The child is protected from over-administration by an increased lockout interval. Parents are encouraged to discuss with the nursing staff changes in their child's behaviour, but the responsibility for administering boluses of analgesia rests with the nursing staff as parents often have understandable anxieties about taking on this role (Park and Fulton, 1991). Nurse-controlled analgesia is still a relatively unusual concept. However, it may become a valuable method of administering a more individualised analgesic regime to certain groups of children.

The use of these less common analgesic techniques may be a source of some anxiety for nursing staff who have the responsibility of caring for the child on a 24-hour basis. Although other health care workers may be available for help and advice, a pro-active approach to the needs of the nurses must be taken to empower them to fulfil their crucial role in paediatric pain management. All change may bring about feelings of insecurity (Matthews, 1987). Pain itself is an emotive concept, but some argue that nurses are exposed to so much pain and suffering during their work that they become desensitised (Akinsanya, 1985), while others suggest that a fundamental role of the nurse is to promote comfort, and failure to do so may lead to feelings of inadequacy (Walker and Campbell, 1988). New techniques should be viewed by all as a positive approach to the child in pain, and not another stressor in an already stressful situation.

Nursing standards that identify acceptable levels of care, in the form of outcomes and the structures or resources which are necessary to achieve these outcomes, may be helpful in identifying strengths and weaknesses within the system, thereby giving direction for further education and provision of resources.

Nursing practice guidelines which have multi-disciplinary agreement, and also refer to existing policies, may provide a means to clearly identify the nurse's role in the care of the child receiving a particular technique. They may include a brief explanation of the technique, how to initiate the intervention, the specific drugs and equipment which may be required and the nursing care required by the child during the use of the particular intervention.

Many hospitals use core nursing care plans to provide an outline of the essential elements of care a particular technique requires. These must be rigorously individualised, and specific care pertinent to the individual child must be included, if the plan is not to become a standardised tool for all children, which in reality is not appropriate for any child.

NON-PHARMACOLOGICAL METHODS OF PAIN RELIEF

The nurse has a vital role to play not only in the pharmacological management of the child in pain, but also in the non-pharmacological management. Techniques such as hypnotherapy, massage therapy, reflexology and aromatherapy may be beyond the nurse's ability, but her role in ensuring the child's physical comfort, and the use of distractional therapy such as story-telling, games, colouring, singing songs and of course cuddles and psychological comfort, are the essential elements that make a nurse who cares for children 'special'. Her ability to care not only for the child, but also for his family is essential in providing reassurance and comfort to them all in a potentially stressful and anxious time. The value of nursing actions as a method of non-pharmacological pain relief should not be underestimated. The nurse should be given positive reinforcement from her co-workers, and the value of her therapeutic use of 'self' should be acknowledged and applauded.

There can be little doubt that pain management is a complex area of nursing, and that when the patients involved are children the issues become even less clear and the solutions to the problems even less obvious. Paediatric pain management is an imprecise science. No two children are the same, no one child is exactly the same on two different occasions, and a flexible approach to the issues which are raised, a realisation that rarely does one problem have only one solution, will help the nurse to explore the potential ways of solving the problems which confront her when caring for children in pain. Most important must be a desire to work with the child and his family, to find the most effective solution together, and to acknowledge the contributions that all members make to the team approach. The nurse must also realise that only when an holistic approach to pain management is made, which acknowledges the child's physical, psychological, social and spiritual needs, will the child be likely to receive truly effective pain management.

REFERENCES

Akinsanya C Y (1985) The use of knowledge in the management of pain: the nurse's role. *Nurse Education Today*, **5**, 41–6.

Barr R G (1990) Pain in children. In Melzack R and Wall P (Eds) *Textbook of Pain*. 2nd edition. Edinburgh: Churchill Livingstone.

Beyer J E and Wells N (1989) The assessment of pain in children. *Pediatric Clinics of North America*, **36**(4), 837–53.

Beyer J E *et al.* (1990) Discordance between self-report and behavioral pain measures in children aged 3–7 years after surgery. *Journal of Pain and Symptom Management*, **5**(6), 350–6.

Boelen T (1990) Paediatric pain. *NAWCH Update*. Autumn, 7.

Bragg C L (1989) Practical aspects of epidural and intrathecal narcotic analgesia in the intensive care setting. *Heart and Lung*, **18**(6), 599–607.

Bucknell S and Sikorski K (1989) Putting patient-controlled analgesia to the test. *Maternal and Child Nursing*, **14**, 37–40.

Darbyshire P (1985) Happiness is an old blanket. *Nursing Times*, 6 March, 40–1.

Doyle C (1991) How to ease a child's pain. *Daily Telegraph*, 5 February.

Gauntlett I S (1987) Analgesia in the neonate. *British Journal of Hospital Medicine*, **36**(6), 518–19.

Gedaly-Duff V (1989) Palmar sweat index use with children in pain research. *Journal of Pediatric Nursing*, **4**(1), 3–8.

Haralambos M and Holborn M (1990) *Sociology Themes and Perspectives*. 3rd Edition. London: Unwin Hyman.

Lambert W E *et al.* (1960). In Seers K (1988) Factors affecting pain assessment. *The Professional Nurse*, **3**(6), 201–6.

Marlow D R and Redding B A (1988) *Textbook of Paediatric Nursing*. Philadelphia: W B Saunders.

Matthews A (1987) *In Charge of the Ward*. Oxford: Blackwell Scientific Publications.

McCaffery M and Beebe A (1989) *Pain Clinical Manual for Nursing Practice*. St Louis: C V Mosby.

McGrath P A (1990) *Pain in Children. Nature, assessment and treatment*. London: Guilford Press.

McGrath P J *et al.* (1985a) CHEOPS: a behavioral scale for rating postoperative pain in children. *Advances in Pain Research and Therapy*, **9**, 395–402.

McGrath P J *et al.* (1985b) The clinical measurement of pain in children: a review. *The Clinical Journal of Pain*, **1**(4), 221–7.

McLintock T T C and Hodsman N B A (1987) Patient-controlled analgesia. *Intensive Care Nursing*, **3**, 8–13.

Park G and Fulton B (1991) *The Management of Acute Pain*. Oxford: Oxford University Press.

Piaget J (1930). In Hurley A and Whelan E G (1988) Cognitive development and children's perception of pain. *Pediatric Nursing*, **14**(1), 21–4.

Rigge M (1990) Pain. *Which? Way to Health*, April, 66–8.

Rosen H F and Calio M M (1990) An epidural analgesia program: balancing risks and benefits. *Critical Care Nurse*, **10**(8), 32–41.

Ross D M and Ross S A (1988) Assessment of pediatric pain: an overview. *Issues in Comprehensive Pediatric Nursing*, **11**, 73–91.

Royal College of Surgeons and College of Anaesthetists (1990) *Commission on the Provision of Surgical Services. Report of the Working Party on Pain After Surgery*. London: RCS.

Sofaer B (1984) *Pain: A Handbook for Nurses*. London: Harper & Row.

Tackett J J M and Hunberger M (1981) *Family-centred Care for Children and Adolescents*. Philadelphia: W B Saunders.

Walker J and Campbell S (1988) Pain assessment and the nursing process. *Senior Nurse*, **8**(5), May, 28–31.

Wallace M R (1989) Temperament: a variable in children's pain management. *Pediatric Nursing*, **15**(2), 118–21.

Whaley L and Wong D (1989) *Essentials of Pediatric Nursing*. St Louis: C V Mosby.

Whaley L and Wong D (1990) *Clinical Manual of Pediatric Nursing*. St Louis: C V Mosby.

Zborowski M (1952) In Walding M F (1991) Pain, anxiety and powerlessness. *Journal of Advanced Nursing*, **16**(4), 388–97.

FURTHER READING

Aradine C R *et al.* (1988) Children's pain perception before and after analgesia: A study of instrument construct validity and related issues. *Journal of Pediatric Nursing*, **3**(1), 11–23.

Berker M and Hughes B (1990) Using a tool for pain assessment. *Nursing Times*, **86**(24), 50–2.

Beyer J E and Wells N (1989) The assessment of pain in children. *Pediatric Clinics of North America*, **36**(4), 837–53.

Beyer J E *et al.* (1990) Discordance between self-report and behavioural pain measures in children aged 3–7 years after surgery. *Journal of Pain and Symptom Management*, **5**(6), 350–6.

Ellis J A (1988) Using pain scales to prevent undermedication. *Maternal Child Nursing*, **13**, 180–2

Gauvain-Piquard A *et al.* (1988) Pain in children aged 2–6 years: A new observational rating scale elaborated in a pediatric oncology unit – Preliminary Report. *Pain*, **31**, 177–88.

Gedaly-Duff V (1989) Palmar sweat index use with children in pain research. *Journal of Pediatric Nursing*, **4**(1), 3–8.

McGrath P J *et al.* (1985) The clinical measurement of pain in children: A review. *The Clinical Journal of Pain*, **1**(4), 221–7.

McGrath P J *et al.* (1985) CHEOPS: A behavioral scale for rating postoperative pain in children. *Advances in Pain Research and Therapy*, **9**, 395–402.

Ross D M and Ross S A (1988) Assessment of pediatric pain: an overview. *Issues in Comprehensive Pediatric Nursing*, **11**, 73–91.

Savedra M *et al.* (1982) How do children describe pain? A tentative assessment, *Pain*. **14**, 95–104.

Walker J and Campbell S (1988) Pain assessment and the nursing process. *Senior Nurse*, **8**(5), 28–31.

Wong D L and Baker C M (1988) Pain in children: Comparison of assessment scales. *Pediatric Nursing*, **14**(1), 9–17.

11
Sibling Care

Janet Mikkelsen

INTRODUCTION

When a child develops a life-threatening illness, it is a devastating experience for the whole family. This chapter looks specifically at the well siblings in these families and how the illness affects them. The experience of the Auckland unit in establishing sibling information and support sessions and the feedback received will be discussed. Although this experience is focused on children whose siblings have cancer or leukaemia, research has shown that the same problems arise for children whose siblings have any chronic illness. In a similar way children whose parents have cancer or any other long-term illness also experience changes in family functioning (Koch-Hattem, 1985; Blumberg *et al.* 1988; Heiney *et al.*, 1990; Lewis, 1990; Gallo *et al.*, 1991). The experiences discussed here could well be relevant to people working in a wide variety of health care areas.

PREVIOUS RESEARCH

Sibling relationships are very complex, long-term and, especially in childhood, quite intense. Carr-Gregg and White (1987) examined these relationships and concluded that:

'They are obligatory relationships where, for better or worse, the children spend more time together than any other family subsystem .... They may assume a variety of roles with each other: mentor, supporter, comforter, protector and socializer.'

When a child in the family develops cancer or any other life-threatening illness, it rocks the entire family structure. Initially, it requires an immediate change in their daily routine and roles within the family suddenly change. Of necessity, parents focus their energy on their sick child, but this can often be to the detriment of their other children.

EFFECTS OF CANCER ON SIBLINGS

As childhood cancer has become more 'curable' and attention is starting to focus more on long-term effects than on developing more effective treatment, people involved in this field are also widening their focus from the child with cancer to his/her family. Over recent years research into the psychosocial issues around childhood cancer has been focused on the effect on well siblings and there has been an increasing awareness of the vulnerability of this group. The importance of this emphasis is supported by a study (Walker, 1990) which showed there is 'less adjustment and greater need on the part of the siblings than any other family members'.

Early studies on the effect of cancer on well siblings found a majority of them exhibiting abnormal behaviours such as headaches, bedwetting, school problems, abdominal pain, fire-setting, feelings of rejection, fear and guilt, and significant anxiety about their own bodies and health (Carr-Gregg and White, 1987; Walker, 1990; Bendor, 1990). In America Martinson *et al.* (1990) looked at the disturbance in family relationships due to the absence of parents, substitution of parent surrogates and the increase of energy spent on the needs of one member of the family. Most studies identified that the well siblings felt isolated from their family and friends and remained anxious and confused for long periods of time.

In Bendor's (1990) study children were asked whether they ever wondered about getting leukaemia themselves:

'the answer was a resounding yes, with two children adding: "I often think it might not be so bad. Then at least you would get all the presents and would not be blamed for everything." '

Young children can often feel guilty and feel very responsible for their sibling's current illness. This guilt results from the egocentric and magical thinking of the young child.

Rollins (1990), in her analysis of children's drawings, concluded: 'on interview and in the drawings, mothers in these families frequently appeared exhausted and unavailable to their children.' When studying older children, their school performance can be a good indicator of stressors at home. Walker (1990) felt that a drop in school performance in children could be interpreted as a maladaption to stress, whereas Heiney *et al.* (1990) preferred to interpret it as an inability to concentrate on school work due to worrying about what is happening at home or the hospital.

As cancer treatment involves months or years of treatment and follow-up, the change in family dynamics can become semi-permanent. Some studies suggest that this seriously compromises the long-term needs of well siblings such as educational planning and goal-setting, as well as their daily emotional and physical needs receiving low priority (McKeever, 1983). This constant, ongoing devaluing of their importance can leave these children at high risk of developing severe psychological problems in the future.

SIBLINGS OF CHILDREN WHO DIE

A further group at risk are those children whose brother or sister dies. 'Many become forgotten children. All the sympathy is directed at the parents' (Blake, 1990). They are often left out of the terminal phase of their brother's or sister's death, are not involved in funeral plans and, once again, are told to be understanding of their parents and to look after them! Lauer's (1985) study compared siblings of children who had died at home to those who had died in hospital, and showed that those who participated in home care had a significantly different experience. They were prepared for the impending death, received consistent information and support from their parents, were involved and did not see death as a particularly frightening experience. Those whose sibling had died in hospital felt isolated from the dying child and his parents, unclear about the circumstances of the death, felt useless in terms of their own involvement and described death as a major fear. This same report indicated that 88 per cent of 40 families experienced serious problems with effective family functioning after their child's death.

The feelings of one sibling towards her brother's impending death are captured in the following poem. The title in itself indicates how her role as his sister is perceived as unimportant.

ONLY A SIBLING

How do you tell someone you love
You don't want them to die
How can I try to be normal
When I hold you I know I will cry

How do I cope with my anger
At life, at God and sometimes even you
How can I put a smile on my face
While my insides are ripping in two

How can I tell you I'm frightened
Of the skeleton my brother's become
Tired and thin from your battle
A war that I'm scared can't be won

How can I tell you I love you
When all our lives it's gone unsaid
How do I stop you from drowning
When the water's already over my head

Every wince stabs me too, with pain
Why can't I tell anyone how I feel
When I feel like I'm going insane

How can I think of my future
When it's possibly a future without you there
Why do I feel so damn helpless
And my problems too insignificant to share

How do I tell you big brother
That I'm scared of what's happening to you
Why can't anyone seem to understand
That your dying is killing me too.

(Tammy McGowan, reprinted from *Candlelighters*)

THE AUCKLAND EXPERIENCE

The collective experience of workers within the Auckland unit reinforces the findings of the current research. The well siblings worked with are often jealous of the attention received by the child with cancer and one certainly hears about children who, when asked what they want for Christmas will say 'leukaemia'! This response is particularly true if they have been excluded during the initial hospitalisation stage and have been 'protected' from hearing how serious their brother's or sister's illness is. Often, after a few weeks, their sibling is home again and may go off to school and appear quite well. Yet for years to come, the 'sick' child may get extra presents and attention from every relative or friend, even if the parents have tried to keep the relationships within the family as 'normal' as possible.

Well siblings of children at the Auckland unit have, until recently, been left out of any information or educational sessions. They have had to rely on their own knowledge or past experience to reflect on reasons as to why this has happened to their brother or sister. This consistently appeared to lead to massive confusion and consequently misconceptions about cancer and its treatment.

In the groups currently running, the well siblings often express resentment about having to be good all the time, and being constantly told to be quiet and understanding. Older siblings frequently have to take on added responsibility for the family in the form of child-minding, preparing meals and generally keeping the household functioning. These adolescents express resentment of the extra burden and then feel guilty, assuming that they are being selfish. They are wanting to get on with their own lives and to complete their own developmental tasks which, in adolescence, include becoming more independent of the family.

Most well siblings experience considerable anxiety which may not be recognised as a child's expression of anxiety or fear. This anxiety and fear may take different forms. They may have difficulty communicating verbally their feelings and distinguishing and labelling their emotions. Younger children tend to use immature coping skills such as attention-seeking behaviour which, for a tired parent with limited energy, is more likely to be perceived as general naughtiness than a plea for normality and reassurance. All the siblings in the Auckland groups have focused on the worrying they do about their brother or sister with cancer and about their parents. They find it particularly frightening to see their parents upset and scared. Parents are meant to be able to cope and make everything better! It is important that all health professionals recognise that even though parents are going through a particularly traumatic time, they at least have had some experience with dealing with crises in their lives. Most children have had limited experience with any kind of major trauma and therefore have not developed any useful coping mechanisms. Without guidance they are at risk of developing inappropriate and ineffective ways of dealing with stress which they could easily carry on to adulthood. Even when they have developed coping mechanisms they may not engage them without adult support.

THE PROGRAMME

So what can be done to help these very vulnerable groups of children? Most of the research emphasises the need for information and communication and this is where it was felt the Auckland team could start. 'One dominant theme for the siblings was the need for information, a problem definitely within the scope of nursing intervention' (Martinson *et al.*, 1990).

The Auckland Unit

The Oncology Unit in Auckland is the only paediatric oncology unit in New Zealand. It has ten inpatient beds including two bone marrow transplant rooms. The unit has approximately fifty new patients a year and runs its own daystay and outpatient service. The area it services covers the north half of the North Island and the Pacific Islands, e.g. Samoa, Tonga, Fiji, the Cook Islands. On the unit a major emphasis is education and psychosocial support of the children with cancer and their families. It is felt by the team that, generally, the children with cancer/leukaemia and their parents are well cared for. Indeed, a significant amount of time is spent teaching the parents and the children about the various facets of disease and treatment. The large multi-disciplinary team attached to the unit as well as organisations such as the Child Cancer Foundation and Canteen are able to provide social and financial support. The unit team consists of ward grandparents, social workers, whanau (family) workers, chaplain, play specialist, dietitian, dentist, occupational therapist and physiotherapist. There has been, however, little specific support for well siblings apart from being 'nice' to them and including them whenever possible. In January 1991 it was decided something must be done to fill this gap in the support programme.

Sibling Questionnaires

Questionnaires were designed and distributed to well siblings of past patients asking what they wished they had known before their experience and what could be included. Suggestions were given such as a visit to the laboratory, a visit to outpatients, a tour around the oncology unit, a talk on cancer/leukaemia and a discussion on how other family members are affected by cancer. The usefulness of the sessions has been summarised in Table 11.1.

Table 11.1 Results from questionnaires sent to siblings of past patients (1991) (n = 8)

	Very Useful	A Bit Useful	Not Useful
Visit to:			
Lab	7	1	0
Outpatients	3	4	1
Inpatient unit	4	3	0
Talk on:			
cancer/leukaemia	6	1	0
how family members			
are affected	6	2	0

In the questionnaire, there was space for other comments. Some of these were: 'A visit to the theatre'; 'Maybe outings, just brothers or sisters, without the parents, and patient'; 'Go through to the radiation unit'; and 'A talk on how the brother/sister may play on their sickness. And how to avoid getting angry'.

Other hospitals were approached and asked what they offered, if anything. Unfortunately, few responses were received. Added to this the literature offers little practical advice on what health care workers can do to support the well siblings of children with cancer.

A large percentage of the patients seen at the unit are in the toddler age group. Consequently, many of their siblings are also under 5, which makes it difficult to include them in group sessions. The hospital play specialist tends to work with these young children with cancer on an individual basis and involves the well siblings as she/he is able. There is some evidence that because of the long-term nature of the family disruption, siblings would derive great benefit from involvement in an information programme even months and years after the initial diagnosis. Information can be presented in a different way as they grow older and their coping mechanisms change with their developmental level.

Meeting the Needs of Maori and Pacific Island Children

Another issue specific to the work in New Zealand is a recognition of the unique needs of Maori and Polynesian children. Childhood cancer is less common in Maori children than in Pakeha (non-Maori). There is, however, a higher incidence in some Polynesian groups, specifically Samoan. A commitment to providing holistic care means encouraging mutual respect of values and beliefs between cultures. It also means providing information in a culturally appropriate way with the uniqueness of other cultures taken into consideration. The Auckland Children's Hospital is working towards developing a bicultural policy of partnership where traditional Maori and traditional European attitudes and beliefs are regarded of equal value in policy formation and decision-making. A fundamental basis of Maori culture is the extended whanau (family) and recognition is made of whanau support during times of illness or hardship. The hospital has established a special unit called Te Whanau Atawhai, in which Maori people provide support for all families in a culturally appropriate, practical, emotional and spiritual way. Whanau workers are incorporated as invaluable members of the unit team. They provide support for families and give guidance to other non-Maori members in providing culturally safe care for their ethnic group.

In an educational setting, which is primarily how the sibling information and support sessions could be described, it has been important to acknowledge culturally different ways of learning. For example, in Polynesian culture 'children would go to where old people were and ask to be told legends, but, once seated in the presence of the elders, they must give respect and not ask questions. Furthermore, to ask a question implies that you do not understand and that would be shameful so the learning mode is one of wide-eyed silent watchfulness' (Ritchie and Ritchie, 1985). The Western style of learning, therefore, is not appropriate. For Polynesian people to question what they do not understand would be considered rude. Learning in Polynesian cultures tends to be traditional with an emphasis on authority rather than participant active learning.

Also, in traditional Polynesian society, young children (0–3 year olds) are solely looked after by their parents and rarely left alone. After about 3 years of age, however, their primary care givers and role models tend to become older siblings. The siblings in these families may develop a particularly close relationship and so need even more support to deal with a life-threatening illness.

Sibling Information and Support Sessions

The sibling information and support sessions are offered to two age groups, 5–9 year olds, and 10+ years. These sessions are run every 6–8 weeks, depending on need, and have had up to eight children. The programme lasts approximately 4 hours and is run differently for the two groups, so the discussion is age appropriate. These age-appropriate sessions will be discussed separately.

What is Cancer/Leukaemia?

The format for the session for 10+ year olds includes: a discussion with the charge nurse on the physiology of cancer/leukaemia, a visit to the laboratory, an explanation of treatment and side-effects, a session with the child psychiatrist, and a visit to outpatients, radiotherapy, theatre and the treatment room. The charge nurse in her presentation, explains about normal cells – how they function and how they differ from cancer cells. The lack of knowledge of these children continues to amaze those facilitating, especially the siblings who have had a brother or sister with cancer or leukaemia for years. Often they have appeared to be well informed. One 11-year-old who came to this group has since written: 'I found this interesting because I never knew what cancer was exactly.'

The charge nurse as part of this session asks them if they know what causes cancer. Many of the children mention different foods, lack of exercise and sitting in front of the television for too long. One pleasing cause many identify is 'the sun' which, although not a major cause of childhood cancers, supports the effectiveness of the melanoma awareness campaigns in New Zealand.

Laboratory Visits

The children visit three laboratories, these are: haematology, biochemistry and microbiology. At the haematology laboratory a blood sample is taken from a volunteer (or the facilitator if no one offers!) and the children are able to put the blood through the blood cell counter. A 7-year-old who attended this session wrote: 'It was fun. I liked it when D. put the blood on the thing that sucked up the blood.'

They then look at peripheral blood films and at bone marrow through a microscope. The haematologist explains further the role of different cells and how malignant cells differ from normal cells. In the biochemistry laboratory they, once again, put blood samples through the various machines and receive an explanation of the importance of different substances in the blood. While at the microbiology laboratory they look at culture specimens, and learn about testing for antibiotic sensitivities. The fun time is when they are allowed to fire up the bunsen burners and wipe 'bugs' on to the culture mediums. They are also shown inside the incubation cup-board. The laboratory staff are very sensitive to these children's needs and the way they carry out these visits adds greatly to their success.

Treatment and Side-effects

The content of the session on treatment and side-effects depends on who is in the group. For example, if the group consists mainly of children whose siblings have leukaemia, the discussion will centre more on chemotherapy than the other treat-ment modalities. Videos are often shown to highlight the focus of the session. 'An Explanation of Leukaemia and its Treatment for Older Children' by Victoria Publi-cations (Newcastle upon Tyne), for example would be shown to the group previously mentioned. Usually after the video the group discusses aspects of the care such as che-motherapy, radiotherapy, surgery and bone marrow transplantation. Once again, this is a good forum for clarifying the sibling's many misconceptions. A 12-year-old sibling said of this session: 'Everything about cancer and leukaemia is really inter-esting.'

Family and Feelings

A discussion with the child psychiatrist on feelings and families is the next part of the day. By this time the children are generally comfortable with each other. Doughnuts and juice are part of this session which helps create a more relaxed, informal atmo-sphere – they are received with great enthusiasm! These sessions with the psychiatrist have been wonderful – the children have been far more open than expected about their fears, anxieties and angry feelings. A 10-year-old wrote the following comment on this session: 'I liked this session because Louise understood how I felt about having a sister with cancer. She knew that I had trouble about talking to K. and how I felt.' Another younger (7-year-old) child who attended this session wrote: 'I really enjoyed it. The best part I liked was painting those pictures, but I don't like having a sister with cancer.'

Common issues that are brought up include: resentment of their brothers and sisters getting so many presents; of having to be quiet and good all the time; not being allowed to fight; having always to eat what the sick person wants; having to do more around the house; and having to look after younger siblings all the time. They often express feelings of isolation, particularly from their friends who they believe do not understand. To go and play with their friends however without feeling guilty was important.

An anxiety not uncommonly expressed is that related to their parents. Seeing their parents visibly upset and/or exhibiting other signs of shock and grief can cause signif-icant anxiety in these children. They are unsure how to help and it threatens the sense of security they generally receive from their parents. One unexpected finding for the team has been the perception the children make of their parents' mental status. When there was concern about parents whose anxiety levels had precluded them from coping effectively at all, it was expected that their children would also express concern. This was not so. They generally perceived their parents as coping really well. One explanation for this is that there was no change in parental behaviour; this was the way their parents had always coped with stress.

Tour of Important Areas

The day finishes with a tour. They visit the outpatients clinic, the theatre, radiotherapy and the treatment room in the unit. These are all places where the children with cancer are likely to spend some time, and it was felt important that the well siblings could envisage these areas. A large percentage of the patients from the Auckland unit are treated as outpatients, so it is very relevant that this area be included on the tour. The standard procedures performed on children with cancer in the outpatients area are weighing and measuring. They then have a consultation with a doctor. On the tour discussion with the well siblings often centres around why this measuring is necessary. They are encouraged to use the equipment and to explore the doctor's rooms.

All lumbar punctures and bone marrow aspirates are done under general anaesthetic, so the operating rooms are a vital part of the tour. The sibling group go into the check-out room, experience a trolley ride around the theatres and past the recovery room. The staff receive them with the same enthusiasm and respect as any child going for a pre-operative theatre visit.

A tour of the treatment room on the unit is included as it is an important place for children with cancer. Their bedrooms are encouraged to be 'safe' places so any painful, invasive or distressing procedures are carried out in the treatment room. All central line care, injections, insertion of intravenous lines and so on are done in the treatment room. Some well siblings have never been in the room but may have either heard distressing sounds emanating from it or have seen the anxiety some of the children with cancer attach to it. For them, an opportunity to explore it, discuss what happens in there, what the machines are and how they are used, is an important demystifying experience.

The final part of the sibling group tour is to the Radiotherapy Department. Although not all the children with cancer will require radiotherapy, it was felt to be an important aspect of care for the children who do. The staff there are extremely welcoming of the well sibling group and give them a full tour of the department. They show them how cranial masks are made and the computer room where planning is carried out. They then spend time letting them explore the actual radiotherapy machines. The children sit on the radiotherapy table as the machine is raised and lowered. It can be very exciting as the machine is moved around them and the laser lights are switched on. As one would expect, this is one of the highlights of the day.

Younger Siblings

With the 5–9-year-old sibling group a slightly different format is used. Sessions that are the same as for the older age group are: the 'What is cancer/leukaemia' session with the charge nurse; the visit to the laboratory and the tour. The majority of their time, however, is spent with the play specialist. From the session with the charge nurse they learn, as one of them put it, that 'cancer is a cell that has no brains and doesn't know what it is doing'. Another stated: 'I also learned that having leukaemia is no joke.' One 6-year-old, after visiting the laboratory, wrote: 'It was great to look through the microscope at all the white cells. I took my drawing of white cells to school to show my class and explain about' (sic).

Play Therapy

The time with the play specialist appears to be the most useful session for this age group. They give injections to dolls, play with IV equipment, drip stands and so on, and generally get a chance to learn about their brother's or sister's illness through play. It is also a place that they can express some of their feelings about the situation they are in. One interesting observation made by the play specialist was the initial reluctance of the young siblings to become involved in medical play. Most children with cancer are only too eager to deal with their experiences through medical play but their well siblings appear to need permission to do so. Perhaps this is due to the siblings being told not to touch equipment when they do come to hospital and having constant reminders at home about leaving medicines and central lines alone. One 6-year-old who attended this session wrote: 'I thought this part was the best part of all but I wouldn't have liked to be a doll. I am glad that it is N. who has to have all the injections and not me. I thought when the dolls had the real drip in, it was really fun' (sic).

Before they leave, the well siblings are given a copy of either 'When your Brother or Sister has Cancer' by Laura A. Rudolph (for the older age group) or 'When your Sister or Brother has Cancer' by John Silkstone and Allyson Hague (for the younger children). Both of these books are a useful resource for them to take home. They cover in a clear and age-appropriate way the following topics: cells and their function; what is cancer; what happens in hospital; feelings they may have; and ways to feel better. Apparently a number of the children have found them valuable and have even taken them to school for their friends to read.

The children are also asked to evaluate the sessions. The feedback received has invariably been positive: 'It was good fun I liked it all'; 'Very interesting and I learnt a lot'; 'Interesting to see what your brothers/sisters go through'; 'Really good good session'; 'I found out all about cancer and meeting other children'; 'Please keep up the donuts. They were great!!!' The verbal feedback we have received from parents also indicates that the children are not only learning about their sibling's care but also enjoying the days. There have been many requests from parents for the children to come back for further information and support sessions. As one parent stated: 'It is the best thing that has been done for him since S. was diagnosed. He is still talking about it a year later.'

Parents are often aware that their well children need help to deal with the situation but need guidance on the best way to do this. The sibling sessions provide peer support, something that parents are unable to offer. The children find out that there are others who are experiencing similar problems to themselves and that their feelings are quite normal and common. This is particularly important for adolescents whose desire for normality can be quite overwhelming.

The team also feels that these sessions are of considerable value. It improves the relationship individuals on the team have with the well siblings and provides important insights into family dynamics that may have been inaccessible previously. These sessions extend the team's commitment to family-centred care.

Looking Ahead

What is needed now is evaluative research to show that these sessions are in fact benefiting the children in the long term. Also strategies need to be developed to involve the children whose parents appear to see no value in the sessions and do not allow their children to take time off school to attend. At present about 60 per cent of the well siblings invited do come along.

The reasons for non-attendance include transport difficulties and conflicts with school activities, neither of which are insurmountable problems. Volunteer drivers for transporting children are available from the Child Cancer Foundation. The team is also endeavouring, when possible, to run the sibling information and support sessions during school holidays.

Follow-up procedures also need to be established. At present any siblings who appear to be having severe adjustment problems are followed up individually by the child psychiatrist. It is believed that the stressors can be evident in the siblings for many years, so there is a need to develop some sort of ongoing support that can change with their developmental level.

Sibling information and support sessions are one way of helping these children. All team members are constantly attempting to deal with the needs of well siblings at whatever level they are involved with these families. For parents whose energy is being totally sapped by their sick child, team members often suggest that another adult could usefully take responsibility, though temporarily, for meeting the well sibling's needs. This may at least in part engender a feeling of being special and important to someone. As Carr-Gregg and White (1987) note: 'Extended families are a valuable asset.'

The importance of school is very much considered by the team in their advice to parents. Carr-Gregg and White (1987) note that: 'Since the first manifestation of distress often occurs at school, it is important for a team member to enlist the child's school teacher as an additional source of information, and to maintain that liaison.' The Child Cancer Foundation in New Zealand has recently become committed to setting up a school reintegration programme which it is hoped will improve the relationship and communication of the team with schools and thus provide further support for the well siblings. The programme will enhance the existing system where the primary nurse of the child with cancer talks with teachers at schools and kindergartens before the child returns. It could be appropriate to include the siblings in this meeting as well.

CONCLUSION

In conclusion, well siblings of chronically ill children have been recognised as being at risk of developing future psychological problems. A concerted effort has been made in

Auckland to meet the needs of these children. A specific programme has been developed to provide them with appropriate support and information. It is only a start but so far the signs are that it is a positive innovation. The team involved in the programme believes it is an investment in the future and part of their commitment to family-centred care. Running sibling information and support sessions needs to be seen as only a small part of the process – all team members involved with these families are also teaching parents about the problems their other children may encounter. They too help the parents devise strategies to cope with these problems. It is an effort involving all who come into contact with a child with cancer. The well siblings of these children are very much critical to a positive outcome. They are part of how the family maintains its function and relationships, and the way the unit adapts to a major event in their lives. It is encouraging to note that 'the fact that many siblings of chronically ill children do not develop symptoms that dictate professional intervention may reflect their capacity to function effectively under stress' (McKeever, 1983). The siblings need and deserve, however, special consideration and this programme attempts to do this.

REFERENCES

Bendor S (1990) Anxiety and isolation in siblings of pediatric cancer patients: the need for prevention. *Social Work in Health Care,* **14**(3), 17–35.

Blake T (1990) A death in the family. Helping brothers and sisters to mourn. *The Australian Women's Weekly*, May, 114–17.

Blumberg B, Burklow J, Cosgrove M, Adams-Greenley J and Kranstuber M (1988) Responding to the information needs of young people whose parents or siblings have cancer: a description of a National Cancer Institute booklet journal. *American Pediatric Oncology Nursing,* **5**(1 & 2), 16–19.

Carr-Gregg M and White L (1987) Siblings of paediatric cancer patients: a population at risk. *Medical and Paediatric Oncology,* **15**, 62–8.

Gallo A, Breitmayer B, Knafl K and Zoeller L (1991) Stigma in childhood chronic illness: a well sibling perspective. *Pediatric Nursing,* **17**(1), 21–5.

Heiney S, Goon-Johnson K and Ettinger R (1990) The effects of group therapy on siblings of pediatric oncology patients. *Journal of Pediatric Oncology Nursing,* **7**(3), 95–100.

Koch-Hattem A (1985) Siblings' experience of pediatric cancer: interviews with children. *Journal of Health & Social Work,* **11**(2), 107–17.

Lauer M, Mulhern R, Bohne J and Camitta B (1985) Children's perceptions of their sibling's death at home or hospital: the precursors of differential adjustment. *Cancer Nursing,* February, 21–7.

Lewis F (1990) Strengthening family supports. Cancer and the family. *Cancer,* **65**, 752–9.

Martinson I, Colaizzo D, Freeman M and Bossert E (1990) Impact of childhood cancer on healthy school-age siblings. *Cancer Nursing,* **13**(3), 183–90.

McKeever P (1983) Siblings of chronically ill children: a literature review with implications for research and practice. *American Journal of Orthopsychiatry,* **53**(2), 209–17.

Ritchie J and Ritchie J (1985) *E Tipu E Rea. Polynesian Socialization and Psychological Development.* University of Waikato, Hamilton, NZ.

Rollins J (1990) Childhood cancer: siblings draw and tell. *Pediatric Nursing,* **16**(1), 21–6.

Silkstone J and Hague A (1985) *When your Sister or Brother has Leukaemia.* Lederle Laboratories Ltd, Hants.

Walker L (1990) Siblings of children with cancer. *Oncology Nursing Forum,* **17**(3), 355–60.

FURTHER READING

Birenbaum L (1989) The relationship between parent–sibling communication and coping of siblings with death experience. *Journal of Pediatric Oncology Nursing*, **6**(3), 86–91.

Brett K and Davies E (1988) What does it mean?' Sibling and parental appraisals of childhood leukaemia. *Cancer Nursing*, **11**(6), 329–38.

Davidson G and Carr-Gregg M (1983) Grief, death and bereavement among New Zealand's Polynesian people. A community affair. *The New Zealand Nursing Journal*, July, 12–15.

Davies B (1988) Shared life space and sibling bereavement responses. *Cancer Nursing*, **11**(6), 339–47.

Trahd G (1986) Siblings of chronically ill children: helping them cope. *Pediatric Nursing*, **12**(3), 191–3.

12

Ethical Issues in Paediatric Nursing

Gosia Brykczyńska

In a perfect world all children would be wanted, there would be no disease or infirmity, parents would provide all that is necessary for a child's growth and development and there would be no need for paediatric nurses. In a perfect world there would also be no moral distress and therefore no need for moral deliberations; people, should they so choose, may still take time out to philosophise, but there would be no need to consider moral problems in the light of moral distress, since all courses of action would be in harmony with the moral agent's moral identity. (Augusto, 1984). The world, however, is not an idealised place. The world into which children are born today and in which paediatric nurses work is often all too cruel, rejecting and uncompromising.

The history of childhood illustrates very well the unwelcoming attitude that the world traditionally has reserved for children (Mause, 1974). As Liz Ullman commented in reference to rights of childhood 'most children are born not with rights but with threats' (UNICEF, 1989). None the less, since the end of World War II, after the initial declaration of the Right of the Child by UNICEF, the proclamation of 1979/80 as the International Year of the Child, and in 1990 the publication of the Children's Convention by the United Nations and UNICEF, which culminated in September 1990 in an International Children's Summit, at the United Nations in New York; perhaps the International Community is beginning to pay more than just lip service to its most junior and vulnerable citizens.

The Children's Convention is a list of 41 articles encapsulating the most important rights to which each and every child in the world is entitled. At this point, perhaps an explanation concerning rights, needs and wants, especially in conjunction with obligations and duties towards children, requires some elaboration. Moral philosophers refer to rights as claims that demand respect (Hare, 1981). Historically, people have voiced claims pertaining to individual liberties or concerning the violated liberties of others, e.g. concerning slavery or child labour. Rights, as Beauchamp and Childress (1989) point out, are significant because they have in recent years become part of our symbolic language and because of their legitimate role in ethical theory. The authors define moral rights as 'claims that are justified by moral principles and rules – an entitlement validated by moral principles and rules'. This distinction is important, as we shall see when looking at children's rights and the ethical implication of these for paediatric nurses. A need in contrast to rights might be a requirement for specific food or education or health care but unless specified more precisely, may not automatically also be a right. This is most evident with certain 'emotional' needs. Thus a child has a need for love and security in order to develop into a well-adapted and healthy adult. However, it is hard to see how this need can be translated into a 'right' – even though in popular language and thought there is little disagreement that a child has *the right* to a 'loving' environment. In summary, whereas all rights represent children's basic needs and wants, not all 'wants' are basic needs, and therefore not all 'wants' are rights, that is, they do not represent justifiable moral claims. This is of great significance to health care policy-makers who require precise understanding of human rights language, if they are to facilitate the occurrence of some basic child needs. Human rights, therefore, represent in a rather loose (some would say clumsy) correlative fashion, human moral obligations (Beauchamp and Childress, 1989). In order to override a human right, one would need to justify the alternative moral device or action, the same way one would need to justify overriding a prima facie moral obligation (ibid.).

As mentioned, there are some serious moral problems with notions of rights, obligations and interests, namely that their very enforceability is dependent on freely accepted moral conditions and the moral agent's moral identity (Augusto, 1984).

Kuhse (1985) categorically states: 'All beings capable of suffering and enjoyment can be benefited and harmed … and hence [can be] the proper focus of moral action; they have interests which ought to be taken into account.' The problem of enforceability of child (or human) rights may stem from a blurring of the distinctions between moral and legal rights. Most legal rights are based on ethical principles, but whereas legal rights are backed up by the judiciary system, moral rights can only ultimately demand enforceability by recourse to the moral agent's moral identity.

The fact that children's rights are being violated and infringed is hardly newsworthy, but this in itself does not absolve paediatric nurses morally from being ignorant of the nature of children's moral rights, nor does it tacitly condone a moral position of minimum obligation of beneficence towards children. Those who have freely chosen to work with children such as paediatric nurses, more than other members of society, have an obligation to internalise the content of child-centred moral obligations, i.e. identify with the children's rights and be prepared to go beyond the minimal acts of beneficence, as required by law, in order to see that the moral rights are assured. The Nobel laureates' meeting in Paris in 1988 declared:

If mankind is to realize the full potential of this planet, and to pursue the dream of a future free from hunger, disease and fear, then it is imperative that we, as adults, recognize the needs of children and acknowledge our responsibility to provide for their survival, for their protection and for their future development. (UNICEF, 1989)

There is finally the distinction to be made between positive and negative rights – where positive rights impose an obligation on another individual to provide a particular good or service, while a negative right is a right acknowledged as owing to that person, not to have a particular good or service or interference by the state (Beauchamp and Childress, 1989). On balance, for adults, it is easier to ensure negative rights than positive rights but in the context of children's rights this is not necessarily the case. Thus, it is difficult for a child to request not to have treatment, or not to be moved from one foster home to another. The burden of *rational* choice in decision-making falls on the child disproportionately more frequently than on an adult.

The Rights of Children contained in the Children's Convention, are therefore minimal, universal, moral *and* legal rights necessary for the existence of a child. They attempt to allow a child to be a child, for the duration of its childhood, and not to be an exploited breadwinner, or an abused sexual object, or an uneducated, sickly and unwanted extra pair of hands. Frank's statement: 'I've wasted my childhood on being a man – my childhood was stolen from me' (Channel 4, 1989), should never be heard again. Some of the rights in the Convention can only be adequately overseen and guaranteed by a morally conscientious family member, but some rights will need additional societal backing and professional support.

It is the aim of the Convention to provide an internationally accepted moral and legal framework to achieve the targets set by the Special Task Force for Child Survival! The Task Force which met in 1988 in Talloires, France, set the following heath care targets to be achieved by the year 2000:

1. The global eradication of polio.
2. Virtual elimination of neonatal tetanus.
3. A 90 per cent reduction of measles cases.
4. A 70 per cent reduction in deaths due to diarrhoea in children under 5.
5. A 50 per cent reduction of infant mortality rates.
6. A 50 per cent reduction in maternal mortality rates.

(UNICEF, 1989)

These targets have serious implications for British paediatric nurses who will be working with young children and mothers. As the Canadian Ambassador to UNICEF stated:

'The convention is an important action by the International Community for Children, it is for all of us – Governmental, Non-Governmental and Inter-Governmental organizations – a set of common goals and a framework for common action.' (ibid.)

In view of this statement, will paediatric nurses of the 1990s be sufficiently competent to advise mothers about vaccination programmes, are they expert enough to influence the child morbidity and mortality figures? The Centre for Diarrhoea Research insightfully comments that 'The single most important correlate of child survival is not, as might be expected, the family's wealth, or the availability of medical facilities, but the mother's educational level' (ibid.). Are the paediatric nurses of the 1990s prepared for this *moral* challenge?

Ten governments have already ratified the convention and have therefore officially backed its content making it equivalent to international law. Paediatric nurses are now faced with the consequences of implementing child-centred health care programmes that address the children's rights enshrined in the Convention. In this fashion there has been a move from 'global targets to global obligations' (ibid.) for 'Governments which formally accept and sign the Convention have the responsibility of meeting its provisions' (ibid.). The United Kingdom was one of the ten countries to ratify the Convention, together with Poland, a country which ten years ago, during the International Year of the Child, put forward the initial proposal to draft the new Children's Charter.

The Convention is based on three identifiable principles, the first, that children need special safeguards beyond those provided to adults, second, that the best environment for a child's survival and development is within the family, and third, that governments and the adult world in general should act in the best interests of children (ibid.).

For the purpose of this chapter, I now wish to focus on three of the articles from the Children's Convention, and discuss how an increased awareness of the ethical implications contained in the rights may affect the paediatric nurse of the 1990s, for:

'The way a society treats children reflects not only its qualities of compassion and protective caring but also its sense of justice, its commitment to the future and its urge to enhance the human condition for coming generations.' (ibid.)

In final analysis, it is in the interest of nations to be concerned about children for 'there can be no peace without justice and justice begins with children' (Freiberg, 1989).

CONVENTION ON THE RIGHTS OF THE CHILD

Article 12

'The child has a right to express an opinion and to have that opinion taken into account, in any matter or procedure affecting the child.'

Of all the ethical principles, the moral reasonings surrounding the principle of autonomy seem to be more crucial to the understanding of moral behaviour. Autonomy refers to the notion of self (*autos*) and of rule or control. Thus autonomy includes in its sphere of reference, concepts concerning self-determination, self-worth and self-sufficiency. Initially, the Greeks used the term to refer to the type of governments entertained by self-governing city-states of ancient Greece. These city states were not only politically and economically self-determining and had a developed concept of self-worth (i.e. a sense of unique identity derived from a particular sense of history, language and culture) but also had a measure of self-sufficiency. Mutual co-operation and economic dependency on other independent states determined for the ancient Greeks a pattern of political activity that has subsequently evolved into modern democracy (i.e. literally rule of/by the people) and modern consensus governments. From this initial politico-economic understanding of the word 'autonomy' stem subsequent derivations that now include such notions as individual rights, choice, liberty (personal and political), privacy, confidentiality and most relevant to health care workers – the idea of individuality – that is, that each human individual is in control of his own person. From the concept of the individual state being autonomous we have moved to the position where each person is seen as an autonomous being – self-determining, with a sense of self-worth, personal dignity and self-sufficient.

In the domain of moral philosophy, the concept of autonomy is important, because it refers to an ethical concept or principle which underlies various moral reasonings, which is an important enough consideration (Beauchamp and Childress, 1989). Autonomy and the understanding of autonomous decision-making is also vital to an appreciation of true moral identity. For only a person truly in control of his life and behaviours can act in accordance with their moral-self, i.e. in harmony with moral identity and moral cognition. That is, there will be a better reflection of moral unity if the moral agent's actions reflect their moral reasoning (cognition) due to the internalisation of moral principles which lead to an acquisition of moral virtues. In such instances their moral identity is harmonious with their moral conduct. This may be because 'morality is more a characteristic of the agent than either action or thinking; the ultimate source of goodness lies in good will, and good will is at the core of what a person is' (Augusto, 1984).

Thus a person can only manifest his autonomy if he is indeed autonomous, whether the moral conduct is seen as good or bad is irrelevant if the moral agent is not responsible for his moral behaviour. Autonomy, therefore, is the core principle behind all ethical conduct and underlies all ethical debate. As Augusto (ibid.) points out, 'it is impossible to understand the moral quality – positive or negative of an action without resorting to the agent's judgement' and nothing is more central to a person's true identity than the true nature of their moral judgements. Personal moral autonomy is best displayed when moral identity and moral reasoning can meet unimpeded by social and cultural vagaries.

Traditionally, philosophers accepted the premise that an autonomous human being and a person were synonymous entities and they used the terms interchangeably.

More recently, however, moral philosophers and bio-ethicists have been dwelling on the perceived differences between the concepts 'human being' and 'person' and this has had immediate import for the health care professions and therefore also for nursing. On analysis, the description 'person' is given by society to those human beings who possess the maximum amount of 'autonomy' and are most likely to fulfil the criteria for autonomous living. The fate of the human being who is also a person will then depend upon whether the autonomous 'rights' of that individual have prior claims to recognition over the rights to autonomous decision-making of another individual. The more immature, frail, marginal and insignificant developmentally, socially, economically and physically a human individual will appear, the less likely it will be for that individual to be seen as a whole autonomous person. For personhood to be recognised, you need individuality, i.e. autonomy and agency – which is the socio-cognitive mechanism for moral conduct, indeed any action, to be made manifest (Henry and Tuxill, 1987; see also Piaget, 1932; Piaget and Inhelder, 1958). The implications for such philosophical and social deliberations on the thinking and therefore conduct of health care workers are quite significant (Lanara, 1982; Pinch, 1985). For a review of a wider debate on the interrelationship between moral deliberations and moral conduct (which I cannot enter into here) I would refer the reader to the writings of Hare (1981).

Additionally, much research is still needed in the area of child growth and development and the area of contributions of aspects of personhood to the developing foetus, before we can confidently talk of a substantial body of knowledge concerning the nature of the child, especially the unborn or premature infant. Increased knowledge of the early developing child would then help formulate logical, research-based premises from which to base philosophical assumptions. This would be in contrast to much philosophical bio-ethical writing currently available, which is based on intuitive thinking. In order to be able to talk about the growing powers and spheres of influence that a child's autonomy may represent, we need first to be able to establish that a child is indeed a person with full moral and legal rights of personhood and therefore entitled to those rights and protection guaranteed to other more 'developed' mature autonomous beings (Henry and Tuxill, 1987).

In the context of paediatric nursing, the practising professional rarely has to decide overtly about the phenomenological nature of her patient. Increasingly, however, neonatal paediatric nurses, who work with premature babies and their families, are finding themselves confronted with a range of existential questions that challenge the very premises with which they operate (Weir, 1989). Twenty-eight-week-old premature neonates are human individuals warranting and demanding a nurse's professional respect. These young patients have a right to a name, culture, religion and health care treatment, but these 'rights assertions' are based primarily on the fundamental premise that these premature infants are persons. However obvious this may seem to the neonatal nurse, this has not always seemed so obvious to some policy-makers and philosophers. Some philosophers would acknowledge that the premature infant has potential qualities of full personhood, especially so if the infant appears to be physically and mentally intact, and most policy-makers would acknowledge growing levels of rights for the infant – but should the infant's rights conflict with an adult's rights, increasingly, the adult's rights would take precedence. Children are still not accorded full human rights as persons, they are seen as only partially autonomous beings and therefore have to fight hard for accretion of any privileges due to them. Certainly the personhood of some foetuses and handicapped children in particular is challenged (Weir, 1989; Fry, 1990).

Of all the emerging medico-moral problems of the 1990s, the evasive problem of determining personhood, and all that follows from that, will figure high on the list. For the profession not to address this issue, will not only not promote the best interests of the child, but all subsequent discussions concerning the autonomy of the child will be rendered pointless. How can doctors and nurses look after a pregnant woman and facilitate intrauterine surgery on a 30-week-old foetus unless they perceive the foetus as human and a person – however small and immature? Human society which condones research and therapy for ever younger members of its species should, at a minimum, also be consistent in its decisions as to whom it considers a person. It should thus appear from a brief survey of the situation in obstetrics and neonatology that age of an infant or foetus does not assure personhood *per se*, not to mention the bestowing of autonomous rights of a person (Kuhse, 1985).

The child as a growing individual acquires rights of autonomy – but as demonstrated with the weakest and most insignificant of our children – the premature infants – these developing rights will only be acknowledged in so far as adults undertake co-relative responsibilities for becoming aware of them.

The child has a right to such level of autonomy that his or her opinion or say on a matter is significant. As already demonstrated, in order to take into consideration a child's opinion and wishes, we must first accord the child the status of an *autonomous* person. The child's autonomy will be truly respected if, and only if, we also accord the child our professional care. Thus, unless a child is brought up in an atmosphere of security and warmth, where basic needs are provided for, and the child is encouraged to develop socially, cognitively, physically and morally, it is useless to encourage self-expression, self-determination and/or aspects of self-sufficiency. Paradoxically, the more we wish to acknowledge the intrinsic autonomous nature of the developing child, the more we must work with and for the child. It is by acknowledging the basic dependency and vulnerability of the child that we can best respect the child's autonomy.

The opinions and expressions of a child should be meaningful and significant for us. The more we respect the child and all the child represents, the more we will respect what the child has to say. Thus Martina's statement: 'My greatest pleasures are music and having people accept me as I am' (Channel 4, 1989) is all the more relevant, as Martina is a handicapped youngster.

Some preferences or opinions of children can be anticipated in advance and the nurse is obliged as a sensitive moral agent to provide for some of these needs and wants, even if they are never overtly expressed. Finally, there are those wants which are also anticipated needs, for example, a mother's presence in the hospital ward. If the absence of this wanted need is seen as detrimental to the child, its necessity transforms the need into a child's right. Those in society who are most concerned with children have considered various children's rights, and have deemed that a child's need to express himself autonomously to be a child's *basic* right (UNICEF, 1989). The child's right to autonomous decision-making carries with it the correlative responsibility for adults to listen to children – to know what children are thinking, wanting, needing and saying. Operationally, in order to manifest positive moral behaviour towards the growing child, and to be seen to be according ever increasing levels of autonomy to the child, society, which includes paediatric nurses, will have to spend greater amounts of time, energy and monies on child-care schemes, child health projects and child-centred social activities. Even the training of paediatric health care workers to higher levels of moral appreciation will require the use of precious human resources. None the less if Article 12 of The Convention on the Rights of the Child is to be more than just a pious platitude, paediatric health care workers will have to be more cognisant of child growth and development, more aware of a child's level of autonomous decision-making capabilities, and more willing to truly share with a child and its family, the child's private understanding of his reality – his world. (Piaget and Inhelder, 1958; Harris, 1985; Green and Stewart, 1987.)

Article 19

'The state has an obligation to protect children from all forms of maltreatment perpetrated by parents or others responsible for their care, and to undertake preventive and treatment programmes in this regard.'

Article 39

'The state is obliged to ensure that child victims of armed conflicts, torture, neglect, maltreatment or exploitation receive appropriate treatment for their recovery and social-integration.'

Recently, much has been written and spoken concerning abuse, torture, exploitation and maltreatment of children (UNICEF, 1989). The very concept 'maltreatment of children' in professional literature is fairly recent with its interest to the majority of paediatric workers dating no more than thirty years (Fontana, 1973). Maltreatment of children as a sociological problem, however, is nothing new – and as a social phenomenon is known all over the world – but some of its more glaring aspects are found where the extended family is disappearing and there is an increase in social and cultural mobility (Mause, 1974). Articles 19 and 39 of the Children's Convention actively suggest that those individuals responsible for children are obliged to protect them from all forms of maltreatment. The ethical obligation to protect a child from harm stems from an interpretation of the moral principles of beneficence, fidelity and justice.

Unfortunately, it is not only close associates and family members or strangers who in various ways maltreat children. Health care workers can also contribute to children's distress by inflicting unwarranted harm, by not adequately protecting and caring for children entrusted to their care, by neglecting children's legitimate needs and not being familiar with their basic rights. Health care workers have been known to abuse children physically and sexually and in different ways exploit them, however improbable this may appear, for there is the genuine belief that paediatric physicians and nurses 'wouldn't do something like that'. This approach, albeit understandable, all too often leaves children most vulnerable to abuse, where vigilance ought to be highest. Children deserve more rational and sensitive protection than such benign and misplaced trust in *all* carers.

A far more common type of maltreatment of children, however, by health care workers is that which manifests itself in political and professional neglect and abandonment, or as Eliot eloquently stated, abuse due to 'things I've done and done to others' harm, which *once* you took for exercise of virtue' (Eliot, 1963). This is in part due to the underfunding of health care posts which leads to a lack of qualified paediatric personnel to deal with ever-growing case-loads. All too often children who are known to be in unsafe environments are left in these inadequate environments. Not enough effort is made to ensure that children at risk from exploitation and abuse are reasonably cared for. Children are often sacrificed for the good of a hypothetical family life or to conform to adult wishes (Harris, 1985; Green and Stewart, 1987). Such haphazard approaches to protection of vulnerable children can, unfortunately, lead to unnecessary hardships for children (Harris, 1985). Apart from such thoughtless 'care' of children, where protecting the child from known potential or real harm is apparently minimal, there is the more subtle form of abuse that health care workers, as much as anyone else in society, are guilty of – namely, the abuse perpetrated on children by society's attitude towards the child's global environment (Agakhan, 1984). By not providing an adequate, suitable environment for children to grow up in, an environment free from unnecessary pollutants, free from excess noises, noxious fumes, toxins in foods and under- or overstimulating of children – nurses too are guilty of inflicting a particular form of maltreatment on children.

In the hospital context, this environmentally-based maltreatment of children may manifest itself by exposing children to needless noxious stimuli, for example, too many needless injections or superfluous x-rays, or repeat studies with contrast dyes, or exposing children to the many 'hospital noises' that health care personnel appear to become deaf to, e.g. the constantly playing radio or television. Understimulation of children is also a form of maltreatment and can occur where toddlers or infants are not exposed to adequate forms of play or sufficient meaningful human interaction, which fortunately is less evident in the United Kingdom, but still quite a problem in some countries. For the extent to which a country can become oblivious to its responsibilities in regards to protecting children from environmental abuse, one need look no further than the child health policies of Romania in the 1980s.

It has been suggested by child psychologists that hospital environments by their nature are harmful to children. Therefore, all needless hospitalisations of children should be examined in the light of the message contained in the Children's Convention.

There is finally a form of child maltreatment peculiar to hospital and health care institutions – namely, research on children. Obviously, not all research with children is a form of maltreatment; however, many a research project, even if it has been passed by an Institutional Review Body such as a Regional Ethics Research Committee, has an element of 'harm' or 'risk' in it and children should be protected from exposure to all superfluous, non-essential research studies. Protection of children from researchers and research projects is becoming an ever more important aspect of the paediatric nurses' role in the 1990s in spite of Redman's (1986) study.

All these forms of protection from environmentally and professionally induced harm appear fairly logical. The moral basis which provides the ethical argument for suggesting that society, and this includes the paediatric nursing community, 'protect children from *all* forms of maltreatment', rests on the moral principles of beneficence, fidelity and justice, but these principles tend to wane in significance when nurses are confronted with the complexities of moral realities.

Beneficence states that we are obliged to do good, avoiding harming others (sometimes referred to as nonmaleficence) because by doing good we are maintaining a positive balance in interpersonal relationships. We also do good because it tends to increase total amounts of good and pleasure in the world (a form of utilitarian argument) and we do good and avoid harm in respect to children precisely because they are frail and vulnerable (an overlap with the principle of fidelity). Beauchamp and Childress (1989) state that 'no [moral] arguments or reasons can be persuasive unless they can be stated in the language of rights' and, as we have already shown, it is a child's right because of their common humanity with us and their autonomous status not to have harm inflicted upon it (a negative right) and to be the recipient of good, protective and safe care. The moral principle of beneficence is not exclusive to adults or those who have achieved a certain cognitive level of development; it refers to all members of society and binds all members of a moral community.

References to the principle of justice are also fairly fundamental to moral reasoning in that, if treating people with goodness and concern (i.e. in accordance with the principle of beneficence) were an arbitrary act, then the unpredictable nature of the moral actions would itself prove extremely stressful, thereby negating any good done. There needs to be some overriding assurance of stability and uniformity of moral approach and distribution of moral resources, i.e. justice, in order for society to feel that justice is indeed taking place.

Harris (1985) comments about an ultimate form of abuse within the health care community, i.e. 'failure to recognise that a body of knowledge concerning child abuse exists and is expanding'. She adds, 'Research on child abuse is in need of replication and advancement. Parenting, by individuals or by the state, costs money and effort'. In view of all these ethical issues, the health care moral agent can do no other than humbly recognise that she too sometimes contributes to a child's distress, and take heart from Lanara's conviction that 'No external condition can really hinder the nurse's effort to provide truly humane care if she chooses to do so ... True responsibility lies within the individual and includes commitment to fulfil one's trust and accountability for one's actions' (Lanara, 1982).

Article 23

'Handicapped children have a right to special care, education and training designed to help them to achieve greatest possible self-reliance and to lead a full and active life in society.'

The third area I wish to explore is that of care extended to children with chronic diseases and/or children with multiple handicaps. In our present medical climate of pursuit for perfection, children with handicaps have additional hurdles to overcome in order to qualify for medical and nursing care. Article 23 of the Children's Convention states that 'handicapped children have a right to special care, education and training designed to help them to achieve greatest possible self-reliance and to lead a full and active life in society'. The question that needs to be addressed is, to what extent do paediatric nurses, in the course of their nursing practice, maintain the covenant relationship with handicapped and chronically ill children – that is, to what extent is the moral ambience of paediatric nursing consistent with the moral identity of handicapped children and their families?

First, one has to address the issue of pursuit for perfection in respect to the human individual (Ramsey, 1985). Apart from increased knowledge concerning the physiology and anatomy of the foetus, medical science has progressed sufficiently so that it is now possible to determine in some cases the foetus's genetic make-up. Thus it may be possible to know whether or not the foetus is carrying a particular known, identifiable genetic disorder. Professional knowledge of the genetic disorder carries with it the subsequent problem of choice – does one in consequence of such knowledge counsel the mother to terminate the pregnancy on utilitarian grounds, i.e. that it will be better if such a child should never be born, or does one allow the pregnancy to proceed providing all the support and love available?

To a large extent, decisions concerning the nature of elected care for children with handicaps will depend on the nature of the specific detected defect. The degree of deviation from the expected normal growth and development pattern and degree of projected future handicap all play a part in the mother's and medical society's determination to allow the foetus to develop to term. Underlying the vast bulk of these moral positions is a utilitarian argument which proceeds as follows.

Adding to the parents' and child's pain and distress (by allowing the child to be born) and to society's worries by delegating the child's burden of care onto concerned members of society is surely a position to be avoided. However unpleasant in the short term, a termination of pregnancy would be of more lasting societal benefit and utility, producing more lasting good than any other option. It is not a frivolous digression to address this issue, for the care of handicapped children in Western societies has become an increasingly more difficult financial, social and emotional proposition – which is only partly explained by the underlying societal assumption that many of these children should not have been allowed to be born in the first place.

Societal care extended to these children is reluctant and generally speaking highly marginalised. Even children who acquire their handicaps after birth or develop subsequent chronic conditions are tainted with this essentially utilitarian philosophical approach. How do paediatric nurses maintain *their* moral identity in an atmosphere where the very nature of their work is being challenged and severely undermined (Pinch, 1985)?

The moral identity of paediatric nurses as a professional group is characterised in part by a respect for all children, whatever the nature of their medical or nursing problem and a commitment to care for all children to the full extent of their professional ability. Laudable virtues based on principles of autonomy, justice and fidelity seem unquestionable in the care of the acutely ill child but do not go unchallenged however, when nurses, committed professionals and family members attempt to apply them to the care of the chronically ill and/or handicapped child. Unless the nurse looking after a handicapped child has internalised and therefore made as part of her moral identity the pervasive theories of autonomy and justice, there will be a certain degree of moral disharmony – or as some ethicists prefer to call the phenomenon, moral distress (Jameton, 1984). In order for there to be moral harmony there must be moral accordance between personal moral values manifested in moral identity, professional moral orientation, usually encapsulated in a Code of Conduct, e.g. the UKCC Code of Professional Conduct (1992) and societal expectations and moral directives. Needless to say, some tension is inevitable and this does not of itself mean moral disintegration. In fact, precisely because we are aware of moral disharmony, ideas and approaches to the care of the handicapped child can be evaluated and refined. Much human (and professional) progress has taken place due to a positive approach to moral distress. The problem we are facing in our present deliberations concerning the care of handicapped children, refers not so much to whether or not there is moral disharmony in an absolute sense, but what is the basis for the disharmony.

In the delivery of care to a child and while working with a child and its family, precisely because the child, due to its handicap, is inherently additionally frail and vulnerable, it is important to return to the original UNICEF postulation that all children are important in their own right. Children matter not only for what they represent to adult society in future years, not only for any potential future economic gains they may represent, nor even for what they ought to be or may become, but because they are significant beings here and now. They are autonomous beings, sharing with us a common humanity. A child does not need to reflect an adult's appreciation to be valued, nor does it need external evaluation to be capable of maintaining its own central self-worth. A child who is ill and in need of paediatric nursing care receives the care appropriate to its needs. This care is not contingent on who they might become or who their parents are, or their potential future economic worth. Likewise, a handicapped child is entitled to our care and love solely because like any other child that care and love are needed for the child's well-being.

It is quite another issue 'to overtreat' a profoundly multiply-handicapped child, where the child may be referred to as an object of moral concern in order to justify an inappropriate non-person centred ethical position. It is as morally questionable to use a child, even severely mentally handicapped, as a means to an end, e.g. as a depository of potential organs for transplantation, as it would be questionable not to offer any care whatsoever (Fry, 1990). Paediatric nurses do care for children, and the better the quality of care the more involved and complex the moral commitment between carer and child becomes. Caring for a handicapped child ought thus to incorporate special knowledge of caring for children with the specific handicap, it should include special education for the child (e.g. by physiotherapists, speech therapists and other professionals) and should be designed to help the child to reach *its* fullest potential.

There ought not to be an intrinsic disequilibrium between the moral identity of the nurse, requirements of the profession and directives from society. None the less there are many areas of concern, some due to the moral development of the nurse who is not immune to the various value influences which life can offer. There are also potential problems with the somewhat theoretical-sounding moral directives of the profession, which per definition are general and do not take into account individual cases (UKCC, 1992) – but by far the greatest disquiet arises from an apparent mismatch between the moral virtues of the profession and society's expectation of the health care team as regards to care of handicapped children (Weir, 1989).

To overcome some of these moral problems nurses will have to listen carefully to what society is really saying. What do parents *really* want from the health care team? At the same time the care that is offered to children and their families must be practical, appropriate and sustainable, otherwise the profession is making a mockery of the principle of fidelity. There is as much an ethical responsibility to care for a handicapped child in an institution as there is to ensure quality care for a child in his own home. The moral obligation to deliver appropriate care does not therefore limit itself to a checklist from a paediatric textbook. Political activity may also be required to achieve an ethical outcome in the name of justice and the fiduciary relationship between the child and the health care team – as the ever more vocal agitation of parent groups can witness.

Finally, care of handicapped children, if it is to become more central to paediatric nursing and its ethic less questioned by some sections of society, will have to be incorporated more into general paediatric nursing care. Speciality hospitals for handicapped children will always exist to provide expert and excellent centres of referral, especially for long-term care, follow-up care and rehabilitative care. But the more often that physically handicapped youngsters and multiply-handicapped children are cared for on general paediatric wards, for surgery such as removal of wisdom teeth or for an array of acute medical and surgical conditions, the less likely that these children will become marginalised and stigmatised.

Not only does the nursing profession and the health care team need to listen to what society has to say, but, however reluctantly, the health care team, precisely because of its increased knowledge about these children, should see as part of its care for these children, education of public moral awareness. Hence the message of Article 23 of the Children's Convention. Ethical care of the handicapped child is an expensive financial and emotional proposition and requires much thought and determination. The price of not adequately caring for handicapped children is the formation of a society that is so intent on perfection that it disregards its weakest and most vulnerable members. As Ramsey so aptly stated: 'we must seek our rendezvous with some Nevers, and the good reasons for them', for 'the good things men do can be made complete only by the things they refuse to do' (Ramsey, 1985). Paediatric nurses cannot afford to neglect handicapped children.

In conclusion, paediatric nurses have much to be aware of in the new Children's Convention, which will soon become international law. There is much hope for the health and well-being of future generations of children, but the present-day practising nurse would do well to heed the Chilean poet, Gabriela Mistral, who proclaimed:

'Many things can wait.
Children cannot.
Right now their hip bones are being formed,
their blood is being made,
their senses are being developed.
To them we cannot say tomorrow.
Their name is today.'
(UNICEF, 1989)

REFERENCES

Agakhan Prince S (1984) We need a more human perspective. *Int. Nursing Review*, **13**(3), 82–4.
Augusto B (1984) Moral identity: Its role in moral functioning. In *Morality, Moral Behaviour and Moral Development*. New York: John Wiley & Sons.
Beauchamp T L and Childress J F (1989) *Principles of Biomedical Ethics*. 3rd edition. Oxford: Oxford University Press.
Channel 4 (1989) *Stolen Childhood – the Rights of the Child*. London: North South Prod. Ltd.
Eliot T S (1963) 'Little Gidding'. *Collected Poems 1902–1962*, London: Faber.
Fontana V (1973) *Somewhere a Child is Crying – Maltreatment – Causes and Prevention*. New York: Macmillan.
Freiberg R Y (1989) *Statement at 33rd Annual Committee for UNICEF*. London, 8 November.
Fry S T (1990) Outlook on ethics: Brave New World: Removing body parts from infants, *Nursing Outlook*, **38**(3), 152.
Green J and Stewart A (1987) Ethical issues in child and adolescent psychiatry. *Journal of Medical Ethics*, **13**, 5–11.
Hare R M (1981) *Moral Thinking: Its levels, method and point*. Oxford: Clarendon Press.
Harris Jean (1985) Child abuse and neglect: ethical issues. *Journal of Medical Ethics*, **11**, 138–41.
Henry C and Tuxill A C (1987) Persons and humans. *Journal of Advanced Nursing*, **12**, 383–8.
Jameton A (1984) *Nursing Practice: the ethical issues*. Englewood Cliffs, NJ: Prentice Hall.
Kuhse H (1985) Interests. *Journal of Medical Ethics*, **11**, 146–9.
Lanara V A (1982) Responsibility in Nursing. *International Nursing Review*, **29**(1), 7–10.
Mause Lloyd de (Ed.) (1974) *The History of Childhood*. New York: Harper & Row.
Piaget J (1932) *Moral Judgement of the Child*. London: Routledge & Kegan Paul.
Piaget J and Inhelder B (1958) *The Growth of Logical Thinking from Childhood to Adolescence*. London: Routledge & Kegan Paul.
Pinch W J (1985) Ethical dilemmas in nursing: The role of the nurse and perceptions of autonomy, *Journal of Nursing Education*, **24**(9), 372–6.
Ramsey P (1985) The issues facing mankind. *Ethics and Medicine*, **1**(3), 37–43.
Redman R B (1986) How can children be respected as 'ends' yet still be used as subjects in non-therapeutic research? *Journal of Medical Ethics*, **12**, 77–82.
UKCC (1992) *Code of Professional Conduct*. 3rd edition. London: UKCC.
UNICEF (1989) UNICEF/UK Information Sheet No. 8. *A New Charter for Children 3/88*.
Weir R (1984) *Selective Non-treatment of Handicapped Newborns*. Oxford: Oxford University Press.

FURTHER READING

Brykczyńska G (Ed.) (1989) *Ethics in Paediatric Nursing*. London: Chapman and Hall.
Brykczyńska G (1992) Caring – a dying art? In Jolley M and Brykczyńska G (Eds) *Nursing Care: the Challenge to Change*. London: Edward Arnold.

13

Advances in Paediatric Surgery

Virginia Colwell
with
Rachel M Fretwell, Rebecca Sury
Linda E Davies, Janette S Budd
Brigid T Carr

INTRODUCTION

The 1990s will continue to see new developments in paediatric surgical nursing. Some of these will be in response to new techniques developed by other disciplines, while others will be evolved by the nurses themselves or in liaison with the many disciplines involved with their patients' care.

A variety of recent changes in management have greatly influenced the nursing requirements of this group of children. The introduction of subcuticular sutures, diminishing use of wound drains and intramuscular premedications have helped reduce the child's fear of a surgical admission. Improved nutritional status both prior to and during the hospital stay with the use of alternative forms of enteral feeding and intravenous parental nutrition have influenced their speedy recovery, while the use of prophylactic antibiotics, improved management of post-operative pain and many other innovations have all contributed to improving the care and well-being of these children.

This chapter includes just a few of the recent innovations in paediatric surgical nursing. The subjects were chosen and written by ward sisters, the experts employed by this Special Health Authority. They were asked to write in detail regarding one particular innovation that had greatly influenced their sphere of work. The subjects although diverse, are of their choice.

PATIENT-CONTROLLED ANALGESIA

One of the main changes governing paediatric surgery is the latest developments in pain control. Management of pain in children is one of the primary concerns of paediatric nurses. Their ideas and interpretation of pain and the use of various analgesics, together with pyschological intervention, strongly influence the management of a child's pain. In the paediatric area, various methods of pain control administration are carried out. These encompass bolus intravenous or intramuscular pain control, continuous analgesia infusions, and of late the piloting of epidural analgesia and patient controlled analgesia (PCA) infusions.

Used in conjunction with these methods are psychological interventions for pain management such as relaxation techniques, using guided imagery desensitisation and distraction techniques with puppetry, and age-appropriate pop-up books and cassette tapes. The method of pain control most recently used on the orthopaedic ward is patient-controlled analgesia (see chapter 10), used in association with children undergoing spinal fusion.

It has been observed on the orthopaedic unit that the use of continuous infused analgesia such as morphine sulphate gives a much more constant pain relief than the peaks and troughs induced by bolus analgesia, which gives only intermittent pain control. Thus, there has been a natural progression to patient-controlled infused analgesia. This initially proved to be immensely successful in the treatment of adults, and PCA is now being considered as a preferable alternative for selected children.

The children selected on the ward for the use of PCA were chosen under the following criteria:

1. Age, preferably over 10 years.
2. Development level appropriate to age.
3. Ability to manipulate equipment.

Once selected, children, together with their parents, are instructed pre-operatively on the use of the equipment by anaesthetic and nursing staff. They are informed that the infusion equipment is assembled and initially programmed to deliver a bolus dose of analgesia followed by a base rate, which delivers a low continual dose of analgesia. A booster dose can then be administered when initiated by the child pushing a button on a hand-held control. The child and parents are reassured that there is a lock-out feature programmed into the equipment, allowing a maximum dosage per hour and preventing the possibility of overdose.

The aim of piloting PCA is to determine:

1. Whether it is a suitable method for providing safe and effective analgesia for children.
2. At what age and developmental stage the child needs to be before this system can be considered suitable.
3. Its effect on conscious level and vital signs.
4. Whether is is a satisfactory method in the views of child and parents, medical and nursing staff.

To monitor the use of PCA, vital signs are frequently checked paying particular attention to the respiratory rate, although respiratory depression is less likely, due to the elimination of the peaks and troughs induced by intermittent analgesia. The number of successful and unsuccessful attempts at boosting analgesia input by children is automatically recorded by this system, and comparisons regarding overall dosage are made between conventional continuous infusions and PCA.

From piloting the use of PCA in children several advantages have been observed:

1. The emotional trauma often associated with children anticipating and receiving injections was prevented.

2. PCA adequately covered the child's pain using a lower dose of analgesia than more conventional methods. This is probably due to the child feeling totally in control of his/her pain.
3. PCA highlighted the advantages of the child controlling his/her own pain relief prior to any movement/physiotherapy.
4. The PCA saved nursing time.

The PCA method overall was preferred by the child and was considered safe and effective by nursing and medical staff, who were well accustomed to the use of the equipment.

The side-effects are equivalent to those associated with the use of opiate drugs i.e. nausea, vomiting and disorientation. To ensure the safe and effective use of PCA, maximum awareness of changes in both respiratory and neurological status, and how to reverse such changes through dosage adjustment, are of primary importance.

Within the orthopaedic unit PCA has been used on children undergoing spinal surgery, for the first 48 hours post-operatively. It has been found to be extremely successful if supported by mild oral opiates such as codeine phosphate on discontinuation of PCA.

Children undergoing two-stage spinal surgery requested the use of PCA during the second stage, thus confirming the child's satisfaction with the system.

It can be concluded that, through the use of PCA, increased pain control is achieved. The child maintains ultimate control and is not subjected to the interpretation of his/her pain by the medical and nursing staff!

PRE-OPERATIVE AND POST-OPERATIVE CARE FOR THE CHILD WITH TRACHEOMALACIA

Tracheomalacia is a term used to describe an abnormally soft and pliant trachea. The floppy segment of trachea has a tendency to collapse, leading to respiratory difficulty. This is accompanied by a loud expiratory noise indicative of large airway obstruction. As well as this typical noisy breathing, the children present with respiratory difficulty on exertion, especially during feeding. The condition progresses until the child experiences difficulties even at rest and the children are often observed to hold their necks in extension to maintain their airway. Some parents report that their children go blue and even stop breathing, requiring mouth-to-mouth resuscitation; this is known as a 'near death attack' (Filler et al., 1976). These episodes are very frightening for the parents, and some families may be so anxious that they never allow the child to cry for fear of an attack.

Tracheomalacia occurs as a primary condition, but is also associated with vascular rings and tracheoesophageal fistula. Signs of the condition, when secondary to another disease, may start at a very young age, even before 3 months, but it has been reported in much older children. The natural course of the disease is for it to disappear with growth, provided that death does not occur first. Diagnosis is by bronchcoscopy when the trachea is seen to collapse during quiet respiration.

The care described below is for those in whom the condition is a consequence of a tracheoesophageal fistula. In this group the disease may be complicated by other problems such as gastro-oesophageal reflux and oesophageal stricture. These infants are often a very difficult management problem in the pre-operative phase of their care and are a challenge to the skills of the paediatric surgical nurse.

Pre-operative Care

These patients must be admitted to the ward for assessment if the parents describe any of the symptoms described above, as this is a life-threatening condition.

Emergency resuscitation equipment must be available next to the cot. If examination by the medical staff reveals a respiratory tract infection, it should be treated.

The admission history and assessment of the patient must be done by a trained nurse. The nurse must observe the infant while feeding and at rest to determine the severity of the condition and plan care accordingly. The infant is nursed on a head-up tilt (mattress elevated by the head rest or pillows), in a sling (to stop him falling down the elevation), and in the prone position after feeding to prevent further respiratory problems from gastro-oeosphageal reflux. At other times the infant may be most comfortable in a baby bouncer chair. If it is apparent that the infant cannot cope with the volume of feed offered without becoming distressed or cyanotic, then a nasogastric tube must be passed and used to 'top up' when the patient is obviously too tired or distressed to continue. In the event of the condition being so severe that apnoeic attacks are a regular occurrence, the infant must be fed by tube only. It is usual for these patients to be offered a smaller volume of feed more frequently. The infant should be nursed on a respiratory alarm and observations of temperature, pulse and respiratory rate made regularly.

In some cases symptoms will improve with palliative measures such as decreasing the volume of feed offered, increasing the frequency and by keeping the infant upright. In this instance it may be possible to send the family home with the proviso that they come straight back should the symptoms recur or become worse. It may be helpful for some families to use some sort of respiratory alarm, but they should be used with caution as they often increase levels of parental anxiety.

For some infants the symptoms are so severe that to discharge them would be positively dangerous and they must remain in hospital until surgery can be performed.

Surgery

Operation is reserved for those who have apnoea, cyanosis, repeated admissions or who have increasing dysnoea with feeding. The procedure to correct this condition is called an aortopexy (Kiely *et al.*, 1987). The ascending and proximal arch of the aorta are sutured to the sternum thus preventing collapse of the trachea during swallowing or crying. The procedure takes approximately 1 hour to perform and results are often dramatic, the infant returning to the ward breathing quietly. This is especially so when the tracheomalacia has been secondary to another condition.

Post-operative Care

The operation is usually performed through a left anterior thoracotomy; there is no chest drain. Some infants may require nursing in humidified oxygen for a short time. The child will return to the ward with an intravenous infusion which will be discontinued once feeding has been re-established. Feeding is usually reintroduced within 12 hours of surgery. Some surgeons advocate the use of a clear feed at first in case of difficulty swallowing and consequential aspiration. Some infants will require analgesia and a dose of intramuscular codeine is usually sufficient and paracetamol thereafter. Post-operative complications are rare.

For most mothers feeding is no longer a time fraught with anxiety. Discharge home can be arranged as soon as the baby is feeding to requirements and mother has regained her confidence, usually within one week.

GASTRIC TRANSPOSITION

Within this Special Health Authority (SHA) colon interposition was performed on children requiring oesophageal replacement until the early 1980s. However, due to the significant morbidity associated with this form of treatment, it was decided to change to gastric transposition as the operation of choice. This procedure, which involves mobilisation of the whole of the stomach, has the advantage of involving only one anastomosis as opposed to the two required with colon interposition. The results of surgery performed between 1981 and 1986 show a considerable reduction in cervical anastomic leakage; 48 per cent in colon interposition compared to 6 per cent in gastric transposition (Spitz et al., 1987). These changes in surgical technique have resulted in changes in the nursing care required by this challenging group of children.

When a primary anastomosis for oesophageal atresia is not possible, the neonate undergoes formation of cervical oesophagostomy and insertion of a feeding gastrostomy tube. The gastrostomy tube most commonly used in this SHA is a size 10 malecot. Parents are taught total care of the gastrostomy, including hygiene, delivery of the feed and how to change the tube when necessary. At this stage few problems are encountered with malabsorption, and breastmilk is the feed of choice or an appropriate baby milk.

Until a few years ago on reaching the age of weaning various substances were forced down the gastrostomy tube and the child was given the same food for sham feeds as he was for gastrostomy feeds. Feeds have since improved in choice and content and we can now give total nutritional requirements with one liquid feed. The advantages are an improved nutritional state, as the nutritional requirements are easy to calculate, plus easier preparation and delivery of the feed.

Following gastric transposition the child is electively ventilated and has a nasogastric tube, feeding jejunostomy tube and neck drain in situ. The neck drain is positioned at the end of the operation and is inserted through the neck to the site of the anastomosis.

In the immediate post-operative period it is vital to maintain gastric decompression preventing the possibility of respiratory distress. To prevent this, the nasogastric tube must be aspirated as frequently as every 30 minutes. It is important to record both the amount of air and gastric fluid obtained. The absence of air and fluid usually suggests that the tube is not in the correct position and the doctor must be informed.

The most common complication following gastric transposition is difficulty in re-establishing oral feeds and the importance of sham feeding prior to surgery cannot be overemphasised. Parents are taught to sham feed at the same time as they are giving the child his gastrostomy feed. The child should be orally weaned in the usual way.

During the gastric transposition the gastrostomy tube is removed. Routine insertion of a feeding jejunostomy tube has been found to be of great value in the post-operative period. The tube is secured to the abdominal wall by a suture. To ensure patency the nurse needs to flush the tube 4-hourly with water, until full tube feeding is commenced; this normally takes place 2–3 days post-operatively. The milk is given as a continuous feed via a designated feeding pump. Normally, the same milk as the child was taking pre-operatively, is given post-operatively. As the child tolerates the jejunal feeds the rate is increased quite quickly and the intravenous fluids are decreased accordingly.

Occasionally, milk feeds are not tolerated due to the anatomical position of the tube and the associated physiology. The child usually presents with loose watery stools, which on testing may contain sugar; there may be associated weight loss. If malabsorption problems do occur, it is usual for the child to be changed to a short chain feed such as pregestimil. Malabsorption does not tend to be a problem once oral feeds are established and the child can return to his usual formula. Oral feeding is generally introduced 5–10 days following the gastric transposition. Normally this depends on two factors: (1) how quickly the child is extubated, (2) the amount of leakage observed from the drain site.

On commencing oral feeds a combination of oral and jejunal feeding generally takes place. The jejunal feeds are gradually decreased as the oral intake increases. Unfortunately, the commonest complication following gastric transposition is difficulty in establishing oral feeds. This can occur even after previously successful sham feeding. The jejunostomy tube now has two major functions. The first is to provide the child enterally with full nutritional requirements, thus eliminating the need for long-term intravenous feeding. The second is that the child can be fed by this method at home, which reduces the necessity for a prolonged hospital admission. Involvement with the community services is vital if home feeding is required. An increasing number of Health Authorities employ a paediatric liaison person and good communication is necessary so that the child and family receive continuous support at home. Local Authority funding has to be sought for the feeding pump, plus all consumerable items, including the actual feed. This can take anything from weeks to months and can cause prolonged hospital admission.

When problems occur with oral feeding, the child is normally offered oral feeds during the day and supplemented with jejunal feeds overnight. There are two schools of thought on how the oral feeds should be offered. Some believe that the child should be force-fed, and once the child has been shown that he will not be able to refuse to eat, he will start feeding. The other method is to use a desensitisation programme. This may be designed by the speech therapist. The child is allowed to touch and play with food of varying textures and tastes. The nurse encourages this in a non-threatening manner and touches the child on the lips and mouth. Hopefully, the child learns to accept food without the fear or pressure of putting it into his mouth. It is hoped that by following this programme, the child will want to feed rather than being fed by force.

Unfortunately, there is no analysis available regarding these two schools of thought and therefore different professionals will continue to support the method that they feel gives the best result.

There may also be physical problems affecting the re-establishment of oral feeds. Poor gastric emptying can be a complication despite pyloromyotomy or pyloroplasty performed at the time of the operation. The use of metoclopramide has been shown to be effective in some cases.

The oesophago-gastric anastomosis can also cause problems by leakage or stricture. In the case of a stricture, the child may re-present with an increasingly severe feeding problem. Having initially fed well, problems occur with the taking of solids and then, as the stricture tightens, even fluids are difficult to take. Initially, the anastomosis is dilated. However, if problems continue, revision of the anastomosis may become necessary.

Dumping syndrome is another recognised complication following this operation. The symptoms normally occur following feeds. Blood sugars will initially be high but then will drop. The child becomes pale and may sweat profusely, often complaining of abdominal pain. The abdominal pain may be relieved after the child has had his bowels open. The conservative treatment for dumping syndrome consists of dietary manipulation. Small, frequent feeds are given of a low sugar, high starch content.

Despite the improved morbidity using gastric transposition for oesophageal replacement, the surgery continues to carry its own complications. The nurse plays an important role in prevention and recognition of some of the potential risks. In addition, with improved milk formulas, use of jejunal tubes and good communications with the community personnel, the length of stay in hospital can be considerably reduced.

TISSUE EXPANDERS

From the moment of conception, a parent's wish is that their child will be healthy and look 'normal', and from a very early age the child itself is conscious of its appearance and the image that is projected to others. Until fairly recently skin and tissue abnormalities could only be corrected by skin grafting or a variety of flaps being advanced, rotated or moved from one area to another. These methods are still appropriate in correction of some conditions, but it is now possible to generate tissue in an adjacent position to the defect using tissue expanders. This enables the surgeon wholly or partly to remove the defect (Argenta, 1984). Once the defect is removed the skin stretched by the expander can be advanced over the raw area leaving only one scar on the advancing edge. The generation of tissue by a tissue expander was first considered by Neumann in 1959 and developed to its present state by Radovan.

The silicone bags are manufactured or custom-made in various shapes and volumes, and can be used in most areas of the body. Using adjacent tissue provides an ideal skin match in colour and hair-bearing properties, with the tissue retaining skin sensation since the cutaneous nerves are preserved. The whole unit consisting of the bag, the self-sealing reservoir and connecting tube, is buried beneath the skin alongside the defect and consequently leaves no donor site. The bag is gradually inflated over a period of weeks by injection of saline into the reservoir, which is situated just beneath the skin. This is usually performed by a trained nurse. The expander is filled each time to tissue and patient tolerance and dependent on the size of the tissue expander can be anything from 1 ml to over 100 ml. When the expander has generated sufficient tissue the patient can be admitted to hospital to undergo the operation which will actually remove the defect. Multiple prosthesis can be used at any one time depending on the area to be removed, and in which part of the body it is situated.

Two parts of the whole procedure hold great fear for the children and parents. The first is the thought of repeated injections, usually twice weekly. Parents are often already aware of the anguish they faced having to subject their youngsters to immunisations and how the children looked to them for protection when this invasive and painful procedure was carried out. The responsibility of being a parent and having to make decisions on behalf of their children, often looking to the quality of life the child will have, is thrust upon them early on in the child's life and it is a difficult and trying time. It is hard to be rational and practical when it is your own child in question.

The child can only imagine the pain and hurt that will happen if they let this person – a stranger – come towards them with a needle, and understandably they fight against this intrusion. They believe that with the insertion of the tissue expander they have already undergone an operation to remove what makes them different and unacceptable to their peers and so they find it incomprehensible to undergo more than they have already. This is where a paediatric nurse can utilise her skills and form a relationship based not on fear and threats, but on patience, understanding and trust, where the child can still be in control of the situation and where their co-operation is paramount.

Trying to understand how parent and child feel is half the battle. If at all possible, meeting the family on their visit to the outpatient department gives the nurse the ideal opportunity to talk through what is in store over the next few months. This allows time for thought, questions to be answered and fears allayed. If it is appropriate, the family may wish to be put in contact with a family who have been in a similar position. Preparation for the inflation procedure may also require the involvement of an experienced play specialist, who can guide the child's play activities to work through the feelings of anxiety and fear.

Local anaesthetic creams applied topically to the site of injection into the reservoir have been a major step forward. The nurse can truthfully tell the child that the injection will not hurt. This, with the relationship that the nurse has previously built up with the child and family from their first meeting, through to the time that the child spent in hospital having the expander inserted, should enable the injection to be performed on the basis of honesty and trust. Once the first injection has been performed it is important to find out whether the child felt pain, or if there was anything that could have made the procedure easier. If they become particularly upset, it is important to clarify the reason why. Pain should not be experienced with the use of the anaesthetic cream and it may well be both fear of the unknown and of something that they cannot understand.

Some children prefer their parents to perform the task and this can be achieved with careful tuition and support. Occasionally, children like to be involved in the procedure by pressing the syringe and stopping when the tissue has stretched to the point where it becomes uncomfortable. This will depend on the child's age and ability.

The other major problem with tissue expansion is how the inflated expander will make the child look during the time it is in situ. Both child and family will have to endure a few weeks of what appears to be a 'growth' getting larger. For a number of children this means that the teasing and staring that came with their initial problem will now be directed to a new 'abnormality' and may well cause more upset and distress. It is imperative that the child and family understand the implications right from the beginning. This enables them to deal directly with the problems and face them head on, explaining to others what tissue expansion is, and what it involves.

Practical problems can be related to such basic needs as finding clothing that will accommodate the ever-increasing expander, or how to lie comfortably in bed at night so that sleep is possible. Or, if the expander is situated in the scalp area, how hard do you rub when washing hair?

During the period of expansion the children are basically healthy, lively, 'normal' youngsters and can continue their daily routine as usual. However, schools are often concerned about taking on the responsibility of these children. These are all areas in which the nurse can anticipate difficulties and can give advice which will hopefully help solve these problems. Often, head teachers are concerned because of their lack of knowledge of what the expander is, and what they should look for with regards to complications. A visit from the nurse or a phone call, with the parents' permission, is often all that is needed so that the child is able to continue school, and reduce the time that the child will be absent. Physical education and the 'rough and tumble' of the playground should be avoided, but classroom education can continue as long as the child is comfortable. Sometimes families choose to tell the child's friends exactly what to expect over the few weeks the expander is in situ. Knowing beforehand takes away the mystery.

The use of tissue expanders has been a major development in paediatric plastic surgery and has helped to provide an excellent and effective alternative treatment for many difficult problems requiring tissue coverage.

RECENT ADVANCES IN THE MANAGEMENT OF
URINARY INCONTINENCE

There has been a renewed interest over the past two decades in the surgical management of the lower urinary tract, particularly in patients suffering from incontinence. For a high percentage of these children, urinary tract problems are anticipated from birth because of the presence of a congenital abnormality, either directly involving the lower urinary tract such as bladder exstrophy or indirectly as in children with myelomeningocele.

In the past a large proportion of this group needing surgery would undoubtedly have had a urinary diversion, the most common of such procedures being the formation of an ideal conduit or uretero-sigmoidostomy. The main factors which have influenced and contributed to this renewal of interest are:

1. The realisation that for the incontinent child urinary diversion was not the best
    form of management because of complications such as infection, obstruction
    and stone formation, resulting in further deterioration of the upper tracts.
    Altered body image and associated psychological problems experienced as a
    result of the need to wear an external appliance for urine drainage and an aware-
    ness that such procedures could lead to an increased risk of carcinoma.

2. The availability of paediatric urodynamics and urethral pressure profiles have
    provided vital information on bladder capacity, intravesical pressure and outlet
    resistance. This important information allows the urologist to formulate a clear
    picture of the specific clinical situation and to plan the surgical procedure accord-
    ingly. However, this procedure is invasive and requires the insertion of filling and
    monitoring lines into the bladder via the urethra (immediately prior to the
    examination), or supra-pubically (previous day under anaesthetic), plus a rectal
    pressure line. The experience can be traumatic for both the child and parents
    and must be carefully planned and performed to ensure co-operation and valid
    results. This requires the involvement of experienced nursing staff in the psycho-
    logical support of the child both before and during the examination.

3. The introduction by Lapides in the early 1970s of the clean intermittent catheter-
    isation (CIC) technique of bladder emptying has had a dramatic effect on the lives
    of large numbers of children with neuropathic bladders leading to continence and
    reduction of urinary tract infections. For the group requiring surgery the tech-
    nique has allowed the paediatric urologist to create a continent urinary reservoir
    which can be regularly emptied by introduction of a catheter either per urethra or
    via a continent stoma such as Mitrofanoff.

For paediatric urology nurses the introduction of CIC has had a huge impact on
their role with this group of patients. In the past the involvement in the management
of continence with such patients was simply to help them cope by means of pads and
appliances. Now the emphasis has changed to one of positive promotion of
continence by teaching and establishing a regular bladder emptying routine which
is carried out as a clean, but not sterile, procedure (Lapides *et al.*, 1974).

Teaching this procedure to children poses a particular challenge. Careful planning
must take place with sufficient time to prepare the child and parents for the procedure.
This is done with the help of dolls which the children can practise on, diagrams
suitable for both parents and children and sometimes a video. A consistent approach
to teaching coupled with patience and determination is part of the formula for
achievement. At the Hospitals for Sick Children the need for a specialist nurse was
identified, someone who could dedicate her time to this particular group of patients
ensuring consistency, lack of distraction because of other pressing ward commitments and continuity with regard to follow-up and support after discharge.

Pre-operative Assessment

Due to the different indications for surgery it is vital that incontinent children being
prepared for surgical procedures are accurately assessed from presentation. Invasive
investigations should be carefully co-ordinated and kept to a minimum.

The parents' observations and impressions are important and must be taken into account. Occasionally they may not understand the importance of their observations and therefore need clear explanations and exact questioning by medical and nursing staff to provide the precise information required.

In the hospital setting the nurses are ideally positioned to monitor continence patterns. A clear understanding of the normal anatomy and physiology of the urinary tract plus the physiology of micturition and a knowledge of paediatric urology greatly facilitates this task. Assessment should include precise information on the history of micturition and is best completed by the nursing staff involved in the child's care. The accuracy is increased if carried out in conjunction with a daily diary of voiding which is recorded for one week prior to admission and assessment.

The pattern of voiding should be accurately assessed and information should include frequency, timing (day and night), urgency, dribbling (post-micturition or continuous), description of the urinary system and the ability to interrupt flow. Further information should include the history of incontinence and what the contributory factors are, such as standing, exercise, giggling or coughing. Estimated volumes of 24-hour oral intake, 24-hour voided volumes and individual voided volumes are most useful. Any history of urinary tract infections or constipation and their effect on continence, needs to be noted.

Evaluation of the Patient and Parents

This must be done sensitively but accurately, first establishing that all parties involved have a clear understanding of the proposed surgery and its implications for them as a family. If clean intermittent catheterisation is part of the post-operative plan several questions need to be asked:

1. Will the patient's mobility allow for self-catheterisation, particularly in the case of wheelchair-bound female patients?
2. Have they got sufficient dexterity to insert a catheter into the urethra or stoma?
3. Are the family and child motivated towards improvement/continence? Are they prepared to comply with the need to carry out regular catheterisation and accept it as part of daily living?

If these areas are not clarified in the assessment phase, multiple problems may be encountered post-operatively, particularly the need for long-term supra-pubic catheterisation as a result of non-compliance with CIC.

Surgical Planning

The aim of the reconstructive procedure would be primarily to achieve continence and provide adequate capacity by means of a low-pressure reservoir which is non-refluxing.

The surgical procedure adopted will vary depending on the affected area. If the problem is the continence mechanism, the choice would be a bladder neck reconstruction, insertion of an artificial urinary sphincter or formation of a continent catheterisable conduit, such as a Mitrofanoff. When reduced capacity poses the problem the bladder or reservoir would be augmented by means of a colocystoplasty, ileocysto-plasty or gastrocystoplasty. If the incontinence is due to a combination of poor continence mechanism and small capacity, varying combinations of the procedures mentioned above may be used.

Description of the Surgical Procedures

Augmentation is the enlargement of the bladder capacity with a gastro-intestinal segment, the most commonly used segment being ileum and colon, with stomach now being used in selected cases. Potential complications include risk of rupture, excess production of mucus, and the risk of stone formation. To combat these pro-blems patients are advised to empty their bladders regularly, particularly before vig-orous activity, maintain a high fluid intake with restriction on dairy products in the presence of mucus-related problems. The avoidance of long-term supra-pubic catheterisation reduces the risk of infection and stone formation.

Bladder Neck Reconstruction

Bladder neck reconstruction is when fixed bladder outlet resistance is surgically produced by tubularisation of the base of the bladder. Continence is achieved by increasing the urethral resistance while allowing the passage of a catheter per urethra to drain the bladder. Some children manage to empty their bladders by increased abdominal straining.

Mitrofanoff

Mitrofanoff is the creation of a small continent conduit from the bladder to the abdominal wall which allows the passage of a catheter for bladder drainage. This pro-cedure is named after the French surgeon, M. P Mitrofanoff, who first described it. Essentially the appendix is implanted into the bladder in a non-refluxing manner to create the conduit. The procedure has since been modified to allow for the use of dif-ferent vascularised conduits in a situation where the appendix is unsuitable or absent. Such alternatives may be distal ureter or fallopian tube. It is often performed in con-junction with augmentation which ensures adequate urine storage (Horn, 1990). This prevents stomal leakage due to high intravesical pressure. This procedure has proved invaluable where urethral catheterisation is impossible because of urethral stricture, or impracticable because of severe postural disorders. The advantage for the patient is that they are continent with a system that is easy to manage and appliance-free.

Artificial Urinary Sphincter

Artificial urinary sphincter achieves continence by compressing the urethra by means of an inflatable cuff placed around the bladder outlet which is manually deflated to allow bladder emptying. The role of this appliance in paediatric urology is currently being assessed.

Pre-operative Nursing Management

Admission for surgery would be a planned event three days prior to the date of operation. The patients are usually very well and familiar with the ward from the previous admissions. Psychological preparation would have commenced at the time the surgical plan was made but now needs to be continued with the help of the play specialist ensuring that the child and family understand clearly the pre-operative preparations. This includes fluids only, and rectal washouts for two days before surgery. They would also be made aware that bed rest was necessary for 1–2 weeks post-operatively and of the tubes and incisions anticipated on return from theatre.

Post-operative Nursing Management

The child may return from theatre with bilateral ureteric stent catheters which will remain in situ for 10–14 days and require careful management to ensure patency. Supra-pubic and urethral or stoma catheters will be maintained on free drainage and may need regular flushing or continuous irrigation to prevent blockage, particularly in the presence of mucus. These catheters will remain on free drainage for at least two weeks and on the surgeon's instructions clamping and releasing for increasing periods of time will commence. During this important time the patient will be observed for signs which may indicate leakage or intolerance to storage of increasing volumes of urine.

Immediate post-operative pain control is managed by morphine infusion or epidural analgesia with transition to oral analgesia when fluids are resumed. Bladder spasms resulting from the intubation can cause severe discomfort in the weeks following surgery and are usually managed with the administration of Oxybutinon orally. This problem usually improves when the bladder is allowed to fill on commencing clamping of the catheters. Bladder washouts are often necessary during this period. This procedure is carried out in an aseptic manner using normal saline warmed to body temperature. Care is taken to prevent tension on new suture lines by ensuring that each 50 ml or less has returned before further instillation.

Preparation for Discharge

The management on discharge will vary depending on the surgical procedure carried out. Following cystoplasty and bladder neck or outlet surgery, the patient will be discharged with a supra-pubic catheter in situ on clamp and release during the day, aiming for intervals of 4 hours between drainage and free drainage at night. This catheter will need to be changed every 6 weeks either on the ward or under anaesthesia depending on the child. Plans are made on discharge for cystoscopy 3 months from date of reconstruction and at that stage a decision will be made about commencement of CIC. For patients with a Mitrofanoff, CIC commences approximately 3 weeks following surgery. Once this is well established the supra-pubic catheter will be removed.

Careful liaison with the primary health care team and the school needs to take place before discharge, ensuring smooth reintegration into the community. This is particularly important if the child's management has altered in the school setting. Staff may need to be taught how to manage unusual tasks such as catheterisation.

The described advances in the surgical management of urinary incontinence and the recognition of urology as a speciality has had a huge impact on paediatric nursing in this area. It has provided enthusiasm and an on-going sense of progression for the nursing staff. This results in increased job satisfaction and eagerness to help in the development of new techniques which are ultimately beneficial to these children.

REFERENCES

Argenta L C (1984) Controlled tissue expansion. *Reconstructive Surgery*, **37**, 520–9.
Filler R M, Rossello P J and Lebowitz R L (1976) Life threatening anoxic spells caused by tracheal compression after repair of esophageal atresia: correction by surgery. *Journal of Paediatric Surgery*, **11**, 739–48.
Horn S (1990) Nursing patients with a continent urinary diversion. *Nursing Standard*, **4**, 14 February.
Kiely E M, Spitz L and Brereton R (1987) Management of tracheomalacia by aortopexy. *Paediatric Surgery International*, **2**, 13–15.
Lapides J, Diokno A C, Lowe B S and Kalish M D (1974) Follow up on unsterile, intermittent self catheterisation. *The Journal of Urology*. 111–84.
Spitz L, Kiely E and Sparnon T (1987) Gastric transposition for esophageal replacement in children. *Annals of Surgery*, **206**, 69–73.

FURTHER READING

Hosking J and Welcher E (1989) *Post-Operative Pain 1989*. London: Faber & Faber.
Spitz L (1986) Gastric replacement of the oesophagus. In Rob and Smith (Eds) *Operative Surgery*. 4th edition. London: Butterworth.

14

Development and Use of the Partnership Model of Nursing Care

Anne Casey

The true test of an innovation is time. This chapter looks back several years at the development of a simple, practical model of clinical paediatric nursing and attempts to evaluate its usefulness as a tool for describing, discussing and improving the care of sick children. A brief summary of the model is presented and the benefits of its use in practice are discussed, along with some of the issues addressed as a result of its use. Reading this chapter may encourage other nurses to define and develop their practice. It may also convince some of the sceptics that it is possible to develop a realistic model of nursing which will enhance the quality of patient care.

BACKGROUND

The account begins at a time when 'model fever' was at its height in the United Kingdom, at least in nursing education. Some nurses adopted models with the same fervour that they welcomed the nursing process. Perhaps these mainly trans-atlantic 'theories' were seen to give respectability to the sparse recorded knowledge base of the profession. I suspect that the majority of clinical nurses saw nursing models as impractical and time-wasting.

As one of those ward sisters who had been instructed to start the nursing process 'tomorrow', I had much sympathy with busy clinical nurses who no doubt resented the imposition of new and untried working methods. The implication was that your current best practice was somehow not good enough. That unwelcome suggestion was being addressed as nurses began to recognise that nursing care which concentrated on disease and treatment was inadequate. Moves towards the more holistic approach of total patient care were steps in the right direction. Use of the nursing process ensured that each patient received care planned to meet his indivi-dual needs. But we still had no clear description of what those might be and of how nurses could best approach the task of meeting them.

This was certainly the case in paediatric nursing and at the Hospitals for Sick Children in London. There was a consensus among nurses that family-centred care was a good way to work, but no clear definition of what that term meant. In one ward it might mean that parents were allowed to visit all day – the word 'allowed' implying a kind of grudging permission. In the ward next door it might mean that families were welcomed and parents actively encouraged in caring for their child. The differences were evident not only between wards but also between nurses on the same ward. The nurse on one shift might encourage the mother to give medication to her child, while the nurse on the next shift would give it herself. Neither approach was necessarily wrong: there was no evidence to confirm or deny the benefits of one or the other. But because an explicit approach was never discussed there was not much likelihood of such evidence being sought. It was possible that inconsistency in approaches to nursing care could lead to confusion and distress in the child and his family.

So the time was right for the development of a model describing paediatric nursing. Fawcett (1984) defines a nursing model as 'some nurse's private image of nursing'. This definition emphasises the fact that we all have a model of nursing in our heads and for each of us that model represents the reality of nursing as we practise it. The idea of a model as a representation of reality is of paramount importance. There is no benefit in adopting a model which requires practice to be adapted or changed, unless of course there is proof that such a change would improve care. Abstract and ideal models and theories are essential for the development of the discipline of nursing. I hope this chapter will demonstrate that alongside the academic work, real and immediate improvements can be achieved by practising nurses thinking about the nature of their work (see Draper, 1990).

Our search for a model to describe paediatric nursing began with Fawcett's (1984) guidelines for adopting a model for practice. She suggests beginning with a statement of personal (or team) nursing philosophy. This exercise is followed by defining the concepts central to nursing and describing the relationships between them. Then the nurse must analyse and evaluate existing models of nursing and choose one which agrees with his or her philosophy, definitions and descriptions. The final step is to test the model in a variety of situations.

THE PARTNERSHIP MODEL

The original statement of philosophy on which this model was based stated that:

the care of children, well or sick is best carried out by their families with varying degrees of help from suitably qualified members of the health care team whenever necessary.

As the model developed that original statement was added to. But the partnership model remains grounded in a respect for, and valuing of, the parents' expertise in the care of their child. Even the most inexperienced mother can contribute some knowledge and skill, and a commitment to the child's future which the team could not be expected to have.

The second step of defining concepts was more difficult. It was strange to begin by looking in a dictionary for definitions of *child* and *family*. Words like 'dependent', 'developing', 'growing', 'immature' were combined into a statement about the nature and characteristics of a child. I looked at my own children to identify a child's physical, psychological and social needs. Were their needs different if they were ill? Did a child from a different social or cultural background have different needs?

Family was not an easy concept to define and after several attempts the definition became very specific. The paediatric nurse is only concerned with the family as carers of the child. The family are not the 'patient' or 'client' as they might be in a model of health visiting. So while information about the family's structure, dynamics and resources would be relevant, this would only be of use in assessing the family's ability to care for their child.

Definitions were also developed for *health, environment* and *paediatric nursing*. It seemed most appropriate to define nursing in terms of the actions taken to promote, maintain or restore well-being in the child. Orem's (1985) five forms of nursing assistance were the basis for describing these actions. Clarifying these activities and the goals they are intended to achieve (listed in Table 14:1) has perhaps been the most useful part of the innovation, as later examples will demonstrate.

Table 14.1   Paediatric nursing activities

The Paediatric Nurse:
1. Carries out *family care* and *nursing care* to help meet the child's needs, so that he may achieve his full potential.
   (Family care is the care which the child himself or his parents, usually carry out to meet his needs. Nursing care is the 'extra' care he may need in relation to a health problem)

2. *Supports* the child and family by helping them to cope and continue to function.

3. *Teaches* knowledge and skills to help the child and family towards independence from the health care team.

4. *Refers* the child/family to, and consults with, other members of the caring team when appropriate.

It was during the next step of examining the relationships between the five key concepts that the beginning of the partnership model evolved. Words like 'assisting', 'substituting', 'helping', 'replacing' were not adequate to describe the way in which the experienced paediatric nurse works alongside the parents and the child. This concept of *partnership* seemed crucial to defining the best practice that I had seen as a nurse. The child needs to receive consistent handling, the family to remain as a functioning whole and the parents to continue in their role as caregivers if they are to retain confidence and self-esteem. Imagine the inadequacy felt by a mother who has not been able to protect her child from illness. Then these efficient professionals take over her child's care and do everything completely differently, even the most basic things like feeding and changing.

It was the recognition of this important difference in the way paediatric nursing was being carried out that was the deciding factor in rejecting published models as inappropriate for paediatrics. Many of them were difficult to interpret, using terms not in common use in this country. A model represents reality and is used to communicate: to make explicit how nursing is viewed. With a philosophy advocating family involvement any model of paediatric nursing would also need to be understood by parents and children.

Despite its lack of emphasis on the developmental aspects of nursing children, Orem's (1985) model at first seemed most consistent with the philosophy and concepts I had arrived at. The idea of the nurse as 'substitute self-care agent' (replacing the parents in their absence) in some ways emphasised the necessity of maintaining the child's routines as far as possible. It did not, in my view, go far enough in describing the partnership, the negotiation and sharing, which is the essence of the relationship between the family and the paediatric nurse.

Having been through the stages of adopting a model, and not finding one, I was left with something very close to my 'private image of nursing'. This work would have remained an academic exercise if other events had not prompted further development.

CONTINUING DEVELOPMENT

In the nursing world models were being introduced into both education and clinical practice. This national trend was mirrored at the Hospitals for Sick Children. The school of nursing, prompted by the English National Board, was beginning to evaluate various models to discover whether one, or more, would be suitable for use as a basis for curriculum development for RSCN courses. The planning team, which included clinical staff, sought the views of other clinical colleagues, as it was obvious that any model chosen for teaching would need to reflect practice. Disparity would only serve to widen the theory/practice gap already felt by students on clinical placement.

An open-ended questionnaire was sent to all senior nursing staff to try to establish what they thought were the needs of a sick child, what paediatric nursing was, and how they saw it developing in the future. Around forty replies were received and these contributed to further clarification of the definitions in what was beginning to be called the Partnership Model. Discussion with colleagues added further detail and also resulted in a pictorial representation of the model's central ideas (Figure 14.1). These ideas were in turn presented at professional meetings for wider comment.

An example of the benefit of these discussions is the inclusion in the model of the spiritual aspects of a child's nature. My own view of spirituality was rather limited but I was soon reminded that even very young children are concerned with why things happen in life. Human beings need hope in order to survive and babies are no exception. Analysis and criticism by colleagues helped to make the model less vague – what I had thought was plain English became better expressed and thus of more use in communicating ideas.

An aspect of the new model which remained abstract was the nature of Assessment in Paediatric Nursing. It appeared that lists such as 'activities of living' or 'self-care requisites' were sometimes all that were used of a model. The utility of this assessment checklist was taken as the indicator of the suitability of the model for different

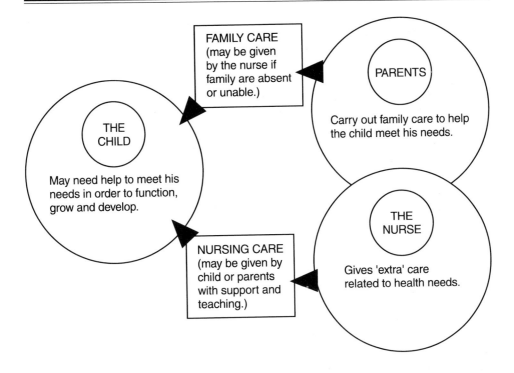

FAMILY CARE
(may be given
by the nurse if
family are absent
or unable.)

PARENTS

THE
CHILD

Carry out family care to help
the child meet his needs.

May need help to meet his
needs in order to function,
grow and develop.

THE
NURSE

NURSING CARE
(may be given by
child or parents
with support and
teaching.)

Gives 'extra' care
related to health needs.

Fig. 14.1 The partnership model. Source: Casey (1988).

practice settings. In order to avoid this situation, developing a list of the child's needs was postponed. However, as the model was refined it became clear that if it were to remain a general model for all paediatric specialities, it should guide the development of assessment tools by nurses in those specialities, rather than restrict them to a single format.

At about the same time as these developments were taking place, the Hospitals' nursing process co-ordinator was beginning to convince clinical staff that it was essential to base the nursing process on a model of care. This would act as a guide to what to look for in assessment, and how to plan, implement and evaluate the care of the child in hospital. Figure 14.2 summarises the key areas to consider when nursing a child using the Partnership Model. The comment by some nurses that 'this is nothing new: this is how we work' seemed to add validity to the model as a realistic representation of paediatric nursing. Thus the model became more than one person's view. It was as a consensus that it was adopted as the underlying framework for new nursing documentation and as the basis for future curriculum developments.

Because previous curricula had been organised along more traditional, medical lines, it was anticipated that there might be difficulties with changing to a curriculum with a truly nursing emphasis. (For a discussion of the implications of using this model in curriculum planning see Casey, 1990.) What was not anticipated was the effect on clinical practice of explicitly stating a partnership approach to care.

ASSESSMENT

The assessment profile
should review:

1. CHILD - presentation,
(physical , developmental,
psychological state);
previous hospital experience;
knowledge about
illness/admission

2. FAMILY - structure,
understanding of child's
illness/admission; if
parents wish to be resident
and involved in 'family' or
'nursing' care

3. FAMILY CARE - who
does what and when; usual
routines; alterations to these
due to illness/admission.

4. REASON FOR ADMISSION
- medical instructions
which affect nursing care.

Also identify: Child and family's
learning and support needs;
Problems requiring nursing care;
Need for referral to other team
members.

PLANNING

Discuss and record:

1. when family care will be
carried out and by whom

2. when nursing care will
be carried out and by whom

3. goals of nursing care
and method of evaluation

4. plan for parent/child
teaching and support

EVALUATION

1. continuously re-assess
child and family's coping/
need for further support
and teaching

2. identify and record care
outcomes/effects of interventions
and plan changes with the family.

IMPLEMENTATION

Includes:

1. continual support and
assistance for the child/family
giving care

2. perform family/nursing care
as agreed in the plan

3. carry out teaching programmes
as planned. Refer to and consult
with other team members as
planned

Fig. 14.2 The partnership model and the nursing process.

THE MODEL IN PRACTICE

As this was a model representing the reality of nursing care it did not seem that it needed 'introducing' into practice other than in formal terms to raise nurses' awareness of this way of describing their practice to others. Opportunities to introduce the model were taken on staff nurse development courses, ENB 998 courses (Teaching and Assessing in Clinical Areas), and study days introducing the new RSCN curriculum. The philosophy and concepts were presented, followed by a discussion of the implications of using an explicit model for practice. It seemed important to ask the question: 'Is this a description of what you do (or would like to do, given time and resources)?' rather than 'What do you think of the model?'

It was unfortunate that this formal introduction of the model was always presented in the context of the new paperwork for nursing records. Every attempt was made to clarify the difference between a model, the nursing process and nursing records. But it became obvious that, to some degree, old antipathies to the nursing process were causing problems with the new records. These records in turn were taken by some to be the Partnership Model.

Following a pilot introduction and subsequent audit of the new paperwork on one ward, it was noted that further education in assessing, planning and evaluating care was needed. This problem remains, and requires addressing at all levels if a planned, systematic approach to care is ever to be a reality. The definition of nursing actions in the model helped especially to highlight deficiencies in planning, evaluating and recording supportive care and teaching of child and parents. If records are used to measure workload and skill-mix, a major part of the paediatric nurse's work goes unrecorded.

The records that were developed to support the model were introduced into most of the wards at the Hospitals for Sick Children (HSC) and were seen as a great improvement. Regular reviews have ensured that changes in practice are accommodated, and as new issues arise, the records have been a way of encouraging change in all clinical areas. For example, discharge planning has been greatly improved with a structured format developed after discussions on accountability (see p. 190 below).

HSC nursing documentation does permit the nurse who is practising partnership care to record that care in a logical way. The assessment format guides the nurse in obtaining information which will help her to care for the child as he is used to being cared for. Because families are encouraged to read the nursing records, it would be difficult to complete the 'care by child/family' section until plans had been discussed with them.

During the development of the records it was recognised that, while 'activities of living' may provide a good assessment structure for children with chronic illness, they may not be so appropriate in intensive settings. Here the distinction between medical and nursing care may blur, and it seems pointless for nurses who think and talk physical systems to record their assessments and care differently. This does not mean that the family cannot be involved in care, or that the child's other needs are ignored. The family requires support and may be very glad of the opportunity to contribute. Once the life-threatening physical problems are controlled, the child can be helped towards recovery with familiar care based on his usual daily routines.

Merely by thinking about whether the Partnership Model suits their speciality, intensive care nurses began to discuss ways of involving parents more. Expertise in this field is evident in an American publication, suggesting a very similar philosophy and practices in Paediatric intensive care in that country (Rushton, 1990).

Another way the model has been used is by nurses wishing to describe their practice to new or prospective members of staff. At a recent interview a ward sister was asked by the candidate whether the ward practised family-centred care. The sister was able to explain in detail how the role of trained staff was very much supporting and teaching parents and children. A discussion followed about the preparation given to new staff to assist them in that role.

It is unfortunate that no quality of care measures were made before the formal introduction of the model. It had been assumed that the model represented reality, but it became apparent that what was described was perhaps an ideal to be worked towards. Some clinical areas were further down the road to an equal negotiated partnership with families than others. However, many positive examples have been reported by staff, suggesting improvements in care directly attributable to using this approach. One example is of a mother labelled as 'difficult' by a ward team. Increasing her involvement and explicitly acknowledging her contribution changed this mother's supposedly aggressive attitude and helped to remove the label.

This model of care is now being used throughout HSC and in several other paediatric units, to guide nursing practice. It is also providing a vehicle and a language for identifying questions for practice which lead to investigation, discussion and change.

QUESTIONS FOR PRACTICE

As an explicit statement of nursing practice, the model highlighted a number of issues which had been of vague concern but were now highly visible. The first of these centred on legal and professional concerns of nurses 'delegating' care to unqualified carers. The Hospitals' management accept vicarious liability for nursing actions, so were consulted to see whether family involvement affected the legal situation. Professional and ethical experts were also approached to inform the debate (see Charles-Edwards and Casey, 1992).

There is no doubt that once a child is in the care of a qualified nurse, that nurse is accountable for ensuring the highest standard of care for that child. When a decision is taken to delegate nursing care, whether to a student nurse, a parent or the child himself, the qualified nurse remains accountable. This is the case if the care is to be carried out in the hospital, with all the facilities available. It is also the case to some extent for care by a family member at home where things may be very different. The Partnership Model helps to identify practical ways in which the standard of care can be maintained.

First, the parent or child needs to be taught the knowledge and skills to perform the nursing task safely. It is a matter of professional judgement when to 'certify' competence and allow unsupervised care. Any teaching given and the learner's competence level should be recorded so that other staff are aware of the skills attained. But teaching alone is not sufficient. Once the family return home there is no longer the safety of readily available expertise. The family must never feel that they have to do the care: this amounts to coercion and would be difficult to defend legally as well as professionally.

Any nurse who delegates care to an 'informal' carer has a duty to ensure that that carer is adequately supported. A parent who is sent home caring for a child having overnight enteral feeds, for example, must know where to get help at a moment's notice. This help might be at the end of a telephone: the amount and type of support needs to be discussed and arranged according to the family's need and the resources available. Given the current political climate, and the pressure on resources such as hospital beds, it is possible for patients to be discharged into the care of relatives who are inadequately supported. That children should kept in hospital for as short a time as possible is a primary goal of paediatric practice. But if adequate support cannot be arranged for parents caring at home, the child should not be discharged.

The next issue which is frequently raised when the model is discussed is the question of parents' views. What about the parents who do not want to stay, who are unable or unwilling to participate in the care of their child? The research carried out by Knafl et al. (1988) into parent (and nurse) attitudes to parental involvement provides some of the answers. One of the problems identified in early reviews of the use of our model was that nursing staff did not discuss the partnership approach with parents. It was sometimes assumed that parents who were coming to the hospital with their child, perhaps for the first time, automatically knew what to expect. In reality, after a period of confusion and uncertainty, the new parent learnt from other parents what the 'rules' were. And if she/he did not conform to the expected pattern, pressure might be exerted by other parents and nurses resulting in guilt feelings and stress.

The basis of the model is negotiation and respect for the family's wishes. If a parent is unable to be present with their child in hospital, the nurse continues the care of the child as the parents would do it, as far as is practicable. If they feel unable to undertake nursing tasks their decision is respected. The partnership does not require equal distribution of tasks. In many cases it is totally inappropriate for parents to take on nursing tasks, particularly technical care which will not be required at home. It is the nurse's responsibility to assess parental needs and wishes and to ensure that the reason for non-involvement is not a lack of supportive care or a lack of understanding of this approach.

It is not uncommon for parents to become exhausted in their attempt to be mother/father and nurse to their ill child. Supportive care in this instance extends to persuading the mother to leave and go home for a rest, while ensuring her peace of mind by attempting to provide the same care that she would give if she were present.

According to a study by Webb *et al.* (1985), parents in one centre were keen to perform various nursing tasks and many had done so. An interesting fact revealed in that study was that neither nurses nor doctors believed parents to be capable of many of these tasks. Because of language or socio-economic background, parents may be labelled as being unable to manage more complex nursing skills. This is a reflection of the attitudes and teaching skills of the nurse, rather than the ability and motivation of most parents. Our experience has been that given time, and a planned teaching programme, almost all parents can become competent, for example, in caring for their child's intravenous central line at home.

One question yet to be researched in depth is what do the children think of all this? How do they feel about their parents carrying out nursing procedures? And what do they gain from caring for themselves? The assumption has been made that this approach promotes independence and feelings of control over what is happening. In adopting a particular approach to care, nurses need to be careful not to impose their view of the world on others. There are few, if any, models of nursing which are supported by research indicating that they are the best approach in any given situation. There is evidence, though, to support the view that some paediatric nurses still have negative attitudes towards parental involvement.

Nursing has struggled to be recognised as a profession and to acquire the power and status that the word 'professional' implies. It might be expected that experienced nurses would resist the sharing of their expertise with laypeople. Inexperienced staff, on the other hand, could be expected to feel threatened and inadequate faced with parents who had become experts in their child's illness and care. Gill (1987) found that experienced nurses were generally very accepting of parent participation, in contrast to more junior staff. This implies that initial nurse training, besides preparing nurses as teachers and supporters, could aim to develop more positive attitudes towards Partnership care.

At present it is not uncommon for a student nurse to carry out the initial assessment of a child and family. Even if the child is only in hospital for a few days, it is possible that they will be cared for by many different nurses. It is unlikely in this situation that anything but the most superficial relationship will be established between nurse and family. The student nurse cannot be expected to have acquired the skills to work in partnership or to be able to cope with the close relationship which may be needed with some families.

One of the first benefits of introducing primary nursing in paediatric settings has been improvements in communications and in the working relationship between child, parents and nurse (Gahan, 1991). Without this method of organising nursing, true partnership care is probably very difficult to achieve. As part of clinical audit we are beginning to measure the level of parental involvement and the quality of the teaching and support being offered. It has been encouraging to find that in all clinical areas families appear to be involved appropriately in many aspects of care. However, resources of time and skills are sometimes inadequate to provide the support that staff identify as necessary. The parents do not report feeling they are left to cope with too much, despite not being 'continually supported and assisted'.

Awareness of what to look for in audit and research has come from the model, which continues to feed into the cycle of identifying issues, investigating and making changes.

CONCLUSION

There are many examples of areas of paediatric practice where improvements could be made. Nurses write wonderful essays about maintaining home routines for the child in hospital and now obtain detailed assessments about those routines. But they sometimes fail to use that information, sticking instead to extremely tenacious ward routines rather than planning nursing care around the child's usual day.

Observations such as these make it even more obvious that the Partnership Model is not after all a description of the realities of paediatric nursing. It has elements of the real world, but much of it would be better defined as ideal. Draper (1990) recalls a correspondence about the value of nursing models. One writer suggested that the theory/practice gap was caused by conservative and unimaginative practice. The reply suggested that the fault lay with abstract and idealistic models and theories. The Partnership Model seems to sit between these two arguments. Developing the model began as a process of trying to describe reality and ended as a generalised ideal view.

Perhaps the difference between this 'abstract idealistic' model and those rejected by the respondent above is that expert paediatric nurses do seem to work this way, despite organisational and resource constraints. When introduced to the Partnership Model many nurses recognise it as a description of what their best practice could be. All the evidence and arguments for family involvement suggest that something like this approach is generally practised and is best for the child, the family and nursing (see Cleary et al., 1986; Callery and Smith, 1991).

Reviewing the process of the model's development, its introduction and use in clinical practice has demonstrated that it does serve as a tool for describing, discussing and improving the care of sick children. The attempt to find an existing model which could be adopted for use in paediatric nursing did not succeed. Instead, a simple conceptual model was created which has led to some visible practical changes, as well as more subtle and far-reaching attitudinal and professional developments at this major paediatric hospital. Interest from other paediatric centres has led to their adopting the model and working through the same issues with the help of the HSC experience. As part of the programme of nursing research at HSC, studies are underway and others planned to add to the growing body of knowledge about the processes and benefits of family involvement in paediatric care.

As this book demonstrates, paediatric nursing has seen some dramatic changes over recent years. Within a changing world, models of nursing should not remain fixed. As new practices and theories emerge so the Partnership Model will evolve. By reflecting on past developments and continuing to search for the best ways of caring, paediatric nurses will be able to provide children and families with the highest possible standards of care.

ACKNOWLEDGEMENT

The author wishes to thank Keiron Spiers and Sarah Mobbs for assistance with this work.

REFERENCES

Callery P and Smith L (1991) A study of role negotiation between nurses and the parents of hospitalised children. *Journal of Advanced Nursing,* **16,** 772–81.
Casey A (1988) A partnership with child and family. *Senior Nurse,* **8**(4) April, 8–9.
Casey A (1990) Nursing models in curriculum planning. In Pendleton S and Myles A (Eds) *Curriculum Planning in Nursing Education.* London: Edward Arnold.
Charles-Edwards I and Casey A (1992) Parental involvement and voluntary consent. *Paediatric Nursing,* **4**(1), 16–18.
Cleary J *et al.* (1986) Parental involvement in the lives of children in hospital. *Archives of Disease in Childhood,* **61,** 779–87.
Draper P (1990) The development of theory in British nursing: current position and future prospects. *Journal of Advanced Nursing,* **15,** 12–15.
Fawcett J (1984) *Analysis and Evaluation of Conceptual Models of Nursing.* Philadelphia: F A Davis.
Gahan B (1991) Changing roles. *Pediatric Nursing,* **3**(10), 23–5.
Gill K (1987) Parent participation with a family health focus: nurses attitudes. *Pediatric Nursing,* **13**(2), 94–6.
Knafl K A, Cavallari K A and Dixon D M (1988) *Pediatric Hospitalisation: family and nurse perspectives* Glenview, Ill.: Scott, Forsman and Co.
Orem D (1985) *Nursing: concepts of practice.* New York: McGraw-Hill.
Rushton C H (1990) Strategies for family-centred care in the critical care setting. *Pediatric Nursing,* **16**(2), 195–9.
Webb N, Hull D and Madeley R (1985) Care by parents in hospital. *British Medical Journal,* **291,** 176–7.

15

The Involvement of Parents in Self-Care Practices

Lorraine Ireland

THE CONCEPT OF SELF-CARE

There is current and widespread interest among health care professionals in encouraging self-care practices. The purpose of this chapter is to examine the concept of self-care, with particular regard to the care that may be given by the parents of the child in hospital. The implications of self-care will be critically appraised and some fundamental guidelines are suggested.

At a time when the Department of Health (DoH) in the 1991 document 'Welfare of Children and Young People in Hospital' is making a strong endorsement of the role of parents as caregivers such discussion is particularly timely:

'Good child health care is shared with partners/carers and they are closely involved in the care of their children at all times, unless exceptionally this is not in the best interests of their child.' (DoH, 1991, p. 2)

To assess the contribution that parents as partners in care may make, a clarification of the concept of self-care may be useful. Levin (1986, p. 285) defines self-care as 'activities that individuals take to restore and promote health, prevent disease and limit illness'. There is potential for such activities to span a range from self-medication to what may be considered 'lifestyle' interventions such as taking care with diet and exercise.

Self-care could further be classified in relation to whether or not the aspects of care are self-initiated or involve compliance with professional care. Segall and Goldstein (1990) suggest that the essence of self-care is self-control, the critical issue being not who initiates the care, but that the care is self-managed, ultimately within control of the individual. This then does not present self-care and professional care as mutually exclusive, but rather as integral and interrelated components of the health care system. Central concerns in translating this concept into practice must be not only the recognition of the validity of lay judgement but also acknowledgement of the primacy of freewill and reasoned action.

The realisation that parents are able to care for their ill children has been slow to be made manifest in the care of the hospitalised child. Contemporary self-care research may be new, but self-care practices are neither new nor reactionary, being the basic health care behaviours in all societies past and present. However, the increased visibility of self-care practices may have been enhanced by factors such as epidemiological shifts in disease patterns from acute to chronic morbidity, a change in focus from cure to care, and public dissatisfaction with the depersonalised nature of medical care. Further change impetus is derived from inherent problems within health care systems and economic constraints, these factors being in addition to a growing body of research related to the care of the ill child and in particular to the effects of hospitalisation (Robinson and Clark, 1980). Children will themselves engage in self-care behaviours, however this is influenced by developmental, familial, cultural and age variables. If the demands for self-care cannot be met by the child, a substitute self-care agent – most often the parents – will intervene on the child's behalf. Self-care demands for the ill child can be met by the child, parent or the nurse. Therefore, partnership as a medium for the enhancement of self-care must become a fundamental value of paediatric nursing.

Several nursing models support a systems approach congruent with visualisation of the family as a unit of care, making explicit recognition of self-care needs and the interface between professional and lay care (Orem, 1980; Casey, 1988), the complexity and function of the family being appreciated and recognition made that the family is the basic system in which health care behaviours are acquired, selected and applied.

Literature and research on the effects of hospitalisation demonstrate the interdependence and interrelatedness of the responses of both child and parents. The consensus of opinion rests firmly with the view that parents should remain with their children as much as possible. In relation to their child's admission parents can experience fear, doubt, separation, anxiety and even perceive the relinquishment of the care of their child to strangers as a form of retribution. Fortunately, parental inclusion in the lives of hospitalised children has become an accepted idea, despite having been a slow process. The findings of the Platt Report (Platt, 1959) recommended the admission of parents with their children and unrestricted visiting. However, the presence of parents did not follow until 1961, following the formation of the National Association for the Welfare of Children in Hospital (NAWCH), which considerably accelerated the impetus for change. Clearly, while parents remained *persona non grata*, their potential as self-care agents remained unacknowledged.

Initially, the entrance of these new participants into the hospital system and the attendant changes in social interaction led to thinly veiled role confusion between parents and hospital staff. The difficulties were well described by Meadow (1969). There was a tension between the mothers' boredom and restriction of their usual roles on one hand, and nurses' perceptions of them as unduly inquisitive, lazy or threatening, especially to junior staff, on the other.

Meadow and other proponents of partnership with parents recognised that a logical solution to these problems would be to allow such mothers to become caregivers for their children. This was not solely construed as occupational therapy for the mothers but visualised as a way of redressing the balance of power between them and the staff, empowering them as informed participants in their child's care. However, it is important to make early acknowledgement of the confusion between intentions that may exist when describing self-care. Self-care may not be 'care' at all without recollection of the concept of self-care being based on the premise of control and choice. It is also crucial to recognise that assumptions of the desirability of self-care rest on a general notion that all individuals will want to be active during the hospitalisation of their child, and raises issues relating to attitude and personality differences.

Each appraisal of parental participation and parental willingness makes manifest the extreme variety of interpretations possible of the self-care concept. Currently in the United Kingdom there appear to be three main categories of interpretation, which are not necessarily exclusive but do embody differing perceptions of the ethos of self-care. The first of these accepts the role of the parent as 'parenting', that is continuing familiar tasks in an unfamiliar environment. This would include the attribution to parents of skills such as play, feeding, bathing and comforting. Thus a demarcation between the roles of professional and lay carers may be clearly elucidated. Viewed in this way parental care may become an option to reduce the children's dependency on nurses. While this may potentially enhance parents' feelings of worth, measured as their usefulness value, and minimise the child's logical distress it is suggested that there is much more to partnership with parents than this.

A second area of parent participation is in the accomplishment of clinical skills such as temperature taking, changing of dressings and the administration of naso-gastric feeds. On many children's wards there is visible evidence of a movement to extend parental roles. Taken to the extreme this again may be a reductionist approach leading to a narrow acknowledgement of self-care behaviours being activities with a clinical bias.

Third, there is the more formalised concept of 'care by parents' (Bivalec, 1976), a concept initially developed in the 1960s in North America. Specifically, units were created for children who were minimally ill in which their parents could deliver care. While this offered a way in which the psychological trauma of hospitalisation could be reduced, additionally and importantly for many families this also provided a pragmatic cost-cutting option. Early care by parent units have been described as 'half-way houses' for children prior to discharge or for those awaiting operative procedures. Latterly, the criteria for admission to such units have increased and now include children who are receiving chemotherapy, and children with serious chronic illnesses. The emphasis is on the nurse's educative supportive role (Orem, 1980) and as a part of primary nursing parents are participants in all phases of their child's care. Prominence is placed on parents learning techniques in the hospital ward which will enable them to care for their child at home, and on the enhancement of the role of the parent as a member of the treatment care team.

In a paper entitled 'Parent Power' Marriot (1990) writes of the focus of self-care activities not merely being bathing and feeding but encompassing skills such as first aid, identification of signals of deterioration and indications for professional support, the emphasis being on empowering skills which could be shared with parents, especially prior to discharge. This appears to reflect clearly the central tenets of the 'care by parent' approach. It is possible that the success of the 'care by parent' units does not solely relate to the provision of a purpose-built hotel-type environment, but is attributable to the negotiation and setting of explicit, mutually shared goals that such an ethos would make fundamental. This highlights the attendant clarification of the philosophy of self-care, required by nurses wishing to involve parents in this way.

THE IMPLICATIONS OF INVOLVING PARENTS AS PARTNERS
IN THE CARE OF THE HOSPITALISED CHILD

The evolution of the role of the parent in relation to the care of the hospitalised child requires a complementary change in role by the paediatric nurse. This is essential if dissonance is to be minimised between nurses and parents. In this discussion two key areas are suggested as being central to the articulation of the concept of self-care into practice. These are clarification of role perception and the control of information, both areas being closely related and indeed interdependent.

The concept of self-care accepted for the purposes of further exploration has the following intentions:

1. The maintenance and restoration of positive levels of well-being for the child and family.
2. Concern for the enhancement of parental roles and increased responsibility in health care decision-making.

Furthermore it is asserted that if the essence of self-care is self-control, from this arises the important premise that empowerment of parents is mandatory if self-care is to become reality.

The parent of the child in hospital is now often expected to contribute significantly to the care of their child. This can include the assumption of clinical roles previously ascribed to nurses. How do parents perceive their role now? And where are the origins of their frame of reference to be found?

To answer these questions it is necessary to examine the existing power alignments within the hospital system. The enhancement of self-care within such traditional structures will involve a recognition and shifting of power bases.

On entering a hospital parents may experience disempowerment. The institution's size and complexity may cause role dissonance, as parents encounter difficulties merely finding their way through the maze of departments, identifying sources of information and attending to their own basic physical needs such as refreshment. To the novice there may be a personal experience of dwarfing and a larger than life first percept of the hospital system, while the rituals and the routines of the children's ward may further contribute to feelings of powerlessness.

Roberts and Krouse (1988, p. 47), writing on the enhancement of self-care, suggest four major influences appear disproportionately to favour the health care provider in the exercise of responsibility and control in health care encounters. Examination of these and consideration of their applicability to parental roles appear essential. First, the position of authority and of power that the health care professional possesses is cited. Second, the language which is employed in communicating with parents could either facilitate or constrain the development of participatory relationships between parent and professional. Third, the nature of the encounter between the parent and professional care provider is very dependent on the interpersonal style of the caregiver. Finally, the decision-making variables of the parent may be dependent on the way in which information is presented.

The authority of nurses and of other health care professionals stems from the concepts of legitimacy and dependence. Legitimacy appears to be strongly based on the parents' conception of nurses as being more informed and knowledgeable about medical problems, this being further validated by an awareness of a long period of professional preparation and visibility of 'badges of office', such as uniform. The children's ward provides a clear context in which the nurse is in a more powerful position than the parent, the location being as known and controlled to the nurse as it is unknown and uncertain to the parent. The parent often resident is removed from his or her known territory and, while 'camping out', the control and privacy possible in one's own home may be severely compromised.

While the nurses may perceive the parent as performing their normal role, if they are bathing, feeding and comforting their child a paradox may exist, unnoticed by the nurses. The strongest impression gained in Meadow's (1969) study from interviews with resident mothers was of anticipating the discharge of their child as of the end of a prison sentence. Even though that study is over twenty years old, Brown and Ritchie (1990) showed that nurses clearly expected parents to attend to their child's activities of daily living if they were resident. They also viewed some parental behaviours such as providing child care, co-operating and being 'pleasant' more favourably than others. In their transcripts of interviews with nursing staff, intense feelings were evident. Conflict of interests was implied when parents did not meet nurses' expectations or exerted some control. However, none of the nurses gave any indication that they explained or reviewed the hospitals 'rooming in' guidelines with individual families.

Dependence on the determination of parental roles appears to rest with the nurse. Dependency results from the vulnerability of the parent in seeking assistance, the stress of having an ill child and the changes in usual role, which entry into the hospital system requires. What has been declared apparent is that there is an assumption that parental participation in care is desirable and should be a feature of children's nursing (DoH, 1991). What is not clear is the extent to which parents and nurses negotiate mutually satisfactory roles in hospital. Such a realignment of roles will not take place without major adjustments by both nurses and parents. For the nurse this means explicit discussion with individual parents about how they would like to be involved in their child's care, and the determination of their respective roles and levels.

Nurses also have an important role as 'information brokers'. Being in a position to control information confers power choices relating to what information is available to whom and at what point, and has significance for the ethical practice of children's nursing. There is a further possibility that parents may be 'informed' but not in an appropriate and meaningful language which they understand (Roberts and Krouse, 1988, p. 47). There is considerable evidence that the failure to receive understandable explanations about the illness and prognosis of their child further disempowers parents and contributes to their feelings of helplessness (Kanneh, 1991).

The decision whether to involve parents in self-care, at its most significant level, addresses the issues of parental autonomy and of the nurse's advocacy role. Brown and Ritchie (1990, p. 32) describe nurses as 'arbiters of information' and 'gatekeepers'. Parents' complaints that they receive too little information about their child's treatment plan and condition, and of their own expected role, may result from the nurse's assumption of control with regard to the families in their care.

This relates to the third influence in the framework for consideration of self-care (Roberts and Krouse 1988, p. 48): the interpersonal style of the nurse. The presumed right to paternalism has origins in the nurse's assertion of professional competence and in functional superiority. Children's nurses who see a demarcation line between the roles of parents and themselves may risk treating parents in this way. Nurses may either underestimate the abilities of parents or rigidly ascribe to them roles which are aspects of the child's care perceived as being basic and non-'nursing'.

Remembering that the grounds for the increased acceptability of self-care practices stem from an economic response as well as in the more commendable notions of improved psychological well-being for the family may further illuminate these differing role perceptions. Even in the United Kingdom care by parent schemes have been implemented in busy children's wards with neither financial assistance nor increases in nursing services. Thus there is a possibility that such initiatives may more readily approximate to a model of self-sufficiency rather than self-care.

The use of interpersonal behaviours that favour an active decision-making role on the part of the parent, or of directive behaviours, relates to the nurse's personal construct of the role of the nurse and that of self-care. For example, Sainsbury (1986, p. 615), describing one ward which was advocating care by parents, comments: 'It is difficult for nurses to find the time to invest in parents when the rewards of this investment are lost to them when the child is discharged.'

Not all families will wish to be involved in the care of their ill child. Particular tensions can be experienced by parents crossing the boundary between parent and nurse roles. From their position of authority, nurses may coerce parents into becoming unwilling participants in the care of their ill child. In particular, this can result if, in discussion of active participation, alternatives are presented in such a way as to control the response. The endorsement of self-care may then not respect the family's free will, which includes the potential for non-participation.

While parents will actively become involved in their child's care, this is not their prime concern. What parents want more than anything is information (Ball *et al.*, 1988; Kanneh, 1991). This must become a priority for children's nurses lest against the background of the increased popularity of parental participation, parents become more concerned in doing what is 'right' and will 'please' the nurse, rather than fulfilling a role as informed care partners. In the acceptance of self-care practices there may be an inherent danger that parents' access to the 'gatekeepers' is further restricted and that parents may be left to get on with it, or perceive this to be the case.

In drawing this discussion to a close it is necessary to declare the writer's perspective as 'devil's advocate' in this exploration of parental participation in self-care practices. This arises not from a fundamental mistrust of children's nurses but from a real concern that in the current wave of enthusiasm for self-care much may be accepted which is undeserving of the previously mentioned hallmarks. Nurses need to examine their attitudes about parental participation and its antecedents such as role interpretations, feelings of power or powerlessness and the primacy of information. Self-care may offer growth for the families in our care and make explicit the nurse's role as educator and enabler rather than leave children's nurses fettered to the 'doing' functions of their role or else narrowly ascribe observable behaviours to parents.

GUIDELINES FOR THE NEGOTIATION OF PARENTAL PARTICIPATION IN CARE

As it is not possible to explore every eventuality of parental participation and possible nursing response here without fear of superficiality, so general guidelines only together with the underlying rationale of each are offered.

Each unit or ward requires specific guidelines and standards in relation to the role of parents. The early communication and documentation of the parents' role in care is essential and should be incorporated in the nursing care plan.

If parents are to share care they need to know what they can and cannot do. Sharing information with parents is a mechanism for counterbalancing the loss of identity that parents may feel on entering the hospital. As practice develops and parents assume greater responsibility for care in hospital, the nurse's potential liability for the acts and omissions of parents assumes increasing significance. Professional staff have a duty to ensure that only appropriate tasks are delegated and that teaching is followed by supervision. Inherent must be the professional duty of care with regard to ensuring harm does not befall as a consequence of instruction or delegation (Dimond, 1990, p. 23).

Each negotiation needs to start with consideration of the meaning that the child's hospitalisation has for the family and exploration of their needs and goals.

Negotiation is a difficult concept to clarify. One meaning that does appear constant however is that negotiation involves more than one party in the pursuit of 'getting things accomplished' (Strauss, 1988, p. 2). However, no distinction is made between ways of achieving desired ends (e.g. coercion and persuasion). It is hoped that the consideration of the previous guideline may lead to the recognition of a concept of more 'active negotiation'. Rather than a unilateral approach, this way of getting things accomplished would allow interaction between parties and emphasise the reciprocity required in making agreements. In this way parental participation has a greater possibility of relating to a spectrum of self-care behaviours.

All health care team members involved with the family need to be orientated to the philosophy of parental participation as a resource for self-care; in particular a shared understanding of the concept is a prerequisite.

It is not difficult to imagine the frustrations experienced by parents when one shift, or certain nurses, allow them to participate in ways that others will not allow. Continuity of care made more explicit by primary nursing and shared perceptions of parental participation by the whole team are essential if self-care which truly empowers parents is to become reality.

Time and information need to be available to enable parents to be involved as contributing members of their child's care team.

Initially, instructing and supervising parents may be more time-consuming than undertaking care oneself. In addition, investment needs to be made in the formulation of relationships which permit questioning and clarification. Information is a medium for sharing power. Nurses need to be knowledgeable about their own practice as well as skilled interpersonally to enable the sharing of this information with parents.

Parents need support and nurturing themselves if they are to be able to give their best for the child's benefit. This includes ensuring facilities are available for their comfort and safety, and renegotiation of their role.

When and if it becomes necessary, nurses need to be available to assume care of the child. Families will need at least short-term relief from the constant duties of caring for a sick child. Care will require daily renegotiation as well as initial negotiation. This will need precise documentation and communication to avoid inconsistencies and assumptions about care delivery.

Inevitable fluctuation in family needs will relate to the health of the child, treatment responses and ongoing developments in family life. The nursing care team will need to accept these variations in coping.

The contexts for negotiation are subject to dynamic change. Issues of territory, anxiety, control and competence may already place parents in a weaker position. Initial validation of the family's coping mechanisms may provide an important step in setting a climate for negotiation.

Ongoing support and education is needed to meet the challenges of parental participation. The opportunity to share care with parents provides enhanced opportunities to make manifest the nurse's professionalism within a creative response to the needs of the child and family.

Acting in a manner which actually enhances parent roles as self-care agents demands self-discipline and autonomy. To do this nurses need the authority to make decisions. The use of unilateral approaches to negotiation or non-negotiation may reflect professional uncertainty or a lack of authority. Empowerment of individual nurses, perhaps by an increased use of primary nursing, could perhaps enable more nurses to choose to negotiate.

Permitting partnership and active decision-making also rests on a clear appreciation of the concept of advocacy and of the responsibilities of the nurse in assuming the role of advocate. Advocacy cannot be narrowly construed as 'rescuing', which usurps parents' responsibility and rights, but as a way of respecting self-determinism.

However, taking priority over the nurse's advocacy role for parents must be the nurse's principal commitment to the health, welfare and care of the child. This role means being alert to safeguarding the child from incompetent or illegal practice, not only by professionals but also by parents. Ways of minimising tension between advocacy roles are dependent on the nurse's awareness of end accountability for the care of the child in hospital. Competence, currency as a valued team member, self-esteem and recognition that practice must be within professional guidelines will underpin this ability.

Hospital policies and practice may need reassessment to enable nurses to be proactive in advocating for the children and families in their care.

This guidance could be a further response to the question, Under what circumstances can nurses develop partnership skills? Family empowerment and parental participation in self-care are incongruent in environments where communication is limited by hierarchical structures and where a medical model of helping prevails. Change may be more likely to occur not only if nurses receive continuing relevant education but also if they practise using empowering models of nursing care. Partnership should be recognised as a distinct skill, which can be learnt in the sharing of situations in which partnership is used as a negotiation model.

In conclusion to this examination of self-care by parents such an approach undoubtedly offers a challenge which is exciting, appropriate and enriching for all care participants. However, analysis of the concept and the requirements attendant on professionals and parents is essential. Many responses to the care of the sick child by the family may purport to be self-care, and as with any change, 'change may be more apparent than real' (Wright, 1989, p. 50).

REFERENCES

Ball M *et al.* (1988) How well do we perform? Parents perceptions of paediatric care. *The Professional Nurse*, December, 115–18.

Bivalec L M (1976) Care by parent a new trend. *Nursing Clinics of North America*, **1**(1), 109–13.

Brown J and Ritchie J (1990) Nurses' perceptions of parent and nurse roles in caring for hospitalized children. *Child Health Care*, **19**(1), Winter 28–36.

Casey A (1988) A partnership with the child and family. *Senior Nurse*, **8**(4).

Department of Health (1991) *Welfare of Children and Young People in Hospital*. London: HMSO.

Dimond B (1990) Parental acts and omissions. *Paediatric Nursing*, **2**(1), February, 23–4.

Kanneh A (1991) Communicating with care. *Paediatric Nursing*, **3**(3), April, 24–7.

Levin L S (1986) The lay resource in health and health care. *Health Promotion*, **1**, 285–92.

Marriot S (1990) Parent power. *Nursing Times*, **86**(4), 68.

Meadow S R (1969) The captive mother. *Archives of Disease in Childhood*, **44**, 362–7.

Orem D (1980) *Nursing Concepts of Practice*. New York: McGraw-Hill.

Platt H (1959) *Welfare of Children in Hospital*. London: HMSO.

Roberts S and Krouse H (1988) Enhancing self-care through active negotiation. *Nurse Practitioner*, **13**(8), 44, 47, 50–1.

Robinson G C and Clark H G (1980) *The Hospital Care of Children: A review of contemporary issues*. New York: Oxford University Press.

Sainsbury C P Q (1986) Care by parents of their children in hospital. *Archives of Disease in Childhood*, **61**, 612–15.

Segall A and Goldstein J (1990) Exploring the correlates of self-provided health care behaviour. *Social Science and Medicine*, **29**(2), 153–61.

Strauss A (1988) *Negotiations: varieties, contexts and social order*. London: Jossey-Bass.

Wright S (1989) *Changing Nursing Practice*. London: Edward Arnold.

16

Environmental Issues in Child Health Nursing

Yvonne Fulton

The health and welfare of children is of paramount concern to child health nurses, and in their contributions to this book they have shown themselves to be resourceful and innovative in providing the best possible primary, secondary and tertiary care within their professional scope. Yet is this perspective now too narrow when placed against the backdrop of mounting concern for the environment?

As the turn of the century rapidly approaches, it may be time for child health nurses to move beyond their traditional sphere of influence into the wider world, and explore what for many may become the cutting edge of their practice; the mitigation of the effects of climate change and global pollution on children's heath.

In June 1992 political leaders of 178 countries met in Rio de Janeiro, Brazil, for the United Nations Conference on Environment and Development, better known as the Earth Summit. The aim was to try to reach some consensus on saving the global environment.

In his closing address to the Earth Summit the British Prime Minister, John Major, said, 'Today we are here, not to argue for a national cause, but for the future of our planet.' These are portentous words, particularly because they are spoken by the leader of the British Conservatives, a group with power, wealth, property and status, and traditionally characterised by their defence of the political status quo.

The Earth Summit had crucial implications for children. Environmental degradation and pollution cause disease and death for millions of children worldwide. Currently, adults are using up the Earth's resources, waste absorption capacity and life-support systems at an ever-increasing rate, and tomorrow's children will reap the consequences.

Analysis of disease trends has shown that the environment is the primary determinant of the state of general health of any population. According to Illich (1976), medical geography and medical anthropology show that food, water and air play the decisive role in determining health.

A growing body of opinion exists which believes that the basic necessities of food, water and air are coming under increasing threat, and the challenge to child health nurses is to become involved as advocates of children in defending these essential requirements. In order to fulfil their fundamental health promotion role they need to understand the threats to the environment clearly and add their voices to those already showing concern.

In their philosophy of care for paediatric nursing the Royal College of Nursing

(1992) states that it 'continually works to identify trends which may threaten the health and well-being of children'. The RCN has also given its support to the United Nations Convention on the Rights of the Child, which in its preamble states that children, because of their physical and mental immaturity, need special safeguards and care, before as well as after birth.

This call for a wider view is also echoed in the International Council for Nurses Code of ethical concepts, which includes the notion that nurses and other citizens share responsibility for initiating and supporting action to meet the health and social needs of the public.

There are many complex and interrelated potential threats to the integrity of the global environment. Global warming, destruction of the ozone layer and pollution from waste, pesticides and motor vehicles are some of the issues which threaten children's health.

Among health professionals sick children's nurses above all understand why there needs to be special concern about environmental effects on children's health. Children are more sensitive than adults to a wide variety of insults due to their small size and physiological immaturity. Disaster epidemiology shows that the highest death rates are among children, often from communicable diseases such as measles, diarrhoea, acute respiratory infections and malaria.

Foetuses, neonates, infants and children are recognised as being vulnerable to the toxic effects of hazardous substances (BMA, 1991). Because of the immaturity of their body systems and protective detoxification mechanisms, the effects of pollutants are amplified. There is also the possibility that a single exposure might lead to a permanent defect.

Neurotoxins, like lead, mercury and cadmium, which poison the nervous system, have greatest impact at times of maximum brain development. In the foetus these effects are magnified still further and children's rapidly dividing cells cause them to be more susceptible. For example, children exposed to atomic explosions at Hiroshima and Nagasaki were eight times more likely to develop cancer than exposed adults.

Their activities and lifestyles, such as the amount of time they spend playing outdoors and their fascination with such dangerous places as waste-tips, increase their exposure to certain risks.

I intend to outline some of these issues from my dual perspective as an environmental campaigner and children's nurse, to show their particular relevance to the health of children, and to make some suggestions for action. There are those in the scientific and business communities who will argue that no action should be taken on these issues until research proves conclusively that life on Earth is being threatened. Rational thinkers will reply that by then it will be too late. Each person who reads this chapter should explore further and reach for their own truth.

GLOBAL WARMING

Global warming is considered to be the biggest environmental threat of the twenty-first century and it has emerged as a major scientific and political issue of the last few years. The build-up of carbon dioxide in the atmosphere from the ever-increasing burning of fossil fuels is responsible for the 'greenhouse effect', and it is now widely accepted that this may lead to immense and socially traumatic changes.

In 1988 the United Nations General Assembly set up the Intergovernmental Panel of Climate Change (IPCC), who reported in 1990:

'emissions resulting from human activities are substantially increasing the atmospheric concentrations of the greenhouse gases.... These increases will enhance the greenhouse effect, resulting on average in an additional warming of the Earth's surface.' (IPCC, 1990, p. 2.)

The IPCC scientists have made the prediction, based on their computer simulations, that if greenhouse gas emissions continue to increase at their present rate, the world average temperature will rise by $1°$ Celsius in about thirty years.

According to Jeremy Leggett (1990), Director of Science at Greenpeace UK, if we carry on with 'business as usual', within less than half a century we will be experiencing average temperatures never before felt while humans have walked on the planet.

There are myriad complex interlinking factors contributing to the greenhouse effect, and some IPCC scientists believe that some of these factors will trigger a feedback mechanism which will cause a spiralling temperature rise.

The IPCC lists some of the implications of this as the desertification of Africa, mass human migration, tropical diseases moving northwards, rivers drying up, mammals and plants facing extinction, food and water shortages, severe winter storms and coastal flooding.

According to Andrew Haines, Professor of Primary Health Care at University College London:

'The primary effects of temperature on human disease are likely to be outweighed by secondary effects on health of climate change. In particular the adverse effects on food production, availability of water, coastal flooding and on disease vectors should be a cause of concern ... the health-impact of climate change will not, however, be limited to the Third World.' (Haines, 1990, p. 149.)

Clearly, no nation will be immune from these effects, and the implication is that children currently within the professional jurisdiction of UK child health nurses will be no exception. It has been painful to contemplate the fate of children in the Third World who are victims of famine and floods. Should UK paediatric nurses stand by, wait until disaster strikes and then find themselves with the responsibility for children's health in a scorched world?

THE OZONE LAYER

Ozone is a gas which is spread thinly in the Earth's stratosphere, about 20–50 km above ground level and its presence is essential to all forms of life. Molecules of ozone at that level act as a filter of high energy ultraviolet (UV) radiation from the sun, and in so doing protect plants and animals from harmful UV-B rays. This natural process can be disrupted by the presence of pollutants. Chlorine, one of the constituents of chlorofluorocarbons (CFC), speeds up the breakdown of ozone molecules, thus leading to a depletion of the ozone layer. CFCs, invented in 1930, are non-toxic, non-inflammable and very cheap to produce. They and related chemicals are used as cooling fluids in refrigerators and in air cooling systems, propellants in aerosol cans, foam-blowing agents for hamburger cartons, house insulation materials and as packaging, and solvents for cleaning electronic equipment and silicon chips.

CFCs decay very slowly; for example, the gas CFC 12 has a lifetime of 139 years. They enter the atmosphere when refrigerators leak or are scrapped, foam is crushed and aerosol cans are emptied. They stay intact for decades, slowly rising into the stratosphere where they break down, releasing chlorine, which in turn destroys the ozone layer.

Additionally, CFCs contribute one-fifth of the warming effect attributed to pollutants in the atmosphere. Each molecule of CFC gas traps 10,000 times more of the Earth's heat than a molecule of carbon dioxide. In the report 'Stratospheric Ozone', scientists from the UK Stratospheric Ozone Research Group drew attention to a large ozone loss above Europe during spring each year, amounting to an 8 per cent depletion.

Increased UV radiation reduces the efficiency of the body's immune system. Plants and food crops show stunted growth when exposed to UV radiation, and animals suffer the same problems as humans. Marine life is also affected with potential disruption to the marine ecosystem.

Even at the low levels that currently reach Earth, UV-B rays cause sunburn, skin cancer and eye problems such as cataracts. Increased radiation of this type would be detrimental to human health. A 1 per cent depletion of the ozone layer may lead to an extra 70,000 cases of skin cancer a year worldwide.

Children are particularly at risk because of the amount of time they spend playing out of doors. They are unlikely to apply sun blocks assiduously to their exposed skin, nor can they be expected to protect their eyes by always wearing sun-glasses. Further, their total lifetime exposure will be much longer than that of the adults of today.

AIR POLLUTION

Motor vehicles generate more air pollution than any other single human activity. The pollutants emitted include carbon monoxide, low-level ozone (formed by photochemical reaction of exhaust fumes and sunlight), nitrogen dioxide, sulphur dioxide, particulate matter, acid aerosols, benzene and lead. Many of these are also greenhouse gases.

There is good reason to suppose that children are especially vulnerable to air pollution (Read, 1991). They breathe more air for a given volume of lung tissue than adults and their airways may be more susceptible to the irritant effects of air pollution. Further, they are likely to spend time playing outdoors, particularly in summer when photochemical pollution is at its height. Various pollutants are linked with asthma, hay fever, chest infections including croup, and childhood cancer.

One in five British teenagers suffers from hay fever and one in seven primary school children has asthma. A 1990 study of wheezing in primary school children by a team at St Thomas's Hospital found that symptoms were on the increase at a rate of about 5 per cent per year.

Professor Stephen Holgate, the Chairman of the Committee on the Medical Aspects of Air Pollution, has urged the Government to sponsor research into the health effects of ozone and other common air pollutants. He believes that an environmental insult in the first year of life, such as exposure to ozone, can sensitise an individual to allergens and lead to the development of asthma (ENDS, 1992).

Road transport is a major source of environmental lead, a neurotoxin which damages the nervous system. There is increasing evidence that low-level lead exposure impairs the mental development of young children, and in recent years removing lead from petrol has been the subject of a prominent campaign relating to children's health.

However, lead in petrol is still responsible for 80 per cent of the lead in air, and for large quantities of lead particles in urban dust. Young children who play in city streets will transfer lead containing dust into their mouths on sticky fingers. Further, car exhausts are placed at the same height as toddlers or children in pushchairs, thereby increasing their chances of breathing car fumes directly.

Britain has a very powerful road transport lobby, and the Government's own figures forecast a 140 per cent rise in the number of privately owned cars on the road by the year 2025. Our present transport system makes much of our environment unpleasant and unsafe; children too are especially at risk of road traffic accidents.

CHEMICAL POLLUTION

Children are exposed to a barrage of toxic chemicals not only through the air they breathe but also through their food and drink. The smaller the child the larger the body burden.

One example is dioxins, a group of extremely toxic compounds, an unwanted by-product of the organochlorine industry. Chemists in the 1940s synthesised the carbon-chlorine bond which is virtually unknown in nature, and thus nature cannot readily break the bond down; it is non-biodegradable. The development of organochlorine compounds led to the manufacture of a vast array of products, including pesticides and plastics. The banned pesticide DDT highlights the problems caused by these poisonous compounds which build up in the food chain and affect the whole web of life (Link, 1991). When organochlorines are burned, dioxins are formed.

The mounting household waste crisis is leading many local authorities to propose incineration as a way of solving the problem. However, there is growing concern in communities threatened by these developments because incineration causes dioxin and heavy metal pollution, as well as requiring landfill of toxic ash residues and restricting recycling. In every part of the United Kingdom there are community groups, backed by environmentalists and health-care professionals, who are fighting the building of incinerators near their homes.

Dioxins are similar to the body's organic compounds so they become incorporated and build up in body fat. Scientific results show that they cause cancer in humans, immunotoxicity and reproductive effects. They mimic body hormones and are a powerful cell disregulator. Because they are so widespread in the environment they are ingested with all food and drink. Dioxins build up particularly in milk because they are fat-soluble and become concentrated in milk fat. British women have the world's third highest level of dioxins in their breastmilk (Link, 1991).

In Bavaria, Germany, mothers who live near a waste incinerator have been advised by their doctors to stop breastfeeding at 3 months because of high levels of dioxin in breastmilk.

British midwives are becoming increasingly concerned about the issue of dioxins and other chlorinated compounds, because of their concentration in breastmilk, and thus their transfer to infants. They have joined a working party set up by The Women's Environment Network to explore chlorine pollution and dioxins (Link, 1991).

Recently, the World Health Organisation relaxed standards for intake, so that the average UK intake now falls within 'reasonable' limits (Link, 1992). However, breastfed babies take in ten times this new relaxed rate, and the foetus is exposed to its amplified effects in utero.

Cow's milk is also affected because cows eat large amounts of grass and foliage on which dioxins have fallen. Because dioxins are fat-soluble they become concentrated in the milk fat. Since children drink far more milk than adults, they receive a much higher dioxin load than adults, at a time when they are potentially more vulnerable to its effects.

Two large research studies in the United States showed that children with higher exposure to dioxin-like substances (PCBs) prenatally showed poor muscle tone and reflexes at birth and lower score on psychomotor scale at 6–12 months. Children exposed to significant doses in utero suffer lower IQs, increased hyperactivity and delayed development of co-ordination, perception and memory (Jacobson, 1990).

It has been estimated that between 1 and 8 per cent of British children are adversely affected by dioxins, suffering diminished potential (Link, 1991).

As these dangerous man-made chemicals build up in children's bodies, they are also exposed to chemicals in food and water, in unknown quantities and with little-understood effects. Much of the tapwater supplied to UK families breaches EC standards for chemical contamination. The contaminants include carcinogens such as trihalomethane, pesticides and nitrates from agriculture, aluminium and lead.

Babies and children are more susceptible to these substances for reasons already outlined, but also because they have a larger water intake in relation to their body weight than adults. In Ripon (Yorkshire) and in East Anglia babies have been prescribed bottled water because of high nitrate levels in drinking water, which can lead to the blue baby syndrome, methaemoglobinaemia (Children's Legal Centre Information Sheet, 1989).

Further, the WHO reports that there are over 1,000 pesticides in over 100,000 commercial formulations used worldwide, and residues will be present in a substantial amount of food and drink (Watterson, 1991).

Toxicologists study the adverse effects of these chemicals on living systems and try to estimate the quantities which may produce adverse reactions in people. Standard toxicity tests study the effects of one chemical on one group of individuals, usually healthy adult male volunteers. Clearly this reductionist approach takes no cognisance of children's special vulnerability nor the additive and synergistic properties of the many thousands of toxic chemicals to which children are exposed.

DISPOSABLE NAPPIES

Disposable nappies are so convenient, what is wrong with them? In reality all those plastic covered parcels of baby waste are dumped into landfill sites – some 10 million each week. They do not rot down, and the untreated waste leaches out with the potential to pollute groundwater and rivers (WEN, 1991).

UK parents use over 3 billion disposables each year, which means felling up to 7 million trees, or approximately 70 square miles of forest. Canada and Scandinavia supply most of the pulp used in Britain, causing diverse forests to be replaced with monoculture plantations which are intensively managed with pesticides and fertilisers. Also, 87 per cent of the pulp imported for disposable nappies is bleached using chlorine gas in a process which causes environmental damage and produces dioxins.

The manufacturers of disposable nappies have claimed that their products are environmentally friendly. However, a challenge by the Women's Environmental Network against this claim was upheld by the Advertising Standards Authority.

WASTE

The Earth's resources are being used up at an accelerating rate, and in a throw-away society metals and minerals are extracted leaving environments scarred; products are manufactured often with polluting processes, and then the products are scrapped, either in landfill sites or increasingly by incineration.

SEWAGE

Children delight in playing on the beach and paddling in the sea, and yet many beaches are polluted by sewage. There is now evidence that this popular form of recreation can adversely affect children's health. A recent research survey, highlighted in Childright (1991), and carried out in Blackpool, discovered that children who had been in the sea were significantly more likely to have diarrhoea and sickness than those who had not.

ACTION FOR GOING GREEN

Having outlined some of the major environmental problems confronting society today, the next step is to give some suggestions for action. When faced with such global difficulties as these it is common to feel overwhelmed and helpless. Individuals often ask what difference their actions could possibly make to problems of this magnitude; yet because these problems have come into being through millions of small individual acts, events can be influenced by changing these same small acts.

'Thinking globally, acting locally' can take place on three levels: the personal, the professional and the political. First, child health nurses can change their personal habits and 'go green'. Second, they can change their professional practice by taking action to 'green' their own workplace, by influencing change within their Health Authority and by educating parents. Third, children's nurses should consider whether they want to recognise their personal power derived from professional knowledge and take political action.

For the individual, going green can begin in many ways. Some start by joining an environmental group such as Friends of the Earth, Women's Environmental Network or Greenpeace. These groups provide their members with high quality information and ideas about how to 'tread lightly on the Earth'.

Going green will involve reducing, composting and recycling waste, making savings in energy and water consumption, using public transport or cycling wherever possible and supporting organic and ethical enterprises when shopping.

These measures will also need to be taken to green the workplace. Some Health Authorities are engaged in improving their environmental performance so the first step should be to ask the Unit General Manager what the environmental policy is.

Friends of the Earth and *Nursing Standard* produced a Green Care Plan in 1989 outlining some of the measures which can be taken, including setting up an Environmental Group and requesting employers to carry out an Environmental Audit.

SAVING ENERGY

Carbon dioxide contributes 55 per cent to global warming, mainly from fossil fuel burning and deforestation. According to Simon Roberts, energy campaigner for Friends of the Earth, if each home and workplace in Britain cuts its electricity use by 20 per cent annual emissions of carbon dioxide would be reduced by 16 million tonnes of carbon dioxide, saving £50 per household per year.

An example of good practice is the world's first low-energy hospital, St Mary's, on the Isle of Wight, which opened in September 1991. Strategies used which save energy are monitoring the use of power, employing heat recovery and recycling techniques, and reducing energy demand.

It is possible to improve the energy efficiency of the workplace while still achieving an acceptable level of warmth, light and cleanliness. For example, replacing a 100W light bulb with a 22W compact fluorescent light bulb would produce just as much light for 80 per cent less electricity and in its lifetime the bulb could save over half a tonne of carbon dioxide from being released.

When choosing new equipment find out about its energy efficiency. In the United States and much of Europe all electrical goods are labelled for efficiency standards and energy consumption, but it is only by persistently asking questions of manufacturers that UK customers will be given this information.

CFCs

There is no such thing as an environmentally friendly aerosol. All the propellants used are damaging to the environment, the materials used to construct the cans are wasteful of resources and polluting to dispose of and no workplace should still be using them. The CFC alternative currently being developed, HCFC, is an extremely potent greenhouse gas and thus needs to be avoided. There are safe alternatives available for all applications and nurses should be vigorous in exposing claims that CFCs are essential in some medical aerosols.

RECYCLING

Recycling was a peripheral issue ten years ago, but now as a result of individual and voluntary group pressure recycling is firmly on the agenda, and almost all local authorities provide recycling facilities. It is estimated that 80 per cent of waste could be avoided, reduced or recycled, and this is fundamental to going green. Waste reduction can be achieved by not performing unnecessary nursing techniques, unnecessary gowning and disinfection procedures, and by avoiding the use of disposable items, particularly those made from PVC, which when burned is a major source of dioxins.

All paper can be recycled, and indeed providing each person in the workplace with a cardboard box to collect scrap paper is a simple way of raising recycling awareness. As well as reducing the amount of waste, recycling paper avoids the destruction of natural forests and habitats, which are felled to make way for fast-growing mono-cultures. Some Health Authorities are beginning to develop recycling schemes, e.g. Salisbury Health Authority collects and sells all wastepaper and buys recycled paper. This latter is essential to complete the chain and provide a market for the wastepaper saved.

Ask that stores provide the workplace with recycled stationery, toilet rolls and handtowels. Paper recycling saves energy and water in its production, but grey recycled paper is the most environmentally friendly because it is made from paper which has been used and would otherwise go to landfill or incineration.

Also start collections for glass, steel and aluminium. Children are great recyclers, so ask them for suggestions. They will enjoy joining in whatever recycling schemes are developed and the cash raised from selling aluminium and paper will be most welcome.

Remember that whatever goes in the rubbish bin will become someone's waste disposal problem. Further, whatever is put down the sink or the toilet will go into the sewer system, travel to the sewage works, and become sewage sludge, which in many parts of the country will be dumped, mainly untreated, into the sea. From there it will find its way onto the beach. Sewage sludge could be composted and used as a valuable resource if it were free from toxic substances.

DISPOSABLE NAPPIES

It is time to consider a return to the reusable nappy as an informed choice. Children's nurses should consider the evidence of environmental damage caused by disposables and share their knowledge with parents. The Women's Environmental Network have produced an excellent leaflet on this subject.

POLITICAL ACTION

Political action begins for many as a result of trying to address some of the issues raised in this chapter. It may begin by writing to a newspaper or an MP, or questioning local authorities. It may lead to campaigning, attending demonstrations and addressing and influencing events within the many citizen groups that are springing up in communities finding their own backyards under threat.

Experience as a voluntary local campaigner against the international toxic waste trade has taught me that the power of the individual should never be under-estimated. The only thing that ever creates change is individual action. Each person who asks leading questions of those in charge of environmental decisions and tenaciously follows the questions through will create a ripple effect that can spread very widely indeed.

CONCLUSION

The chapters of this book illustrate how far child health nursing is travelling in innovative practice. I have outlined some of the problems that the profession may have to address in the future, and suggested that it may now be time to step outside the traditional sphere of our influence and on behalf of the children add our powerful voices to those who are campaigning to stop the planet's life-support system from being dismantled.

The spiritual dimension of children's lives must not be forgotten. What sort of a world will it be when there is no wilderness to dream of: when the last rainforest is felled to make way for a paper plantation and the last watermeadow is buried under a motorway? What sort of a world where children cannot play outdoors without sunglasses and mother's breastmilk is so toxic that they cannot feed their infants?

Those who feel powerless or angry in the face of a seemingly impossible task may find inspiration in this Quaker saying: 'It is better to light a small candle than to curse the darkness.'

Child health nurses may want to act, before what is now regarded as a persistent shadow in the lives of children becomes a gathering storm.

REFERENCES

BMA (1991) *Hazardous Waste and Human Health*. Oxford: Oxford University Press.

Children's Legal Centre Information Sheet (1989) *Children and the Environment*. London: HMSO.

Child Right (1991) Dirty beach poses health risk to children, 75.

ENDS (1992) Government put on the spot on ozone and health. Report 206.

Friends of the Earth (1989) 'Green Care Plan'. *Nursing Standard*, **51**(3), p. 18.

Haines A (1990) p. 149 in *Global Warming the Greenpeace Report*, in Leggett J (Ed) (1990), Oxford: Oxford University Press.

Illich I (1976) *Limits to Medicine.* Harmondsworth: Penguin Books.

Intergovernmental Panel on Climate Change (1990) Report to IPCC from Working Group 1: 'Policymakers' Summary of the Scientific Assessment of Climate Change (June 1990)'. In Leggett J (Ed.) (1990) *Global Warming – the Greenpeace Report.* Oxford: Oxford University Press.

Jacobson J L (1990) 'Effects of in utero exposure to polychlorinated biphenyls and related contaminants on cognitive functioning in young children', *The Journal of Pediatrics,* **116**(1), 38–45.

Link A (1991) *Chlorine, Pollution and the Parents of Tomorrow.* London: Women's Environment Network.

Link A (1992) Press Release, 31 January. London: Women's Environment Network.

Read C (1991) *Air Pollution and Child Health.* London: Greenpeace.

Royal College of Nursing (1992) *Paediatric Nursing: A Philosophy of Care.* London.

Watterson A (1991) *Pesticides and Your Food*, Green Print. Harmondsworth: Merlin Press.

Women's Environmental Network (1991) *Nappies and the Environment*, briefing.

USEFUL ADDRESSES

Friends of the Earth, 26–28 Underwood Street, London N1 7JQ

Greenpeace Environmental Trust, Canonbury Villas, London N1 2PN

Women's Environmental Network, Aberdeen Studios, 22 Highbury Grove, London N5 2EA

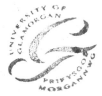

17

Paediatric Oncology

Margaret Evans

INTRODUCTION

One in every 650 children in the United Kingdom develops childhood cancer, and although this figure is much better than for adult cancers, it is still too high. To date, we have been unable to find a cause for childhood cancer, but we have been able to improve our cure rate dramatically.

Childhood cancer was an acute, terminal illness 15–20 years ago. Today, it is a chronic, life-threatening disease, and even in the last few years our overall cure rate has risen from 50 per cent to 65 per cent. These are therefore exciting times in paediatric oncology in terms of our success, but we cannot afford to be complacent.

How then have we made such progress over the last few years? This chapter will highlight factors related to improved prognosis. It will then discuss how facilities and continuing support for families have had to be evaluated, expanded and improved.

FACTORS RELATED TO IMPROVED PROGNOSIS

More Precise Diagnosis and Staging

The spectrum of childhood cancers differs from adult cancers (see Figure 17.1). Although some are the same, for example leukaemia or Hodgkin's disease, different management is likely to be indicated because the adverse effects of therapy on growing tissues must be considered. It is for this reason that more sophisticated means of diagnosis and staging for childhood cancer has been such a bonus, because we are now better able to tailor our treatment more precisely to the stage of treatment. For example, Wilms' tumour used to be treated by intensive chemotherapy and radiotherapy, thus compromising fertility and spinal growth. Today, certain stages of this cancer can be treated with single agents, like Vincristine.

Early Diagnosis

Better education and understanding in relation to childhood cancer allows doctors (and especially GPs) to be alerted to the disease at an earlier stage.

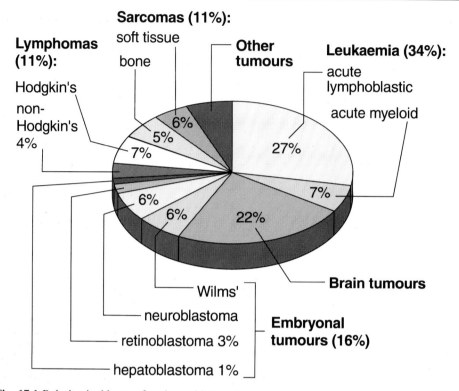

Fig. 17.1 Relative incidence of various childhood cancers shown as a percentage of all child-hood cancers. Source: Stiller and Bunch (1990).

Multi-disciplinary Approach

All nursing and medical staff in the major centres in the United Kingdom meet at regular intervals to share expertise and pool resources. In this way they are able to be more consistent in their approach.

New Forms of Treatment

Although more sophisticated techniques in surgery and radiotherapy have contributed to the overall survival figures, the variety and intensity of chemotherapy regimes have played the most significant role.

When cytotoxic drugs were first introduced 40 years ago, single agents were used continuously at increasing doses until unacceptable toxicity or drug resistance occurred. A more rational approach is to combine the most active agents against the tumour, choosing those which do not have cumulative toxicity, but which are an effective combination to improve cell kill. Recent advances in pharmacology and cell kinetics have allowed increasing doses of chemotherapy to be given. The principle on which allografting and autografting take place is to allow as high a dose of chemotherapy as possible to be given. The use of powerful cytotoxic drugs remains hazardous in terms of toxicity to other tissues, but less toxic analogues are being synthesised.

Thus carboplatinum is less ototoxic and nephrotoxic than cisplatinum, and epirubicin seems less cardiotoxic than daunorubicin.

New antibiotics, antifungal and antiviral drugs have led to the survival of more profoundly immunosuppressed patients.

Another exciting development in cancer therapy has been the introduction of techniques for targeting drugs or radiotherapy on a tumour thus sparing normal tissue. Monoclonal antibodies have been raised to a variety of malignant cells and some can be chemically coupled to toxins, radioisotopes or cytotoxic drugs.

Radiopharmaceuticals, for example, meta-iodobenzylguanidine. (MIBG), have been used to treat children with neuroblastoma. This is an analogue of noradrenaline, which is secreted by the tumour cells. It will therefore be taken up by the tumour cells and when tagged to a radioactive isotope allows delivery of radiation directly to the tumour cell.

NATIONAL AND INTERNATIONAL TRIALS

An important factor contributing to survival in childhood cancer has been the development of controlled clinical trials of therapy under the auspices of the Medical Research Council and the United Kingdom Children's Cancer Study Group. Since childhood malignancy is rare, multicentre trials offer the best chance of testing new therapeutic strategies within a reasonable period of time.

Co-operative studies with international oncology groups have been set up for rare tumours.

PREVENTION AND TREATMENT OF COMPLICATIONS

Central Lines

Venepunctures have always been a source of trauma for children. Central venous catheters have revolutionised the quality of life for children receiving intensive treatment. It must, however, be remembered that any invasion of the body is a potential source of infection and infection control must be rigorous.

Anti-emetics

Many cytotoxic drugs induce vomiting and new anti-emetics have been marketed in the last few years. A cannabis derivative, Nabilone, has proved very effective and some children now eat normally during chemotherapy. Anti-emetics are widely used in suppository form because children find these preferable to injections.

Zofran, which can be given intravenously or orally, is still under review but is proving to be a very effective anti-emetic.

Organ and Limb Preservation

Pre-operative chemotherapy has permitted the preservation of organs which in the past would have been removed in an attempt to eradicate disease. For example, limbs can be preserved by local excision of a bony tumour with the insertion of a custom-made prosthesis. These can be lengthened at regular intervals to stimulate the surrounding soft tissue to grow, with leg lengths therefore remaining equal.

Regular Monitoring of Side-effects

Children are carefully screened for toxic side-effects of drugs like cardiotoxicity or nephrotoxicity and drugs reduced or changed if necessary. Long-term follow-up has become more vigorous to minimise compromised growth and development as a result of treatment.

Alkylating agents have been implicated in the development of second malignancies, but primary treatment protocols are being revised in the hope of decreasing these late effects.

IMPROVEMENTS IN FACILITIES AND SUPPORT

It is clear that in the light of so much progress many changes have had to take place in the field of paediatric oncology. The three main areas we have had to address have been to upgrade our facilities, to provide community support, and to review our education and support for families.

SUPPORT AND EDUCATION FOR PARENTS

The psychological and social impact of cancer is devastating for parents and requires skilled assessment and follow-up by all members of the multi-disciplinary team. Parents experience numbness and shock, and for some time their behaviour closely resembles a grieving process described by Kubler-Ross (1970) as shock–fear–anxiety–helplessness–isolation.

The acute stress and anxiety experienced by parents makes it difficult for them to absorb information, although in most cases they crave as much as possible. It is therefore important to repeat information and advice and to choose an appropriate time and place to impart it. It is also vital to take account of the individual needs of each family and to tailor all education and support with this in mind. Booklets and videos are often helpful but should always enhance, not replace verbal communication.

Assessment in cancer care can make or break the team's relationship with a family. Thus, it is essential to understand family dynamics: to know whether there is an extended family nearby; how many family members there are; where the child fits into the family structure; culture; background and the status of parents. The increase in single-parent families in our society has exacerbated the stresses associated with childhood cancer as single parents battle to keep many balls in the air. Grandparents play an increasingly necessary role in such families, and may suffer a double grief – both for their own child and their grandchild.

Despite the many stresses associated with cancer, parents find strength to care for their children and are increasingly taking on the role of care-giver. The improvement in knowledge and control which this facilitates is seen as positive by most parents. It is, however, essential that parents are encouraged to take time off, and nurses have a responsibility to dispel the inevitable guilt which they feel when leaving their child. It may be necessary to remind them that they are needed by other family members because there is no doubt that childhood cancer is enormously disruptive to the family – siblings feel left out, and because mother usually looks after the child, husbands do also. Unless support and guidance are offered at an early stage, it is not uncommon for families to break up or for siblings to suffer psychological setbacks. Social workers and psychologists play an essential part in helping families to cope with a multitude of unexpected problems.

It has been widely accepted in paediatric nursing that a parent should sleep alongside or close to the sick child and many units are now able to make provision for the whole family to be resident. Parents may still need to travel long distances and this additional expense, as well as perhaps loss of earnings or higher phone bills, can be crippling for families. The social worker should be able to find help and usually makes every effort to do so.

Paediatric oncology demands a high level of commitment and this is best provided by a multi-disciplinary team approach. This approach encourages communication and dissipates some of the stress for the members of the team who must all make themselves accessible to families.

The key to good education and support lies in providing an environment where trust is built and continuity of care is encouraged.

ACUTE CLINICAL CARE

Attention to detail and early anticipation of problems are the essence of the nursing care of children with cancer. To involve parents in the care of their children will potentiate this philosophy, but it must not be seen as a cost-saving or compulsory exercise. Parents do, however, know their own child and to enlist their co-operation and listen to what they say enhances nursing care.

Surgery, radiotherapy and chemotherapy are used to eradicate childhood cancer. Children usually cope well with recovery from surgery and radiotherapy poses fewer problems in terms of short-term side-effects than chemotherapy.

Radiotherapy

As with chemotherapy the child may experience bone marrow suppression, perhaps nausea and vomiting and, if cranial irradiation is used, hair loss and a period of sleepiness about 6–8 weeks after treatment. Skin reactions may occur unless parents are warned to avoid perfumed soaps, talc and ointments containing zinc or lead, all of which can increase sensitivity to radiation.

Chemotherapy

Cytotoxic drugs act by interfering with cell division and metabolism, but unfortunately, cannot be selective. They are, therefore, poisonous to all rapidly dividing cells, the most crucial being the hair follicles, bone marrow and gastro-intestinal tract. Alopecia is often more traumatic for parents than children in the younger age groups, but for teenagers it can be a devastating threat to their body image. The fact that the hair will grow back is little consolation. Bone marrow supression means that the child may be anaemic, thrombocytopaenic or prone to infection. The effect on the gastro-intestinal tract may be debilitation due to nausea and vomiting, diarrhoea, poor appetite or mouth ulceration. There are other side-effects specific to individual drugs, but it is impossible to itemise them all in this short chapter (see pp. 230, 232, 235).

Thus whether the child is newly diagnosed, in the midst of toxic treatment, newly relapsed or receiving a bone marrow transplant, the nursing care of the child receiving chemotherapy presents a unique challenge to the nurse. The core care plans at the end of to this chapter identify some suggested key factors in that care. It must, however, be remembered that each child should be treated as an individual and a full assessment made to make additions or amendments to the plan. (The care plans were based on a Partnership Model designed by Anne Casey, Charles West School of Nursing, Great Ormond Street.)

Bone Marrow Transplantation

Bone marrow transplantation is viewed with trepidation by those who are unfamiliar with it. There is no doubt that ablative therapy and possible graft versus host disease can (but do not always) make the child extremely ill and the challenge to nursing care in that event may be immense. The idea behind bone marrow transplantation whether it be an autograft or an allograft is to administer as much treatment as possible and the consequences of that are to render the child severely neutropenic. In terms of nursing care, then, the child is treated in the same way as any neutropenic child except that his resistance to infection is further compromised and extra precautions to minimise risk must be instituted.

It must also be emphasised that the child and parent are in isolation for a long period of time and the resources of all members of the multi-disciplinary team, must be at their disposal to alleviate the psycho-social consequences of this stressful time.

This treatment is viewed as a last resort and the associated anxiety weighs heavily with all members of the child's family. If a sibling has donated the marrow he has made a wonderful contribution to his brother's or sister's recovery. Equally, however, he is shouldering an enormous burden of responsibility which must be acknowledged, especially if the ill child should die.

COMMUNITY LIAISON NURSES

Paediatric nursing encourages a philosophy of family-centred care and early discharge. To complement this philosophy paediatric liaison nurses have become established in many centres.

The nurses form a relationship with the family at an early stage and assist with education and support, which they continue at home, bridging the yawning gap between hospital and home which parents find so terrifying. They are very much a part of the multi-disciplinary team and it is for this reason that their base should be in the hospital setting. They are also a part of the community and liaison with community colleagues is therefore vital for the smooth functioning of their role. It is particularly important that they liaise with school nurses and teachers to facilitate the child's return to school as soon as possible after discharge. 'Normal living' is an essential component of the child's recovery process.

Central lines have revolutionised the care of children with cancer and have made it easier for drugs, such as antibiotics or diamorphine during palliative care, to be administered in the home. Now that it has become more acceptable for parents to be involved in care, many of them feel happy to accept this responsibility, knowing that the community nurse is available if they encounter problems.

Blood tests also are easier to manage using a central line. Families can be saved a visit to hospital, when the community nurse is able to take blood and deliver it to hospital.

There is no doubt that community liaison nurses provide a valuable service, not only in terms of cost-effectiveness, but also in terms of a better quality of life for the child. Their presence is particularly beneficial to families during palliative care when they are able to facilitate home care.

THE DYING CHILD

If in the end our efforts to cure a child are unsuccessful, parents face the agonising decision to agree to withdraw treatment. Perhaps more than at any other time, they need support and guidance to reach a decision which feels right for them and their child. Once the decision has been reached there is often a sense of relief and parents will find the strength to make the quality of remaining life for their child appropriate and rich.

Just as home is the natural place for a child to live, so it is the natural place for a child to die. Various studies have suggested that home care is more acceptable to families, provided they are given regular support – and that family adjustment following the death is healthier (Kohler and Radford, 1985; Martinson et al., 1978; Lauer et al., 1983).

There are, of course, circumstances when a child may have to be admitted to hospital and the door should never be closed. Hospices provide respite care for dying children. It is however rare for a child with cancer to die there, as their terminal phase is usually short.

Children under 6 years have a limited capacity to appreciate the permanence and irreversibility of death. Very young children have no fear of death, but as they grow older they naturally become afraid of separation from their parents.

It seems that many children know intuitively that they are going to die; the difficulty lies in finding someone in whom to confide when no one has actually told them. This is particularly true for teenagers, who, aware of their parents' grief, are afraid to upset them more. By avoiding all discussion on the subject parents may actually increase the child's distress and loneliness, and cause themselves unnecessary anguish. It is always better to be honest with children and to give them a chance to talk, and most important of all to say good-bye.

Turning to the more practical aspects of nursing care, parents should be reminded to carry out regular pressure area care, mouth care and general cleanliness and also reminded of the importance of avoiding constipation when the child is on opiates and eating small amounts.

Avoiding unnecessary discomfort for the child is fundamental to care and, of course, includes the use of regular and effective pain relief, anti-emetics and perhaps hypnotics or anti-depressants. The community nurse may need to give platelets as a prophylactic measure to prevent haemorrhage. Blood transfusions are usually with-held unless parents feel that their child would benefit from a top-up to enable him to do something which is important to him.

Linked to the fear of death itself is the anxiety over practical arrangements, and the community nurse should be able to help to overcome these difficulties.

Family friction often arises during the terminal phase due to the many stresses of this painful time. Siblings will feel neglected and may behave badly as a result. They may also resent being sent to school, and school teachers must therefore be made aware of the sick child's imminent death.

The death of a child is probably the greatest anguish a parent will face. Bereavement support following the death is usually by a social worker who will continue for as long as is necessary.

SHARED CARE

Since paediatric oncology is a relatively small speciality it is entirely appropriate that intensive treatment, particularly during the induction phase of treatment, is carried out at a major regional centre. It would be entirely inappropriate and dangerous for this to happen elsewhere – not because district general hospitals are inefficient, but simply because it would be impossible for them to maintain the expertise and necessary equipment to look after these children. It would also be extremely costly and in these times of resource management such issues must be taken into consideration.

Shared care works well when it is carried out in close liaison with the main treatment centre. Following induction the child returns to his local hospital for follow-up treatment and, depending upon his requirements and the facilities available, he may rarely return.

Fundamental to the success of shared care is good communication and regular updating for those in the outlying centres. Although such a scheme is often more convenient for parents it is usually difficult for them to break their ties with the main treatment centre. It has, in the past, been common for them to be unduly critical of shared care, requesting to return to the regional centre where 'people know what they are doing'.

Macmillan paediatric nurses play an essential role in facilitating this service which could be of great benefit to families.

TEENAGERS WITH CANCER

The teenage years are a unique and turbulent period of life when the young person experiences many physical and emotional changes. Ambivalence between childhood and adulthood is common and conformity to peer group norms in appearance and behaviour is common. The resulting conflict with parents and other adults accounts for much of the misunderstanding experienced by this age group.

Recognition of the very specific needs of the teenager with cancer is fundamental to their care and to their future quality of life. Staff must have developed a clear understanding of how to manage this age group, because multiple issues will be confronted during the course of treatment. These issues include threats to body-image, self-concept, interpersonal relationships, future plans and life itself. It is little wonder that at a time when the young person is emerging into adulthood and looking forward to new challenges, a diagnosis of cancer poses such a threat to all his developmental tasks. Major changes in daily living must be faced as the teenager tries to adjust to the shock of debilitating disease and treatment. (Changes in appearance such as hair loss, weight loss, perhaps muscle-wasting or pallor are particularly difficult to face.) These changes exacerbate his inherent ambivalence and the associated stress is intensified.

Many parents have great difficulty coping with the increasing mood swings of their offspring and have a tendency to encourage child-like behaviour in their efforts to diminish the pain of the cancer experience. The teenager may, however, see his parents as having double standards, because he has been encouraged to conform to adult behaviour prior to his illness. Families often require help to encourage mutual understanding during this stressful and difficult time.

It is fundamental to the care of the teenager to maintain open lines of communication and to treat him as an equal in an environment of mutual trust and honesty. This means including him in all decision-making and discussions. The teenager needs to be involved and to understand the implications of what is happening to him. He needs to be able to take control – to know what options are available to him, so that he can make choices and seek information when he requires it. Knowledge is power for the teenager and helps to restore his independence which is so vital to his coping strategies. There are, however, times when a teenager may use denial as a coping mechanism and it is important that nurses respect this and allow him to progress at his own pace. Sometimes the teenager will give vent to anger, frustration and sadness – especially when he is confronted with so many insults to his body-image. Donovan and Pierce (1976) observe that it makes all the difference in the world if painful facts about oneself are first realised in a friendly and accepting atmosphere.

Oncology units must be flexible with treatment protocols to allow the teenager to resume as normal a lifestyle as possible.

For most teenagers missing school is of most concern, and those who have reached the end of treatment always recommend return to school as soon as possible for those embarking on it. School life allows a sense of normality and autonomy and if at all possible the teenager should be encouraged to return. This poses a challenge both for teachers and peers, but good liaison by the community team should facilitate it. Tutors may be required to allow the teenagers to catch up with work, but should not replace school.

Finally, the question arises as to whether teenagers should be nursed on a teenage unit where the environment is tailored to the very individual needs of this age group. It would also be interesting to consider whether involving teenagers in their own treatment and care would enhance their coping strategies. Research is required in both areas, to establish whether these measures would be appropriate.

The challenge of nursing teenagers with cancer is unique – they need boundaries and they need freedom, to keep their independence intact. As one young man said: 'Just treat us like regular human beings.'

LONG-TERM FOLLOW-UP

As more and more children survive childhood cancer, the long-term effects of treatments are becoming evident. Oncology centres are now seeing many more children with long-term effects and are setting up clinics to monitor their growth and development carefully. The introduction to this chapter identified the steps which have been taken to prevent and reduce toxicities in terms of organ and limb preservation, regular monitoring of side-effects, and the synthesis of less toxic analogues of effective chemotherapeutic agents. This progress must continue, but in the meantime the aftermath of previous damage must be dealt with as effectively as possible, and, in the future, early recognition and prompt management will pre-empt many of the problems we see today.

It was probably the rather cavalier use of radiotherapy in the past which caused such problems as muscle-wasting, compromised growth and impaired endocrine and intellectual functioning. Chemotherapy has caused such problems as compromised growth, high-tone deafness, cardiotoxicity, nephrotoxicity and infertility. The alkylating agents, although useful, appear to be a contributory factor in the development of second malignancies (Shalot et al., 1977).

High doses of radiotherapy and chemotherapy are now being administered to patients undergoing bone marrow transplantation and centres must be particularly vigilant with these patients.

Psycho-social Consequences

Koocher and O'Malley (1981) note that 'even with the passage of many years and the high probability of survival for these children, the parents are still very much worried and anticipate possible loss in the future'. Thus families continue to live with the fear of childhood cancer, and parents may be unable to cease over-protection of the affected child long after he has completed treatment.

He/she will probably always be treated as 'special', which for younger children may be equivalent to spoiling. This causes untold behavioural problems both for the child himself and also for siblings who continue to feel 'different' and less important.

For teenagers embarking on a career, finding employment and insurance cover may pose a problem as many people are quite ignorant as to the effects of childhood cancer. Much perseverance is required to overcome these difficulties.

The problem of infertility requires careful handling as it may not have been appropriate to mention this at the time of diagnosis when the child was too young to appreciate its significance. Sensitive guidance and support are required for these young people and alternative suggestions made, such as adoption or in vitro fertilisation. If at all possible boys should be offered the facility of sperm-banking.

Thus, long-term follow-up clinics are an essential part of the paediatric oncology service. Patients' and families' needs are very different from those who are undergoing treatment, and require an approach which takes account of this.

SIBLINGS

As more and more children survive childhood cancer our experience of the disease and its side-effects increases. We have, however, been slow to recognise the special needs of the siblings of children with cancer, and it could be argued that we have only paid lip-service to the philosophy of family-centred care. It is understandable that parents in their distress unwittingly ignore siblings and concentrate their energies on the sick child. It is unforgivable if health professionals do likewise, and our record to date indicates that there is room for improvement.

Little research has been undertaken on the needs of siblings and most of that is American. Spinetta and Deasy-Spinetta (1981) have suggested that siblings suffer more than patients in terms of unattended emotional needs. Research has consistently identified psychosocial problem areas, which include confused feelings of resentment, anger, guilt, anxiety, depression, jealousy, fear of their own and the patient's death, isolation from parents, and a wide variety of behaviours aimed at obtaining parental attention.

As with the sick child, the way in which siblings express their emotional unrest is dependent partly on their developmental stage. Maladaptive behaviour, depression and school problems are ways in which children express emotional needs. Spinetta and Deasy-Spinetta (1981) found that infants and toddlers are at greatest risk, because they are unable to verbalise their concerns and interpret parents' absence as rejection; but all age groups undoubtedly suffer some form of resentment, and a lack of structure or boundaries.

Parents are often completely unaware of the isolation they are causing siblings or indeed the acute anxiety and confusion they are suffering. Even if they are aware, they feel that their neglect is unavoidable, and that they must hope for the best with regard to the sibling.

Nursing staff have a responsibility to support and educate parents, offering constructive help as to the problems they may encounter with siblings and why they must receive attention.

An honest and open approach within the family is fundamental to sibling support. Siblings should, as far as possible, and according to age, be included in decision-making and discussions, and certainly appreciate honesty. They should be encouraged to visit the ward and should be shown around. In this way, they will feel involved and might even be able to help with the care of their brother or sister. Involvement with the ill child's treatment helps to resolve the strain of separation and a feeling of confusion.

Siblings do not always share their anxieties in an effort to protect their parents. Kellerman et al. (1980) describe how group meetings were set up to provide peer support. This helped siblings to talk about their feelings in a safe environment.

They also find literature specifically aimed at them helpful, because they feel that they too play an important part in the care of the child.

It is vital that more attention is paid to the very specific needs of siblings in terms of healthy adaptation to maintain their future stability. This is particularly relevant, if in the end their brother or sister should die, when they will be better able to cope with the sadness.

PLAY THERAPY

Cancer causes many stresses and associated behavioural problems for the affected child. Childhood development depends to a large extent on a stable physical, emotional and social environment. Repeated hospitalisation, absence from school, lack of contact with friends, and much attention focused on survival will all affect development. It is also inevitable that parents will want to spoil the child, discipline him less, and worst of all praise him if he produces a good blood count or a clear x-ray. The immediate and long-term effect of this can be potentially destructive to the child. Although it is difficult for parents, the emphasis must be on treating him as a normal individual to allow healthy growth and development.

It has become increasingly clear that play and school activities within the hospital setting make a major contribution towards balanced growth and development. Play specialists and school teachers are therefore essential members of the multi-disciplinary team.

For the child, play represents a sense of normality, fun and relief from boredom. It also has an important therapeutic function and play specialists require specialist training to meet the needs of the ill child and his siblings. Through play the play therapist uses her expertise to help children understand frightening procedures such as blood tests or insertions of lines. She also helps parents to cope with behavioural problems experienced by the child and his siblings, by using play as a medium.

Missing school is traumatic for most children especially when exams must be faced. School teachers provide work in hospital, liaise with schools and perhaps arrange tutorial support. It must be emphasised, however, that return to school should be encouraged. The longer it is left, the harder it becomes, and school represents normality – an essential component of healthy adaptation for the child.

STAFF SUPPORT

Caring for children with cancer is emotionally demanding and therefore extremely exhausting. In order to meet the needs of families, nurses must learn how to maintain their energy levels, by finding ways of coping with their inevitable stress. There are three fundamental support mechanisms to facilitate coping – management, colleagues and self.

Management must recognise the requirement to reduce stress levels by providing adequate staff, sufficient equipment, a good working environment and a clear understanding of the emotional needs of their staff.

Peer support is essential to good team work, and ranges from being positive about others' contributions to participating in a mutual support group. Maintaining a regular staff support group is difficult. It must be programmed into the working day; it must be safe and confidential and it is probably best run by a non-nursing member of the team. Social workers are often well equipped to facilitate this, and it is a great advantage if they are also able to take on individual support, when necessary.

Self-support means taking care of oneself and nurses are notoriously inept at this. They must stop taking on the role of 'martyr', and learn to be more assertive. Proper relaxation and holidays help to recharge batteries. Primary nursing is contributing to better total patient care and improved communication with clients. In paediatric oncology, this will encourage a close bond with families, which must be carefully managed. It is all too easy to be drawn into the trap of being a child's 'special' nurse, making it difficult for other carers to take over. It has been demonstrated many times that forming too close a relationship with families causes unnecessary stress for both parties. Children may be hospitalised for long periods, and it is inevitable and indeed part of the nurse's role to become familiar with families. It is, however, imperative that they take a responsible and professional approach to these relationships.

CONCLUSIONS

As yet, the cause of childhood cancer has not been established, but rigorous research to meet this challenge is in progress.

Possible causes have been identified like occupational exposure of fathers, electromagnetic fields and some toxic chemicals. We do know that radiation in high doses causes cancer. It appears that some children have a genetic predisposition and there are very rare examples of an inherited gene (retinoblastoma, a cancer of the eye, is an example of this).

Cure is restoration of complete health and the prospect of living for a normal lifespan.

Not so long ago, our treatments provided cure at any cost. Today, our aim must be to provide cure at least cost, and an undertaking to maximise quality of life for the child and his family.

NURSING CAREPLANS

NURSING CAREPLAN 1

Date	PATIENT'S NAME:	CAREPLAN NO:

PROBLEM/NEED .... is having induction chemotherapy of **UKALL XI**.
Possible side-effects are:

VINCRISTINE	–	constipation, jaw pain, peripheral neuropathy, extravasation, alopecia.
PREDNISOLONE	–	increased appetite, fluid retention BP and oedema, glycosuria.
ASPARAGINASE	–	anaphylaxis, rash, fever, liver toxicity.
METHOTREXATE (Intrathecal)	–	mouth ulcers, stomatitis, bone marrow depression, CNS effects i.e. dizziness, malaise, blurred vision.

SHORT-TERM GOAL   To ensure that the chemotherapy is administered correctly and

that .... has minimal side-effects.

LONG-TERM GOAL   That any long-term side-effects are monitored and prevented.

NURSING CARE	CARE BY CHILD & FAMILY
To explain chemotherapy and related problems to .... and parents. Wear gloves when handling nappies and bedpans. Measure accurate intake and output with 12 hourly balance at 08.00 hrs and 20.00 hrs. Discuss hair loss with .... and family and advise accordingly – e.g. wig, hat, etc. *VINCRISTINE* – monitor bowel actions and report signs of constipation and give any medications as prescribed. *PREDNISOLONE* – test urine daily glucose and report. *ASPARAGINASE* – give only when a doctor is on the ward and observe for reaction – have hydrocortisone and piriton available. *METHOTREXATE* – ensure regular mouthcare and inspect mouth each shift for ulcers and soreness. Teach parents mouthcare and importance.	

Signature ....   Counter-Signature ....

NURSING CAREPLAN 2

Date	PATIENT'S NAME:	CAREPLAN NO:

PROBLEM/NEED .... is to have a transfusion of blood products.

.... does/does not require cover with platelets.

SHORT-TERM GOAL   That .... receives his/her transfusion with no adverse reactions.

LONG-TERM GOAL   That .... haemoglobin and platelet count return to normal limits and that no further transfusion is required.

NURSING CARE	CARE BY CHILD & FAMILY
Explain procedure fully to .... parents and give reassurance as needed. Maintain accurate fluid balance and observe for signs of fluid overload, i.e. decreased urine output, puffy eyes. Check CMV status prior to starting infusion. **BLOOD** Record hourly temp., pulse and resps., and inform doctor of any significant rise in temperature and stop infusion until further notice. Observe .... for any other signs of reaction – rash, rigors, loin pain. **PLATELETS** Observe for signs of reaction – rash, fever, breathing problems, facial oedema. Inform doctor and stop infusion until further notice. If necessary – ensure cover is prescribed and given as ordered prior to platelet transfusion.	

Signature ....   Counter-Signature ....

NURSING CAREPLAN 3

Date	PATIENT'S NAME:	CAREPLAN NO:

PROBLEM/NEED .... is having chemotherapy during his/her
intensification module of UKALL XI.
Possible side-effects are:

ETOPOSIDE (VP16)	–	hypotension (with fast infusion), alopecia, bone marrow depression.
CYTARABINE	–	nausea and vomiting, fever, rash, mucositis, sore eyes, diarrhoea, bone marrow depression.
DAUNORUBICIN	–	red urine, cardiotoxicity, nausea, local red flush (peripheral).
VINCRISTINE	–	constipation, jaw pain, peripheral neuropathy.
THIOGUANINE	–	nausea, diarrhoea, bone marrow depression.

SHORT-TERM GOAL   To ensure that chemotherapy is administered correctly and that

.... has minimal side-effects.

LONG-TERM GOAL

NURSING CARE	CARE BY CHILD & FAMILY
Explain drugs and related side-effects to .... and parents. Ensure mouth and teeth are kept clean. Check mouth each shift and give mouth washes as ordered. Give Nystatin when neutropenic. Wear gloves when handling nappies or bedpans. Change nappies regularly. Measure accurate fluid balance with BD totals at 08.00 hrs and 20.00 hrs. Observe for nausea and vomiting and give antiemetics as prescribed and monitor their effect (especially with Daunorubicin and Cytarabine). *VP16* – record baseline BP and take 2-hrly during infusion. *CYTARABINE* – observe eyes, give eye care as necessary and give Predsol eye drops as ordered. Observe for diarrhoea and report if severe. *VINCRISTINE* – observe bowel actions and report any constipation or signs of anal fissures.	

Signature ....   Counter-Signature ....

NURSING CAREPLAN 4

Date	PATIENT'S NAME:	CAREPLAN NO:

PROBLEM/NEED .... has a cuff cath central venous line in situ.

Potential problems: – air embolism

disconnection

infection

occlusion

bleeding

Insertion date ....

SHORT-TERM GOAL   That the central line remains patent and infection free.

LONG-TERM GOAL

NURSING CARE	CARE BY CHILD & FAMILY
Use aseptic technique when disconnecting line.	Parents will learn the technique of flushing the line and changing the dressing as shown by the nursing staff.
Observe neck wound and exit site for oozing or redness and inflammation.	
Apply dressing as necessary. Observe for signs of leakage or disconnection.	
Flush weekly with Hepsal or after each entry into the line to ensure patency.	
IV lines should be changed every 3 days unless child is having TPN or intermittent chemotherapy, when it should be done daily.	
Label line with date of change and check daily.	

Signature ....   Counter-Signature ....

NURSING CAREPLAN 5

Date	PATIENT'S NAME:	CAREPLAN NO:

PROBLEM/NEED .... is neutropenic and has a pyrexia. He/she is
susceptible to further infections.

SHORT-TERM GOAL To relieve .... pyrexia and prevent further
infections.

LONG-TERM GOAL Event-free return of neutrophil count to 1.0×10^9/L for

....

NURSING CARE	CARE BY CHILD & FAMILY
Monitor temperature 2 hourly while pyrexial and report any high temperatures. Give anti-pyretics as ordered and monitor their effects – use of fan as necessary. Give antibiotics as prescribed. Take routine specimens and swabs – MSU, nose and throat swabs, stool. Observe for focus of infection e.g. mouth, IV site, wound site, anal area, etc. Ensure regular mouthcare and take swabs from any possible focal point. Monitor fluid balance and encourage .... to drink mls every 2 hours. Wash hands well before handling .... to prevent cross-infection. Give clean diet and ensure food is freshly cooked and label diet cards accordingly and give parents clean diet guidelines. Restrict visitors, especially young children and anyone with a cold or cold sore while .... is neutropenic.	

Signature .... Counter-Signature ....

NURSING CAREPLAN 6

Date	PATIENT'S NAME:	CAREPLAN NO:

PROBLEM/NEED .... is having high dose Methotrexate and lumbar
puncture with intrathecal Methotrexate (MTX).
Possible side-effects: Bone marrow depression, mucositis, renal toxicity, nausea and vomiting.

SHORT-TERM GOAL   To ensure that the chemotherapy is administered correctly and that

.... has minimal side-effects.

LONG-TERM GOAL

NURSING CARE	CARE BY CHILD & FAMILY
Explain chemotherapy and procedures to . . . . and parents. Give adequate hydration as ordered and check urine output and accurate fluid balance. Test all urine for pH which should be ≥7.5 for each specimen – report if pH drops. Wear gloves when handling nappies or bedpans – change nappies frequently and keep nappy area clean and dry. Ensure mouth and teeth are kept clean and observe each shift for ulcers or soreness. . . . . will have a lumbar puncture after the MTX infusion is completed and may have breakfast before 08.00 hrs and a clear drink before 10.00 hrs on . . . . prior to general anaesthetic. Give folinic acid rescue as prescribed.	

Signature . . . .   Counter-Signature . . . .

REFERENCES

Donovan M and Pierce S (1976) Identity and body image. *Cancer Care Nursing*. New York: Appleton-Century Crofts.

Kellerman J, Zeltzer C, Ettenberg L, Dash J and Rigler D (1980) Psychological effects of illness in adolescence – anxiety, self-esteem, and perception of control. *Journal of Paediatrics*, **97,** 126–31.

Kohler J A and Radford M (1985) Terminal care for children dying of cancer: quality of life. *British Medical Journal*, **291,** 115-16.

Koocher G P and O'Malley J E (1981) *The Damocles Syndrome, Psychological Consequences of Surviving Childhood Cancer*. New York: McGraw-Hill.

Kubler-Ross E (1970) *Death and Dying*. London: Tavistock.

Lauer M E, Mulhern R K, Wallskog J M and Camitta B M (1983) A comparison study of parental adaption following a child's death at home or in the hospital. *Paediatrics*, **71,** 107–12.

Martinson I M, Armstrong G D and Gers D P (1978) Home care for children dying of cancer. *Paediatrics*, **62,** 106–13.

Shalot S M, Beardwell C G, Twomay J A, Morris-Jones P H and Pearson D (1977) Endocrine function following the treatment of A.L.L. in childhood, *Journal of Paediatrics*, **90,** 920–3.

Spinetta J J and Deasy-Spinetta P (1981) *Living with Childhood Cancer*. London: C V Mosby.

Stiller C A and Bunch K J (1990) Trends in survival for childhood cancer in Britain – diagnosed 1971–85. *British Journal of Cancer*, **62,** 806–15.

18

Recent Innovations in the Management of Brain-injured Children

Helen Ainsworth

Following any major head injury or brain insult, children should if possible be referred to a specialised neurosurgical unit.

Initially, the priority is to sustain life, and experts in the management of paediatric accident and emergency and paediatric intensive care will be available to deal with this. The needs of children and their families are unique, and in addition to the management of the injuries sustained (30 per cent of all children over 5 years have multiplicity of injuries, Punt, 1989), the child has to be assessed in the context of development and an incomplete neurological maturation.

Children will not react in the same way as adults, as their central nervous systems are organised differently (Middleton, 1989). Irrevocable harm could be caused by early, insensitive handling by those unaware of the special needs of the child.

Our team approach to the management of brain-damaged children has developed and improved, over the past seven years, to provide a management policy which is obtaining excellent results. The late Jan Williams was instrumental in the setting-up of this service and until her early death was a prime innovator.

The World Health Organisation (Maycock, 1990) defines rehabilitation as 'the combined and co-ordinated use of medical, social, education and vocational measures for training and retraining the individual to the highest possible level of functionability'. We believe that rehabilitation begins in some form immediately following stabilisation of primary and secondary brain injury (Punt, 1989). Here a working knowledge of all aspects of child development is necessary to facilitate a realistic rehabilitation programme.

It is from this sound scientific knowledge base of physical, emotional, cognitive and social needs of the child that the plan evolves.

INTELLECTUAL DEVELOPMENT

Piaget's work on intellectual development proposes that a child goes through three stages of development and, although at varying speeds, each stage must be gone through. By passing through these stages a child acquires knowledge to develop cognitive reasoning, social skills and personal control. From birth to adolescence these strategies are reinforced, refined and learnt (Piaget, 1954; Sylva and Lunt, 1982).

Piaget's theory demonstrates that all learning is progressive. Before a new skill can be learnt, it depends on the foundation of previous knowledge. Following any major insult, memory loss is the most common disorder (Levin and Eisenberg, 1979; Levin et al., 1988; Chadwick, 1985). This will therefore disrupt the complex intellectual learning process and affect general behaviour and social skills.

Kohlberg developed a theory based on Piaget's basic principles proposing three levels of development in moral reasoning. General progression in moral reasoning in children and adolescents can be measured (Kohlberg and Kramer, 1989). Also affected will be the acquisition of perceptual abilities and sensory and motor input; as with memory loss, there will no longer be a store of information on which to build (Laszio and Bairstow, 1985). Added to this is the problem of reduced comprehension ability (Das and Varnhagen, 1986) and we have a child who is frustrated, disoriented, confused and frightened, unable to sustain concentration or focus attention, and with a very high level of distractibility (Wicks, 1990).

Middleton (1989) believes the child may not have the strategies to control his own environment or the ability to predict his own or others' behaviour. This will also affect general behaviour and social skills so we attempt to make the ward as much like home as possible.

Sensory Deprivation

Suedifeld (1979) suggests that emerging from unconsciousness, which is described as a period of sensory deprivation, into a sterile, busy ward environment may create further stress on the child. This impoverished environment will interfere with previously learned or organised processes and could result in inappropriate behaviour. If parents are relaxed and welcomed as the most important members of the team, their co-operation is invaluable in the management of the child and his care. As we gained experience in care of brain-injured children we realised that the system of rules, as we knew them, would have to go.

Basically, there are no rules. Parents make themselves at home, with free access to a well-equipped kitchen to prepare their own and their children's meals, if they wish. Having a large Sainsbury's nearby has helped enormously. All are made welcome, at all times. The beds have duvets and co-ordinated bed linen and curtains. Parents are encouraged to bring in personal belongings and the bed area becomes a bedroom. Once admitted, the child is not removed to another area, unless they themselves request it.

FAMILY-CENTRED CARE

Visits are encouraged from schoolfriends and family pets. Pets are often the child's closest friend and a link with home (Ainsworth, 1989). Freud and Breuer believed that hysterical symptoms were often preceded by great fear (Sylva and Lunt, 1982).

Therefore, if the child has disobeyed his parents by climbing a high tree, playing on a forbidden playground or running across a busy road he may see his hospitalisation as a punishment and rejection. For this reason we tell parents and carers to sit with the child, gently stroking his hand and repeating over and over again what has happened, where he is and that he is loved. Separation from a favourite pet may also be perceived as a punishment. When he is given an animal to care for, many parents say that it is the child's sole responsibility and he must take care of it. This must play some part as the child lies in a hospital bed worrying who is caring for his pet, who is feeding it. By allowing free visiting for cats and dogs and having smaller animals to stay by the bedside we believe we alleviate this fear.

This method of ward management is a natural extension of planning individual care, where we adapt to the patient's needs and do not expect them to adapt to ours.

We aim to create a state of security, trust, love and well-being, and do away with a sterile, alien environment. As well as being humane, we aim to reduce stress response and the adverse effect this has on homoeostasis and recovery. In any stressful situation, caused by such incidents as emotional disturbance or pain, the body's physiological and psychological systems overlap to produce the stress response. If there is intense stimulus of a long duration, homoeostatic regulation breaks down. Relaxation, massage and aromatherapy are some ways of coping with stress and we are at present exploring their beneficial uses.

For the past four years the nursing staff have not worn uniform. Parents are our partners in care and it eliminates barriers (Ainsworth, 1990). Nursing needs thinking, understanding, reflective nurses who will challenge accepted stereotypes. For this reason primary nursing was introduced to the ward and an individual style of caring developed where child and parents are fully involved and informed.

As the child's normal development has been disrupted the programme of rehabilitation is based on their specific needs. Before implementation the schedule is discussed with the family and they play a major part in planning and performing stimulation therapy. They also derive a feeling of satisfaction by doing rather than just sitting. It helps to increase their understanding (Quine, Pierce and Lyle, 1988), and returns to them the parental control of their child. It is they who know the child best and with whom the child feels safest.

SENSORY STIMULATION

Following any major brain insult, many synapses are ineffective because of oedema. Recovery of motor, sensory and cognitive function takes place within the 1–2 weeks it takes the oedema to subside. In addition, there are 'silent synapses' which are activated by the lack of input from other normally functioning inputs and regenerative sprouting from injured axons which form new synapses on other neurons in the area. Denervated neurons attract side sprouts from nearby uninjured axons (reactive synaptogenisis) (FitzGerald, 1985).

The brain has therefore a capacity to reorganise itself after injury and this process may facilitate recovery. In young children there is a greater cerebral plasticity. This enables new connections to be made and new areas to adopt functions previously controlled by the damaged areas (Goodman, 1989). The loss of millions of neurons can have little or no detrimental effect provided the overall pattern of inter-connections remains intact (Finger and Stein, 1982). Not all the connections will be correct and the establishment of misconnections could cause intellectual or behavioural problems. For this reason we are aiming to offer a follow-up service, with frequent periods of assessment as some problems may resolve while others are created.

The nurse can only help the child to reach their maximal potential with in-depth knowledge of the mechanism of brain injury and the pathological changes which are responsible for the complexity of the resulting disabilities. This reinforces the belief that children should be referred to specialised units which benefit from having: clinical neuropsychologists who are able to describe the function of the site which has been damaged by injury, physiotherapists, occupational therapists, speech therapists and an educational team. Our team meets weekly for case discussions, where strategies and progress are considered. This information is shared with the child and family.

A co-ordinated team approach of the many facets of child care experts is achieved with all disciplines basing their care on scientific knowledge and theory. The nursing process makes use of this, and the nurse is the centre on which all converge. She is then in a position to co-ordinate care, which is the foundation of primary nursing. Only nurses have 24-hour involvement with the child and his family and although not assuming any greater importance than any other team member, do become the natural pivot for co-ordination.

Management will be dictated by the child's condition. All disciplines work together to facilitate a return of normal function or to restore as much as possible and then teach the child and family how to cope physically with any disability which remains.

The therapists devise a variety of activities to prevent or overcome problems. The nurse needs to be aware of the theories underpinning these programmes to maintain 24-hour support. These can only be achieved by co-operation and close working relationships based on respect for each other's expertise. If there is a lack of co-ordination the various multi-disciplinary activities will fail to function as one unit and the team approach will break down (Hicks, 1987).

Active sensory rehabilitation begins immediately the child is stable by using the coma kit. This aims to activate the reticulolimbic system as it has multiple efferent and afferent connections with all other systems of the central nervous system and so acts as a stimulator (Moore, 1980; Finger and Stein, 1982). The reticular formation passes through the brainstem and is important for regulating the general arousal level of the brain by activating the cortex. The ascending reticular activating system acts to detect the arrival of external stimuli and then produces immediate and wide-spread activation of the whole brain.

Coma arousal is a scientifically-based therapy, so should not be used imprudently. All incoming stimuli must be explained to the patient to assist their interpretation. Unknown stimuli can confuse the reticular activating system and hinder progress. Only a certain range of stimulation can be tolerated, and disorganisation response can occur by exceeding or falling short of the range (Hebb, 1955). To prevent habituation to stimuli, sessions should be brief and each form of stimulation changed frequently. Multi-sensory stimulation is introduced gradually as improvement in alertness is seen. The aim is to promote homoeostasis of the autonomic nervous system (Farber, 1982).

Stimulation begins with the subcortically integrated senses of touch, movement and olfaction. It appears from animal lesion experiments that these areas have a greater number of multi-sensory connections and may not be as damaged by the trauma as the more cortically-located systems (Moore, 1980). Treatment is focused on these areas and progresses onto the cortically-oriented systems of vision and hearing.

Pre-recorded tapes from schoolfriends are obtained. Some schools are especially helpful and allow a tape-recorder to run during a normal classroom session, so providing known sounds which help reduce the unfamiliar hospital and ward noises. The Hospital radio volunteers compile tapes of favourite tunes and familiar sounds specific to the child's needs.

Videotapes of home and familiar people and places, together with favourite television programmes, are shown to provide visual stimuli. Again, these sessions are short, as no useful purpose is served by hours of continuous television or listening to tapes. Anything which is painful or too intense should be avoided and assessment made by observation of the patient's emotional and physiological status.

Pain is controlled, as this is an unknown and disturbing stimulus. It is important to control pain and not merely relieve it when it occurs. Therapeutic touch and massage are at present proving efficacious.

At all times everyone introduces themselves before explaining the procedures which are to be undertaken. Communication is important and during this introduction the opportunity may also be taken to comment on the weather, the time of day/year, what has happened and why they are receiving therapy. A calm atmosphere should be maintained and ideally be free of distractions. Speech should be soft and slow to give time for the information to be processed and adapted to the child's developmental age.

Primary nursing provides another bonus by reducing the number of individuals the patient would normally come into contact with and nurses work smoothly and easily with a patient they have come to know well. Each patient will respond differently and continuous assessment is necessary to build up a picture of progress and the benefit of therapies used.

As soon as possible stimulation progresses on to sensorimotor activity. Active participation and self-initiated self-care or play results in greater cortical activation and integration. It may also improve motivation. Specially adapted toys and computer programs are introduced at this stage.

CIRCADIAN RHYTHM

It has been shown that there are differences between 'morning' and 'evening' personality types. Morning types ('Larks') are generally up early, feel very bright and breezy but are ready to go to bed early. Evening types ('Owls') are still feeling bleary-eyed at mid-morning but enjoy nightlife, often not ready for bed until the early hours.

Children will demonstrate either of these types and we need to ascertain their personality before starting physiological arousal as an evening type will not do well in the morning. This is known as the circadian rhythm (Beaumont, 1988). We attempt to maintain the child's normal sleep pattern and restore a normal day/night pattern. This has necessitated critically analysing our nursing practice and intervention. If the child is stable, should we be doing routine observations? Whose need would it satisfy? The well-known effects of sleep deprivation are contradictory to the establishment of a normal life-pattern.

It is important that the ward is quiet and lights dimmed to promote meaningful sleep which passes through the normal sleep cycles. By observing the patient the nurse can then plan her care for a stage when they are easily rousable.

REHABILITATION

Once the child is no longer comatose we begin a structured programme, based on a normal day's school activities. It is now that some parents have difficulty letting go. Others will be pleased to be able to leave the hospital and understand the need to take the child to the school room in the morning and say goodbye. Brown *et al.* (1981) found that after head injuries, parents tended to be less strict and over-protective. By structuring the child's day around the hours of school, normality is achieved and parameters for acceptable behaviour achieved. Following a severe head injury the child may have behavioural problems, which include attention-seeking strategies (Hill, 1989). This can cause sibling rivalry. The child who is sick will have been given most of the attention and time. Expensive presents are not uncommon. Family life may become totally changed to accommodate the care of the child. It is very easy for the other siblings to feel rejected, especially if they are sent to stay with relatives while the parents are resident in the hospital. For this reason accommodation for the whole family is provided.

The individual programmes of study and rehabilitation can be very tiring so 'rest periods' are put into the timetable. Again, the parents' co-operation is necessary to understand that 'rest periods' are just that and it is advisable for them not to make contact. They can become bored while the child fulfils their busy day and many parents now choose this period not to sleep in but to visit as a family in the evening and join together in normal family activities. Using monies donated from various sources a room was adapted and furnished as an attractive family sitting room. It is small and intimate enough for only one family at a time, or those who have similar problems, and helps simulate normal family 'get togethers'.

As soon as possible the child will begin visits home. This is at a pace dictated by the family. Gradually the visits lengthen and the child becomes a day attender. Progress is monitored and the decision to become a day attender is made by the whole team, including the parents and child. For home visits parents are loaned equipment, bought with money raised by other parents. By involving them in planning and implementation of care the child should then be able to go home sooner and the parents able to maintain care. Home is a familiar place and with visits from friends and neighbours will help prevent further sensory deprivation. The effects of sensory deprivation used against political prisoners are well documented and the plight of those taken hostage results in a greater awareness of problems associated with social annexation.

This service is only available because of the input from the hospital school and the Education Authority, who provide taxis to transport the children.

Any combination of physical, cognitive or emotional problems qualifies the child for entry to the programme enabling a continuation of individualised attention from a team of professionals who work together to ensure immediate liaison and action.

On the child's admission, the school teacher will liaise with the mainstream school and arrange a gradual reintegration. Help is available for the teachers and staff and explanatory, advisory booklets have been produced (Wicks, 1990).

The model for this service was developed following the excellent results we had from our sensory stimulation and rehabilitation programmes. It was devised to prevent regression once the child was discharged home, pick up problems early and deal with them, to continue to support the family and ensure continued lasting recovery. There is a very high investment made in terms of time and money to rehabilitate a child with a complex dysfunction and if they were discharged, unsupported, simply because medical and nursing interventions were no longer required this would be wasted.

The personal cost to the individual and their family who fought so hard for survival and recovery in the early stages is immeasurable. In the long term the cost to society in respect of increased educational support, lost or diminished careers, poor social and emotional adjustment and then later demands on the mental health services is often ignored.

As the hospital school has special school status, the children could, if required, attend until the age of 18. No one has, as yet, required longer than two years. We should, in the future, like to be able to offer assessments on a daycare basis once the child has returned to mainstream school to monitor progress. Woods and Carey (1979) found that language deficits were still present after four years and visuo-perceptual disturbances may continue to be a problem if undetected.

Disabilities could be misunderstood leading to the child becoming labelled as 'naughty', 'failing' or displaying 'unacceptable behaviour' simply because of frustration or emotional disturbances and as the child is developing, there may, as shown earlier, be a tendency for problems to develop. There may also be endocrine dysfunction, which requires further management.

We have never researched the methods we use to confirm our beliefs that they work. It would be difficult to attempt to collect evidence demonstrating the value sensory stimulation programmes play by our instigating clinically controlled trials.

First, we could not ensure that any two children had exactly the same injury, were from the same background with the same environmental sensory input, and second, we would not wish to deny one child the opportunity of maximum recovery by a non-interventionist approach to compare results.

It was easier to accomplish this in the early stages prior to the widespread use of sensory stimulation therapy. By comparing patients with a grade 3–5 on the Glasgow Coma Scale, Le Winn and Dimancescue (1978) reported sixteen stimulated coma patients. All survived and made good therapeutic progress compared to fourteen unstimulated patients admitted during the previous twelve months, also with scores of 3–5 on the Glasgow Coma Scale, of whom eleven died. These comparisons were made by collecting statistics before all hospitals were affiliated to the Institutes for the Achievement of Human Potential, Pennsylvania who began experiments with 'environmental enrichment in coma' before 1955.

By stimulating all five sensory pathways, results were so encouraging that in 1965 special coma teams were developed to design and administer the programme. It is this programme which we have used to provide a comprehensive service involving a multi-disciplinary team approach of individualised child and family care (Ylvisaker, 1985).

Children admitted to the acute neurosciences ward remain here until discharge. Once the acute phase has passed the child's needs will not necessarily require medical intervention on a regular basis. Their needs become one of health and adjustment, with the emphasis on rehabilitation and emotional and social support for the whole family. By necessity the immediate needs of acute patients in life-threatening situations take priority.

If the rehabilitation programme is cost-effective in the long term a further innovation in paediatric care may be patient management by children's nurses, educated to promote holistic care in separate nurse-run units, supported by the multi-disciplinary team.

ACKNOWLEDGEMENT

The author wishes to thank Beth Wicks, Neurosciences School Teacher, Nottingham Hospital School, for help in the preparation of this chapter.

REFERENCES

Ainsworth H (1989) And the guinea pig came too. *Nursing Times*, **85**(39), 54–6.
Ainsworth H (1990) Nurse's Uniform – Social Control or Corporate Identity? Unpublished research.
Beaumont J G (1988) *Understanding Neuropsychology*. Oxford: Blackwell Scientific.
Brown G, Chadwick O, Shaffer D, Rutter M and Traub M (1981) A prospective study of children with head injuries. *Psychological Medicine*, **11**, 63–78.
Chadwick O (1985) Psychological sequelae of head injury in children. *Developmental Medicine and Child Neurology*, **27**, 72–5.
Das J P and Varnhagen C K (1986) Neuropsychological function and cognitive processing. *Child Neuropsychology*. Volume 1, *Theory and Research*, Obsrut J E and Hynd G W (Eds). New York: Academic Press.
Farber S D (1982) *Neurorehabilitation: A Multi-Sensory Approach*. Philadelphia: W B Saunders.
Finger S and Stein D G (1982) *Brain Damage & Recovery*. New York: Academic Press.
FitzGerald M J T (1985) *Neuroanatomy Basic and Applied*. London: Baillière Tindall.
Goodman R (1989) Limits to cerebral plasticity. In Johnson D S, Uttley D and Wyke M (Eds) *Children's Head Injury: Who Cares?* London: Taylor and Francis.
Hebb D O (1955) Drives and the conceptual nervous system. *Psychological Review*, **62**, 243–54.
Hicks A (1987) The role of the medical social worker. *Nursing*, **24**, 912–13
Hill P (1989) Psychiatric aspects of children's head injury. In Johnson D S, Uttley D and Wyke M (Eds) *Children's Head Injury: Who Cares?* London: Taylor and Francis.
Kohlberg L and Kramer R B (1989) Continuities and discontinuities in childhood and adult moral development. *Human Development*, **12**, 93–120.
Laszio J I and Bairstow P J (1985) *Perceptual Motor Behaviour: Developmental Assessment and Therapy*. London: Holt, Rinehart and Winston.
Levin H S and Eisenberg H M (1979) Neuropsychological outcome of closed head injury in children and adolescents. *Child Brain*, **5**, 281–92

Levin H S, Goldstein F C, High W M and Eisenberg H M (1988) Disproportionately severe memory deficit in relation to normal intellectual function after closed head injury. *Journal of Neurology, Neurosurgery and Psychiatry*, **51**, 1294–301.

Le Winn E B and Dimancescue M (1978) Environmental deprivation and enrichment in coma. *Lancet*, **11**, 156–7.

Maycock J (1990) The practice of rehabilitation. *Nursing Standard*, **4**(99), 55.

Middleton J (1989) Learning and behaviour change. In Johnson D S, Uttley D and Wyke M (Eds) *Children's Head Injury: Who Cares?* London: Taylor and Francis.

Moore J C (1980) *Recovery of Function: Theoretical Consideration for Brain Injury Rehabilitation*. Baltimore: University Park Press.

Piaget J (1954) *The Construction of Reality in the Child*. New York: Basic Books.

Punt J (1989) Head injury. *Care of the Critically Ill*, **5**(6), November/December.

Quine S, Pierce J P and Lyle D M (1988) Relatives as lay-therapists for severely head injured. *Brain Injury*, 139–50.

Suedfield P (1979) The medical relevance of the hospital environment. In Osbourne D (Ed.) *Research in Psychology and Medicine*. London: Academic Press.

Sylva K and Lunt I (1982) *Child Development. A First Course*. Oxford: Blackwell.

Wicks B (1990) Unpublished research. Nottingham Hospital School.

Woods B T and Carey S (1979) Language deficits after apparent clinical recovery from childhood aphasia. *Annals of Neurology*, **6**, 405–9.

Ylvisaker M (1985) *Head Injury Rehabilitation: Children and Adolescents*. The Rehabilitation Institute of Pittsburgh, Pennsylvania. London and Philadelphia: Taylor and Francis.

19

Parenting in Public

Philip Darbyshire

INTRODUCTION

What is it like to be a live-in parent? How do parents experience the process of staying in hospital with their child? These seem to be important questions for paediatric nurses to ask. If we are claiming to provide 'family-centred care' or to practise 'holistic nursing' or even if we claim to understand the reactions of parents to their child's illness, injury and hospitalisation then we must try to gain a real insight into the lived experiences of parents.

A review of the literature revealed few such attempts to try to describe or understand live-in parents' experiences. In 1962 the late James Robertson compiled a book of letters sent to him from parents, most of whom described the experience of having their child hospitalised as being extremely traumatic. Meadow's study in the late 1960s, *The Captive Mother* (Meadow, 1969), described the feelings of almost excruciating boredom that many live-in mothers experienced as they sat in enforced inactivity beside their child's bed. More recent qualitative studies by Anderson (1981), Robinson and Thorne (1984), Hayes and Knox (1984) and Knafl, Cavallari and Dixon (1988) have drawn on parents' accounts of their experiences with hospital and care staff. Hayes and Knox (1984) studied parents' experiences from the perspective of parental role stress and suggest that this stress is heightened by parents' and nurses' discrepant perspectives regarding their respective roles. Discrepant perspectives were also implicated by Robinson and Thorne (1984) in their study of families with a chronically ill child. They postulated that parents' relationships with health-care providers follow a three-stage model, where parents pass from the initial stage of 'naive trusting', through 'disenchantment' and finally to the stage of 'guarded alliance'. These researchers recommended that further qualitative research in this area would be valuable.

The study designed to address these issues which I would like to outline here was carried out as part of a Scottish Home and Health Department Research Training Fellowship which I held between 1986 and 1989. The purpose of the study was to gain a deeper understanding of the experiences of parents who either lived in with their child or who stayed with him for most of the day during their hospitalisation. As previous studies had tended to concentrate almost exclusively on the child's experience of hospitalisation, I wanted to discover how parents experienced the process of being a 'live-in parent', and equally important, how paediatric nurses perceived such parents, and what was the nature of the relationship which developed between parents and paediatric nurses. These were the research questions.

METHODS

The nature of this research question indicated that traditional quantitative research approaches would be inappropriate. This was not an issue which could be surveyed, experimented on or counted. The study used a qualitative design and approach based on both grounded theory and phenomenology. The study was undertaken in a large paediatric hospital, using a general medical and burns and plastic surgery ward for the fieldwork. These were selected to ensure a diversity of lengths of parents' stay. Data were collected through an in-depth unstructured interview with 'live-in' parents who agreed to participate in the study. Twenty-six mothers and 4 fathers were interviewed; 10 individually, 4 as couples and 16 in 4 small group interviews. Similarly, 27 qualified nurses were interviewed; 12 individually and 15 in 4 small focus group interviews. Each interview was tape-recorded, transcribed verbatim and subsequently analysed and interpreted using the constant comparative method of grounded theory and the intuiting of phenomenology.

As the work is still in progress, and the analysis still being refined, I wish to share here some of my current thinking in relation to the study and to describe two important aspects of the parents' experiences which emerged from the interview data. First, I will describe the difficulties that parents experienced in making the transition from normal parenting to parenting while living in hospital with their child. Second, I will describe nurses' caring practices and approaches which parents valued and appreciated and which minimised these difficulties. These two aspects will be linked conceptually using the phenomena of exclusion and alienation, and confirmation and connectedness.

I would like to concentrate on the parents' experiences, and in particular, what I have called 'parenting in public', a concept which was derived from the line-by-line analysis of the parents' interviews, and which I believe to be useful in understanding some of the difficulties that parents experienced while living in in hospital. Parenting is taken to be not only a role, with attendant rights, duties and responsibilities but also, in the phenomenological sense, a way of 'being-in-the-world' (Heidegger, 1962). 'Parenting in public' is used to describe how parents experience this transformation, from what is essentially a private and uniquely personal experience, to one which is now to occur in a very public arena – a paediatric ward. Here, I shall discuss only two elements of parenting in public: parental responsibility and parental competence.

PARENTAL RESPONSIBILITY

Being a parent involves a myriad of different child care functions. But perhaps of greatest importance is that they are the people who have direct responsibility for the child and as such they have the right to make decisions affecting every aspect of the child's life. In hospital however, this responsibility becomes shared with the hospital staff. One mother explained:

'You're not the only one that's responsible when they're in here because there are so many other people that are deciding various things . . . you haven't got the same freedom . . . you have to fit in to what their plans are.' (#27, Mother #1, p. 9)

Parents experienced changes in their role in relation to the performance of their usual child care tasks, but there was another important change. The character of their interaction with their child was also affected by the new environment. This was most clearly highlighted by mothers who discussed the problem of discipline while their child was in hospital. The disciplining of your child is one of the most intensely personal aspects of parenting and therefore one which might be expected to be affected when 'parenting in public'. At the time of the child's admission this was not a pressing issue as any 'bad' behaviour would be attributed to the illness or injury and the child was therefore 'excused' from their normal responsibility to behave well:

Mother #4: 'That's one of the things that frightens me about [my daughter], is *her behaviour*, it's *appalling*.'

Mother #2: 'But a lot of that's to do with what's wrong with her too.' (#27, pp. 65–6)

This 'period of grace' was only temporary, however, as parents recognised that their normal disciplinary pattern would have to be re-established at some point. The problem for parents was when and how this should be done:

'You start wondering about how you're going to manage to discipline them and how do you know when they're well enough to start disciplining them ... and then try to get back to normal.' (#27, Mother #1, p. 66)

As the child's condition improved, the parents were faced with the problem of how to continue to use their own disciplinary techniques when these were often seen as being at variance with the professional ethos of the ward and ward staff and as such, were liable to incur staff disapproval at the very least. Paediatric nurse training emphasises a disciplinary ethic towards children, which is based upon calm, reason and explanation. When confronted by children who are being badly behaved, the nurse is encouraged to 'remain unruffled' and of course, as one paediatric textbook emphasises, 'In no circumstances may a nurse hit or smack a child' (Adamson and Hull, 1984). Parents were acutely aware that such a disciplinary ethos was equally applicable to them while they were in the ward and that they were expected to conform to an ideal:

Mother #4: 'because everybody wants to be the ideal mother like they are in the adverts [laughs]'.

Mother #1: 'Yeah, coping with the crises and remaining calm and cool.' (#27, p. 67)

One mother described the ward reaction to her normal disciplinary tactics:

'The first time that I smacked her I was *very conscious* of that, but she'd *really* been naughty ... and the first time that I smacked her hand I felt that everybody had turned round and said ARRRRGH!!! She smacked a sick child in hospital.' (#10, pp. 58–9)

Parents expressed concern that their disciplinary styles were being constantly assessed by nurses and judged to be an indication that they did not care 'properly' for their child. These parents were also afraid that their disciplining of the child could lead to the child being seen as at risk of being abused and even taken into care.

There seemed to be a difference in timescale perspectives between nurses and parents regarding discipline, with parents expressing more concern for the child's behaviour in the longer term while nurses were more concerned with the nature of the present disciplinary action. The parents were very concerned that if children were 'ruined' or allowed to 'get away with murder' while in hospital, this would create serious problems for the family when the child returned home.

PARENTAL COMPETENCE

Another aspect of normal parenting is that parents are seen as being 'the experts' in the care of their child and indeed the nurses in the study often emphasised this point in their interviews. However, parents would describe how there were times when they felt that their competence as parents was called into question.

Tension between the expertise and knowledge of the live-in parents and the professional knowledge of the nurses was apparent in the accounts of both parents and nurses. Parents expressed the view that nurses had an expertise which demanded recognition by virtue of their professional training:

Mother #1: 'it's because you feel in the presence of experts ... that will disapprove of your inadequacies.'

Mother #4: 'They've been trained how to feed and change a baby whereas you just...' (#26, p. 46)

It is notable here that these mothers recognise nurses' expertise as being somehow 'superior' even in an area so 'basic' as nappy-changing and feeding, thus posing a threat to what Silverman (1987) has called: 'parents' moral sense of their own responsibilities by passing on some of their perceived functions to "experts"'.

Some parents felt that their competence was being constantly assessed by nurses as part of a judgemental process, and would become guarded and consequently try to modify their normal techniques of caring for their child in order to better approximate the style of nurses:

'you change her the way the nurses change her rather than the way you would if you were at home doing it ... you know that somebody else is watching you or you think they are, so you've got to, make your patience go longer.' (#4, pp. 25–6)

This mother is alluding to the idea that there is an idealised way of caring for the child, which is exemplified in the procedures followed by nurses. In contrast, the techniques usually employed by the mother are thought of as being somehow characterised by impatience and a less caring manner. This impression that parents gain, that their performance as mothers is being assessed, seems to be particularly acute in the early stages of the child's hospitalisation. One mother explained:

'At the beginning yeah, am I doing the right things? Am I washing her properly? (laughs) ... and sort of silly things like that ... but now I just think ... it doesn't bother me now cos I've got used to it. But at first you're very conscious.' (#10, p. 57)

It seems that parents could achieve this 'normal' and unselfconscious style of parenting within the hospital if they did not perceive that their competence was being questioned, and if they were allowed and encouraged to continue to provide their usual style of care for their child. However, parents' confidence in their ability to provide care in the ward could be shaken when their competence was called into question by hospital staff. One mother described this in relation to an incident where a nurse had suggested that her toddler son would take his lunch better if a nurse were to give him it and if she were to leave the ward for a while:

'it was like the other day, we were told to go away so they could get food into him .. we felt terrible cos we had to go away, felt as if we weren't feeding him right ...' (#25, Mother #2, p. 67)

This was a fairly clear strategy which left the mother in little doubt that her competence was in question. Other more subtle methods included what one mother described as 'the look' of withering disapproval. Another mother described the unspoken disapproval that she received when she initially seemed unwilling to carry out certain aspects of her child's care:

'Because he'd been burned ... and there was a few times I would say, "Look, could you maybe change him or could you give him a wash ... I'm frightened". And they were looking at me as if to say ... Well, you're his mum, are you so stupid you don't know what to do?' (#15, p. 33)

Parents could also feel that their competence was being undermined when their understandings or perspectives were disregarded or belittled by hospital staff. One mother expressed a common view when she said:

'One of the things that really annoys me is when you're asked your opinion ... you're asked about something and say whatever it is and think, "They're not believing a word I'm saying, they're taking no notice of what I'm saying".' (#13, p. 20)

When the professional explanation conflicts with a parent's account of events there is a knowledge value differential which is weighted against the parent. One mother whose baby had severe respiratory difficulties culminating in apnoeic attacks described this process. Having been repeatedly questioned regarding her baby's history, she had lost confidence in her own knowledge of her child:

'I really started to question my judgement, because all the doctors kept asking me if he had been perfectly healthy before, and he had been and he'd had all his regular check-ups. The more people starting asking me the question ... Was he perfectly all right?, in *my mind* implying that he couldn't *possibly* have been. I started to think, I haven't noticed this ... and my judgement counts for nothing, I must just be the worst mother that's ever been.' (#17, pp. 15–16)

It is possible that in situations such as this, where the child's medical condition is the prime focus of professional attention, that parental knowledge is seen to be at its least reliable, for the parent is in the position of entering a field of discourse where professional knowledge and professional language is the accepted currency. For example, a nurse might well find it difficult to evaluate the importance or seriousness of signs and symptoms reported by parents such as the child being 'just no right'.

EXCLUSION AND ALIENATION

There were certain aspects of being a live-in parent which parents found to be difficult; common themes of exclusion and alienation run through the various aspects of parenting in public. When parents give up some of the responsibility for the care of their child, they are excluded from both important decision-making processes and from giving the care which is an integral part of being a parent. When parents feel that their competence is being questioned they may also feel excluded from their child's care and also alienated from the wider community of 'good' parents to which they had previously felt that they belonged. Parents who feel that their moral character as parents is being questioned sense a similar alienation within a system which values particular attributes and characteristics of the 'good mother'.

Nurses' Caring Practices: The Connecting and the Confirming

As the study sought to discover the nature of the parents' relationships with paediatric nurses, the parents were asked to describe encounters with nurses which they had either appreciated and valued or conversely, which they had perceived negatively. I want to finish by describing some of the ways in which the parents described their positive experiences of nurses and the approaches and practices of nurses who they felt had been particularly supportive, caring and helpful. I will also explain how these nurses' caring practices helped to minimise the feelings of exclusion and alienation that parents could come to feel.

Finding Time, Taking Time and Spending Time

Nurses would 'find the time' or 'take their time' or 'spend the time' to help parents or to be with them when they needed someone. One parent described this in relation to her daughter having her medicine:

'They tried to coax her for 10 minutes to take this medicine, they stood very patiently and said "Alice, it'll make you feel better" and ... and I thought after that, What patience! ... they *spent time* you know, they didn't give you a minute and then force it, they gave time ...' (#14, pp. 16–17)

This 'taking time' was also described by other mothers:

'Sally is awfully good with her. She'll sit and talk to her, play with her, sit her up or fix her pillows ... you don't get many nurses that'll do that Philip, 'cos they've not got the time, but she finds time to do it.' (#5, p. 10)

'Taking time' for parents and children confirms for parents that they are not merely names on a Kardex or bodies by a bed but that they are being acknowledged and confirmed as persons, and that their needs, regardless of how 'trivial' these may seem in relation to others, are also important. Parents also appreciated nurses who found and took the time to talk with them about what *the parent* felt was important or who helped them to express their feelings openly and who would genuinely listen in an accepting and non-judgemental way. One mother explained this:

'I suppose that it's somebody that doesn't mind me talking and mentioning all the things and somebody who explains everything to me ... they would all say don't be embarrassed, just if you want to cry just sit there and cry cos you have to get it out.' (#17, pp. 22, 39)

FRIENDLINESS AND WARMTH

Nurses who were warm and friendly in their approaches were also appreciated and often actively sought out by parents. One mother described how nurses' friendliness helped her to feel less alienated and excluded and to regain some of her sense of personhood:

'If there's a friendlier approach you appreciate it more. You're a person then, not just this mother, a parent.' (#13, p. 29)

Another mother described how she particularly valued such approaches at a particularly traumatic time:

'My wee girl had her operation last Monday and I was upset and all the nurses was round me and giving me cups of tea and reassuring me and everything.' (#26, Mother #2, pp. 67–8)

Nurses who were warm and friendly helped to confirm and support parents' sense of both parenthood and personhood not only on an individual level, but by helping to create a ward atmosphere which was more accepting and relaxed, and where parents could more easily 'be themselves' and where parenting in public was consequently less difficult.

SHOWING AN INTEREST

Parents made a special mention of nurses who 'showed an interest' both in them and in their child. This seemed to be a way of describing nurses who were alert and vital in their interactions with the families as opposed to those who might be carrying out similar work but who might seem to be merely 'going through the motions'. One mother described this:

'They took an interest. I mean there's ones that can stand and chat to you, I don't mean that kind ... but the nurses that have took an interest in Alan, have seen to him, they have went over and spoke to him, they *spoke*, they've actually took time and spoke.'

Another mother described how she felt that this showing an interest was a part of the wider context of caring. She had gone to her room feeling unwell and:

'When I came down later there were three nurses came up and asked how I was ... and you know it was lovely ... it was just a bit of caring, just a nice thought really for them to come and ask ... just a bit of interest as well isn't it?' (#2, pp. 23–4)

Parents appreciated and valued nurses who 'showed an interest' or 'took an interest' in both them and their child, for such expressions of interest and concern helped to establish a sense of connectedness between nurse and parent. As one parent noted:

'Some of these nurses, they just click.' (Mother #4, Int #27, p. 53)

Where the parents felt this sense of connectedness with nurses, then concerns and problems could become shared and validated as important. When interest and concern were absent, however, parents' sense of isolation and alienation could be heightened as evidenced by the comments of some parents that 'No one really understands what this is like'.

Supporting, Coaxing, Encouraging and Giving Hope

Another theme which ran through parents' positive accounts of nurses' practices was their appreciation of nurses who supported and coaxed them, giving hope and encouragement. One father's account of his son's serious scalding and subsequent period in the intensive care unit was notable for the number of references that he made to encouraging his son to fight for his life and encouraging other members of his family to hope for the best rather than accept that his son might not survive. This father particularly appreciated nurses who shared his sense of fighting optimism and who would offer hope and encouragement:

'I was just crying at the cot there and holding his hand and praying and saying to him, "Fight it!" and the nurse that was there, she comforted me and said, "Just keep hoping and it'll be all right, he's going to be all right".' (#18, pp. 55–6)

Another mother felt that she had gained strength from the nurses who were so supportive towards her and who had really 'got behind' her baby in his fight:

'There are certain nurses who have cared for him quite often and I feel really care about him ... obviously not as much as I do but who are really behind him ... basically they keep your spirits up, they've kept mine up ...' (#17, p. 22)

Giving of Themselves

Two parents commented on nurses who had given of their own time, over and above their allocated span of duty:

'There was a student who worked on the first bad day and I'll never forget that. She was sitting her exams, but when they thought that he had brain damage ... she was here an extra hour ... she was an awfully good nurse I felt.' (#18, p. 39)

'Like today, there was one nurse who was actually off duty and there was Jill and another little boy and she had bought a video and crisps and things ... Jill was asleep as it happened but she took the little boy to her flat ... that's how good they are.' (#27, pp. 49–50)

These nurses were giving more of themselves than their contracted hours and were willing to make more of a commitment to the children and their parents than might have been written down on the child's nursing care plan. This is also a good illustration of Gadow's (1980) argument, that the professional and the personal qualities of the nurse cannot be artificially separated, as they are inextricably bound together.

CONCLUSION

There were many aspects of nurses' practice which live-in parents valued and appreciated. They wanted to be allowed to speak freely and to be carefully listened to, they wanted to be allowed to express their feelings and emotions in an accepting atmosphere and to have matters relating to their child's care and treatment explained to them in a way that they could understand. They wanted nurses to be genuinely interested in both themselves and in their child, and to express this interest through a warm, friendly and unhurried relationship. They wanted to be involved in their child's care but also to be offered choices as to what they wished to do or not to do and generally to have their needs as parents recognised and responded to.

Nurses whose caring practices addressed these needs were helping live-in parents to 'parent in public'. They were acknowledging, and appropriately enhancing, not diminishing, the parents' sense of their responsibility for their child. They were showing concern and interest for both the parent and the child in ways which confirmed rather than excluded the parent. They were keeping parents informed of and involved in their child's care, thus minimising the parent's sense of alienation and exclusion. They also recognised that, if parents were to be a source of encouragement for their child, they too needed to be given hope and encouragement. Through such caring practices, nurses could help parents to make the transition from normal parenting to 'parenting in public'.

While it would be premature to draw firm conclusions from research which is still in progress, my analysis to date does suggest that nurses and parents may have discrepant perspectives regarding 'what it is like' to be a live-in parent. Some nurses suggest that live-in parents can be helped to adapt to hospital by encouraging them to 'do whatever it is that they would normally do for the child at home', but the parents' accounts show that the hospital-as-home analogy is very difficult for them to sustain. I believe that this study will help nurses to develop a greater understanding of how live-in parents experience being in hospital with their child. Before we presume the arrogance to teach, we must first have the humility to be able to learn. When we make ourselves more open to the experiences and understandings of the parents of the hospitalised child, we will have moved further towards a climate of genuinely shared care.

ACKNOWLEDGEMENT

I gratefully acknowledge the award of a Cow & Gate Paediatric Nursing Scholarship which enabled me to present this work at the International Paediatric Nursing Down Under Conference in Sidney, Australia in 1990.
Philip Darbyshire.

REFERENCES

Adamson E F and Hull D (1984) *Nursing Sick Children*. Edinburgh: Churchill Livingstone.
Anderson J M (1981) The social construction of illness experience: families with a chronically-ill child. *Journal of Advanced Nursing*, **6**, 427–34.
Gadow S (1980) Existential advocacy: philosophical foundation of nursing. In Spicker S F and Gadow S (Eds) *Nursing: Images and Ideals*. New York: Springer Publishing Co.
Hayes V E and Knox J E (1984) The experience of stress in parents of children hospitalised with long-term disabilities. *Journal of Advanced Nursing*, **9**, 333–41.
Heidegger M (1962) *Being and Time*. Oxford: Blackwell.
Knafl K A, Cavallari C A and Dixon D M (1988) *Paediatric Hospitalisation: Family and Nurse Perspectives*. London: Scott, Foresman.
Meadow R (1969) The captive mother. *Archives of Disease in Childhood*, **44**(235), 362–7.

Robertson J (1962) *Hospitals and Children: A Parent's-Eye View*. London: Victor Gollancz.
Robinson C A and Thorne S (1984) Strengthening family 'interference'. *Journal of Advanced Nursing*, **9**(6), 597–602.
Silverman D (1987) *Communication and Medical Practice: Social Relations in the Clinic*. London: Sage.

20

Preparing Children for Hospital

Edward Alan Glasper and Margaret Thompson

Much has been written on the effect of a hospital admission on a child. That the deleterious effect of such an admission was recognised prior to the opening of the first British Children's Hospital in 1852 is surprising and was voiced as a reason for not having children's hospitals. However, the early children's hospitals built in the decade following the opening of the Hospital for Sick Children, Great Ormond Street were happy places full of parents' and children's laughter.

It should be remembered that these early children's hospitals were built in the pre-Nightingale era and prior to the professionalisation of nursing. The Nightingale tradition changed subtly the dynamics of the children's hospitals and military principles developed at Scutari began to be applied. The move away from essentially lay care and the development of professional paediatric nursing care had some disadvantages, namely the gradual exclusion of parents from the direct participation in care. This eventually resulted in the establishment of strict visiting hours where parents were prohibited from visiting at a time convenient to them. Some hospitals only allowed parents to visit once a week or less often.

It is ironic that the current move towards day surgery in childhood, first reported in 1909 by Nicoll, was founded on the premise that the separation of a child from his mother may be harmful. The psychological consequences of a hospital admission have traditionally been ignored when considering the effects of hospital. Until the advent of antibiotics, infection was the only contender in 'the effects of admission stakes'. The often irrational fear of infection made the question of visiting hours a thorny issue. In the Southampton Children's Hospital, for example, at least up until the outbreak of World War I, visiting was allowed from 2–4 pm daily, except Sundays. As the century progressed, it became confined to 1 hour on Wednesday and Sunday afternoons, and then in 1947 was banned completely. Visiting was recommenced in 1950 on a limited basis and parents had to wear face masks!

The recognition that psychological trauma might be perpetrated on children during their hospital stay came about slowly, and in the United Kingdom owes much to the work of John Bowlby and James Robertson. Their work was instrumental in providing the precursors necessary for the creating of the working party under the chairmanship of Sir Harry Platt which reported on the 'Welfare of Children in Hospital' in 1959. The Platt Report recommended sweeping changes in the way children were managed in hospital, particularly in relation to the possible negative psychological effects of a hospital stay. The strict visiting regimes of the pre-Platt era where nurses took over care completely during a child's admission, undermined the role of the parent. This left parents feeling helpless and inadequate. This unhappy state of affairs did not improve substantially following the publication of the Platt Report and the role of parents continued to be denigrated. The creation of the National Association for The Welfare of Children in Hospital (NAWCH) in 1961 accelerated the pace of change and must take much of the credit for the reforms which subsequently took place. This pressure group became the champion of families as consumers of health care. The emancipation of families with children in hospital has been slow and this is regrettable, but the concept of family-centred care is now beginning to gain universal approval.

THE GROWTH OF SURGICAL DAY CARE

The initiatives generated by the Platt Report and NAWCH did eventually do much to mitigate the psychological hazards of an in-patient stay for children. The momentum of change was prohibited from petering out by the concerted efforts of many individuals. While the report recommended that children should not be admitted unless absolutely necessary there was little embodied within the text to promote the concept of day care. This was eventually highlighted by the Court Report in 1976 but the idea spread slowly, and more than a decade later there were still regions not participating in this venture. Politicians of all political parties have described the health services for children as a potent investment in the country's future. Day care surgery provides the minimum of disruption to the family unit and is, therefore, a powerful weapon in the prevention of potential psychological trauma caused by an in-patient stay.

Some hospitals such as the University Hospital at Southampton have purpose-built day surgical units for children. Such units may cater for minor general surgery, orthopaedic surgery, oncology and endoscopy. Day units function in a variety of ways and some keep patients for a full day prior to discharge and others only half a day. For day units to run successfully, a paediatric community nursing service is desirable. Where such a service exists it forms an essential link in the seamless web of the primary health care team and the tertiary service provided by the hospitals. Greater links can only be facilitated when paediatric community nurses are available as part of the child health team. Without the provision of such services, the operative management of children undergoing day surgery is fraught with difficulties. The paediatric community nurses form the caring link between the hospital and home.

Family preparation for day and in-patient surgery may be important in reducing the psychological effects of hospitalisation.

PREPARING CHILDREN FOR HOSPITAL

Modern child health care services require integration between hospital and community. The service should provide for the child as a whole and should meet the social, emotional and spiritual needs of children and their families. The growth of paediatric pre-admission programmes throughout the United Kingdom represents one facet only of this integrated service. Since the publication of the Platt Report, paediatric nurses have developed a reputation for endeavouring to improve the care of their patients and families. Attempting to protect children from the stresses of hospital admission may be partially facilitated through the provision of pre-admission programmes.

Parents of children about to be admitted to hospital hunger for information, but Miller (1979) suggests that people have different coping styles and some seek information while others avoid it. Maddison (1977) among others, has highlighted the importance of seeking the opinion of consumers. Such consumer surveys will invariably demonstrate that parents are in favour of further information. Such information may be transmitted under the auspices of a pre-admission programme. Rodin (1983) has indicated that children who are prepared for hospital procedures cope better than children who have not been prepared. There are still many procedures to which children are subject in hospital which may cause anxiety. Children dread hospital procedures. Needles, tests, anaesthetics and even death may all be associated in the mind of a child with hospital. The benefits of parents may be incalculable when considering methods of reducing anxiety in children about to undergo stressful procedures. Mellish (1969) has pointed out that successful preparation for surgery depends on the attitude of the surgeon, anaesthetists, nurses and ward clerks, etc. He has given credibility to the statement that surgical success cannot be measured through intact wounds alone but must also include intact emotions. It is intact emotions which are the prime motivating source for the development of preparatory programmes for children and parents. It must be emphasised that the child is part of an indivisible unit called the family. Any preparatory techniques employed to prepare a child for hospital must include the other members of the family, in particular the parents. All parents suffer from anxiety when their child is admitted to hospital. Even medical and paramedical personnel and their spouses have been found to be no less anxious despite all their accumulated knowledge. Parental preparation is extremely important and may perhaps be the most important component of any family preparatory programme. Parental reaction crosses socio-economic barriers and it has been suggested that a child's psychological sequelae to hospitalisation are directly related to the parents' emotional reaction. Parental contagion is a major source of concern to those individuals planning any form of supportive programme.

EMOTIONAL CONTAGION

Most children are dependent on their parents' emotional support for help in coping with anxieties. The simplest anxiety is that produced by contagion. This is exemplified in the child who becomes frightened when he is in close contact with frightened adults. If those whose role is one of protection become frightened themselves, then this can be transmitted to the child as quickly as if it were a highly infectious disease. It may be hypothesised that parents who are frightened are unable to contribute to the psychological welfare of a child who is undergoing a stressful procedure.

Campbell (1957) has discussed how emotional states in mothers can be communicated to their children. An investigation conducted in a well baby clinic showed that significantly more infants of mothers who received anxiety-arousing instructions cried before immunisation injections than infants of mothers who received neutral instruction. It is thus important to prepare parents as well as children for stressful events if parental anxiety is mirrored in children. It has been observed that some parents can become frightened about the welfare of their child and that sometimes to the professional observers their reaction appears out of proportion to the event at hand. The quality of interaction between an authoritative person such as a nurse and a hospitalised child's mother can lower the mother's level of stress and can produce changes in the mother's definition of the situation. This in turn has a demonstrable effect on the child's level of stress, producing a change in his social, psychological and physiological behaviour.

Paediatric nurses must learn to recognise the natural resource they have at their disposal in the form of parents and guardians. They must be perceived as equal partners in the traditional nurse–doctor–patient relationship. To this end the National Association for the Welfare of Children in Hospital has committed much of its energies.

If, as has been suggested, a child's psychological sequelae to hospital are related to the parents' emotional reactions, rather than the severity of the trauma suffered, this must be considered when planning any interaction. Mahaffy (1965) demonstrated the benefits of having one nurse attached to a family unit in the pre- and post-operative periods. This early account of primary nursing is interesting in that it highlights the benefits of improved communication between a family unit and a professional.

HOW CAN CHILDREN BE PREPARED FOR HOSPITAL ADMISSION?

Smith (1986) believes that the emotional factor may be an even greater source of concern than the child's physical condition during a hospital admission. On the premise that this may be true, a number of different strategies have been developed to help children and their families cope with hospital admission.

Preparation in the Community

By the age of 5 years, 25 per cent of children will have had a stay in hospital, and one third of these admissions will be caused by accidents. Hospitalisation is, therefore, not an uncommon childhood experience. Brett (1983) has indicated that preparation should begin in the classroom and feature as a component of general education. The needs of children vary with age. It has been suggested that children's fears change with age and cognitive development. Miller (1979) has stated that preschool children are especially frightened of noises, strange persons or events. Schoolchildren are fearful of bodily injury, disease and separation among others.

Vernon *et al.* (1960) have collected data which confirm the hypothesis that children between the ages of 6 months and 4 years of age are most likely to be upset following hospitalisation. This would suggest that preparation might begin in nursery school or play group. Families come in all shapes and sizes, good, bad and indifferent. All appear to profit from a modicum of preparation. Any preparation will be intimately concerned with stress inoculation. Meng and Zastowny (1981) have likened stress inoculation to medical inoculations and indicate that any preparatory programmes should achieve this goal. Stress inoculation may be successfully carried out in school classroom situations and the benefit of this type of approach is that all children can be prepared for the eventuality of being admitted to hospital. The school-age child has a potential greater than his preschool colleagues for coping positively with hospitalisation. This arises because such children are more able to reason, describe and verbalise their feelings than younger children. The school classroom may, therefore, be an excellent environment in which to teach children the skills necessary to cope with hospitalisation. Universal preparation for all children facilitated through preschool or school-based programmes may not be the panacea imagined. Young children are susceptible to fantasy and misunderstanding. Anxiety may even be provoked if ideas of separation from home and family are introduced unnecessarily. Any preparation for hospital must be accurately and sensitively carried out with due prominence being given to the age and level of cognitive development of the child. The role of the primary health care team should also be considered when planning preparatory programmes for children and families. Seventy-five per cent of children under 16 years of age see their GP four or five times in any one year. It is obvious, therefore, that GPs and health visitors are in a good position to supply information about hospitals, especially for elective admissions.

PREPARING CHILDREN AND THEIR FAMILIES FOR HOSPITAL ADMISSION USING WRITTEN AND VISUAL MATERIAL

Rodin (1983) among others has shown that written and illustrated material can be effective in relieving the stresses of hospitalisation. Such authors use highly specific information and they suggest that specificity is required in order to produce accurate expectations. There are a number of books written for children about hospital. They can be read as part of a general educational strategy or can be used by parents and others prior to a child's admission – as always some are good and some are bad. At best they can be perceived as an aid only, but they do fulfil a role as part of an overall preparatory package.

More specifically, it has become custom and practice for many children's units to send out written material in the mail usually with the letter of admission, naturally to save on postage. Such written material in common with the books may be good, bad or indifferent. Some attempt to communicate with the parent and some with the child, some do both. The objective is to provide information, and studies which have examined this reveal much dissatisfaction. Lack of information is the prime cause of anxiety. Anxious parents are less capable of providing support and security for a child during a stressful event. Clearly, attempts to prepare parents and thus children are worthwhile and this explains the growth of mailed information for families.

Parents know their children better than anyone else and should be involved where possible in preparing children for hospital. In the absence of information, some parents say nothing to their children and the first the child knows of his admission is when he walks through the portals of the hospital.

Pre-admission leaflets sent by the hospital for elective admissions vary tremendously in quality. Many are not specifically written for children and their parents, and few give concrete information which helps parents prepare their child for hospital.

Harris (1981) has revealed a desire among parents for more information. She has suggested that specific information sheets appertaining to individual operations be included in the mail-out to parents. In this way the children could be prepared for surgery through the parents who are best placed to achieve this. The children's unit at the University Hospital, Southampton has produced a number of such information sheets.

Visual Material

Some hospitals have produced video films or tape slide programmes, which can be shown to parents and children. The effectiveness of such programmes is such that they are increasingly being developed and used throughout the United Kingdom. Films produced for television may have a general effect in raising the awareness of preparing children for hospital. The cost of producing professionally edited video tapes is prohibitively expensive for most units and they date very quickly. Tape/slide programmes are easier and cheaper to produce with the added advantage that they can be updated periodically with little difficulty.

Pre-admission Programmes

In recent years the various forms of pre-admission preparation for children have concentrated on the development of the so-called pre-admission programmes. Such programmes are conducted either in out-patient departments when children come with their families for an initial consultation prior to admission, or in the hospital at a set time, usually a week prior to admission, but following the out-patient consultation. The changes found in children's behaviour after hospitalisation underpin the growth of such formal pre-admission programmes. There are few National Health Service hospitals providing routine minor surgery which have the financial resources to run pre-admission programmes, but the number is growing. The commonest type of programme in the United Kingdom is conducted in hospital, often at weekends. Jones (1988) found that Saturday mornings were the primary choice of parents in the Southampton area when considering the most suitable day for attending a pre-admission programme. This led to the formation of the Saturday Morning Club, based within the paediatric unit at Southampton General Hospital. In this respect the Club resembled the Saturday Morning Project based at the Queen's Medical

Centre in Nottingham. The project at Nottingham was the first in the United Kingdom, being formed in 1982. The format established by Nottingham has been emulated in a number of children's units, including Southampton. Invitations to the programmes are often sent out in the mail with all the other information usually one week prior to admission. The programmes often consist of a tape/slide presentation followed by a visit to the ward to which the child will be admitted. Therapeutic play programmes and biscuits and juice for the children complete the morning's programme. While the children are playing the parents have coffee, and some units have produced video recordings which portray the lives of children as they pass through hospital. Such recordings may be detailed and include sections on pre- and post-operative management, but they date very quickly. A major benefit of the programmes is that they facilitate interaction between hospital staff and parents, who are encouraged to ask programme workers about their child's admission. In Nottingham the children are given a play-pack at the end of the programme consisting of a paper theatre hat, paints, name band, mask and badge, plus a cotton theatre gown which parents are asked to return on admission.

A factor of great importance for the successful conquest of pre-operative anxiety is the amount of pre-operative preparation given to patients and their families. This is especially true of parents if a reduction in the contagion effect is sought. The pre-admission programmes attempt to achieve this but they have yet to be critically evaluated. The hospital-based pre-admission programmes are not without marginal costs and this may explain their relatively slow growth in the United Kingdom.

The use of volunteer staff should not be overlooked especially in the light of raised parental awareness and expectations. Such volunteers may provide the key for accelerated growth especially in times of financial austerity.

Admitting children to hospital prior to surgery in an attempt to prepare them for what may be a stressful experience has shown positive results. Fassler (1980) indicates that a combination of emotional support and information appertaining to the admission appears to be an effective method of reducing pre-operative anxiety.

The role of theatre personnel in the preparation of children has only recently been given prominence. The growing awareness of the need for infection control practices, following the emergence of antibiotic-resistant bacteria, resulted in the decision to build new district general hospitals with operating theatres well away from the main hospital traffic with clearly defined clean and dirty areas and restricted entry. The consequences of these strategies were far-reaching and in many ways isolated theatre staff from their patients. The difficulties of getting changed to visit patients and their families in the clinical areas effectively prohibit coming and going. The recognition that post-operative anxiety is reduced by better preparation for the ensuing stressful situation has been addressed by some theatre personnel. Bonner (1986) has demonstrated the value of pre-operative visits by theatre nurses and the use of pre-operative therapeutic play programmes in overcoming operation anxiety.

It is apparent that the stress of hospital can be alleviated by giving children and their families adequate information before, during and after anxiety-provoking experiences. Clearly different preparatory strategies must be employed if one is to prepare all children and their families for such events. The differing stages of child development must be addressed if any degree of success is anticipated. Young children especially require more than just verbal explanations. Appropriate child-centred methods such as therapeutic play, story books, games, role play and puppet shows can be successfully employed.

Planning a Pre-admission Programme

Although the role of parents has increased in recent years, for various reasons parents have not taken or have not been allowed to take full advantage of what appear to be new opportunities to become involved in the care of their child during a hospital stay. Pre-admission programmes attempt to exploit that natural resource that exists within all families' desire to help children cope with anxiety-provoking situations.

Utilising the skill of parents in this way helps to establish the trend of perceiving partners in the traditional nurse–doctor–patient relationship. Inspired by the pre-admission programmes at The Hospital for Sick Children, Toronto, and Nottingham, the staff of the paediatric unit in Southampton established a working party to plan and initiate a similar programme. The working party included the course tutor of the NNEB programme at the local College of Further Education. She not only wanted to include the concept of pre-admission programmes in her teaching syllabus, but also offered the use of two student nursery nurses per week during term time to act as helpers on Saturday mornings during the period of the pre-admission visit which was scheduled to run from 10.00 am to 12 midday. The group identified three stages that should be included in any pre-admission programme.

Therapeutic Play

There are considerable differences between adult and child cognitive processes. Many adults use inappropriate language when explaining aspects of treatment to children. This is especially true of hospital staff who are often confronted by a variety of children's explanations of illness. What may be an appropriate explanation for an 8-year-old child may be wholly inappropriate for a 4-year-old. Because children's thought processes and understanding are not just miniature versions of adults' thought and comprehension, child health care workers should be able to offer a variety of explanations that are consistent with the child's level of cognitive development. The 2–7-year-old child often gives life to inanimate objects and this animistic trait can be usefully adopted when discussing aspects of illness with this age group.

Preparation that involves only verbal explanations is insufficient for those children who have immature verbal and comprehension skills. Clearly, methods of preparation which operate at a child's cognitive level may be much more suitable.

Swayed by this argument, the working party decided that a range of therapeutic play material was essential to the success of the enterprise. The acquisition of specialist toys was augmented by the purchase of two Zaadie Dolls, one male and the other female. These dolls, one of a new generation of anatomical models developed specifically for children in hospital, are cloth-covered rag dolls. The dolls have three layers which peel apart using velcro fastenings to expose the vital organs

(N.B. The dolls have several faces and the sleeping face must always be in place before they are opened.) The simple yet effective design facilitates their use among a wide range of children admitted for a variety of surgical and non-surgical procedures. It is believed that children are able to express fear and anxiety through play, and a commitment to this belief is manifested through the increasing numbers of play specialists who are employed in children's wards. Children have a paucity of information about their internal organs. It is widely believed that children's perceptions of their anatomical structures parallel the stages of intellectual development. Any preparatory programme should take this into account. The programme at Southampton utilises Zaadie Dolls, but it must be pointed out that the use of such dolls has yet to be fully evaluated. Nevertheless, when discussing with a child certain procedures involving part of his anatomy, especially if he cannot normally see, touch or hear it, it is necessary to use things he can see, touch, hear and relate to concretely.

The dolls can be catheterised and the female doll is equipped with an injection site on the left thigh and is recommended for use with diabetic children. The female doll also has a removable wig and is, therefore, useful to illustrate hair loss in children receiving chemotherapy. (Further information regarding the Zaadie Dolls may be obtained from the Zaadie Company, 836 Chelmsford Street, Lowell, Ma, 01851, USA.)

Toys that encourage interactive play are now freely available and some have been designed for medico-nursing type play. The 'play people' hospital toys are excellent as are the traditional doctors sets which contain stethoscope, auriscope and fake syringes.

During the early stages of the programme, a number of nurses' old, redundant uniforms and doctors' white coats were transformed into new miniature versions for children. The resulting dressing-up game component of the programme has proved most successful with the children. Through such play, it is believed that children are able to express fear and anxiety. The medium of play knows no boundaries and if it allows children to act out their fears and fantasies, it will only be constrained by that imagination. It is interesting that dressing-up play continues to be popular despite the fact that nursing and medical staff no longer wear uniforms at Southampton.

Narrative Slide Presentation

The flexibility of a narrative slide presentation was considered the most effective method of addressing parental concerns about their child's forthcoming hospital admission. Slides are easy to produce and have the added advantage of being cheap and simple to update. A simple format was adopted consisting of sequential slides covering the hospital stay from admission to discharge. Ideally, a set script should be followed by all participants, but the writing of such proved difficult. An agreed informal approach covering all aspects of hospital admissions was adopted. It was believed that this would ensure full child/parental participation and augment the information mailed to the families in the post.

Tour of Relevant Clinical Areas

Tours of clinical areas by prospective patients and their families generate mixed responses among professionals. After careful consideration the members of the working party agreed that one component of the pre-admission programme should take the form of a conducted tour. The differing needs of the groups (in-patients and day cases) dictated that there should be two tours, prospective in-patients and their families being conducted around the unit, while the prospective day patients and their families watched the appropriate slide presentation and vice versa. The tour was planned to incorporate a visit to the theatre complex where parents could ascertain their role if they wished to accompany their children to the anaesthetic room.

FUNDING

Resource management and income generation leave little room for altruism. The harsh economic climate which prevails in the health service today presents special difficulties for nurses planning innovative programmes for specific client groups. Despite severe cuts, it is sometimes possible to present a cogent case to managers for increases in funding linked to quality of care. If it can be argued that such programmes increase quality of care, then the small amounts of money necessary to fund such innovations can be made available. The amount of staff required was deemed to be two paediatric nurses and one play specialist. This level of staffing was considered to be the minimum number to ensure the viability of the programme. The use of volunteer works in such programmes is extremely valuable and children's League of Friends departments are always worth approaching. Other volunteers may be recruited from within clinical units. Maintaining a steady supply of staff to run programmes, especially on Saturday mornings, is not easy and is a constant source of worry to programme organisers.

ATTENDANCE

Ensuring maximum attendance proved difficult. An evaluation of the Saturday Morning Programme funded under the auspices of a Which? Jubilee Research Award demonstrated that for some parents attendance was impossible for a variety of reasons. Attempts to improve attendance through the mailing of specially designed invitations and information sheets proved partially successful. The key to universal preparation or arranged admissions almost certainly lies in the out-patient department. The out-patient department may provide the key to the successful preparation of many more families as most children for elective surgery are seen there prior to admission. The quality standards of care embodied within the NAWCH recommendations highlight the benefits of preparatory programmes and it should be possible for purchaser units to insist on their incorporation into any provider unit contract.

REFERENCES

Bonner M L (1986) Can my friend go with me? *Nursing Times*, October, 75–6.

Brett A (1983) Preparing children for hospitalisation – a classroom teaching approach. *Journal of School Nursing*, **53**(9), November, 561–3.

Campbell E H (1957) The effects of mothers' anxiety on infants' behaviour – a dissertation presented to the Faculty of the Graduate School of Yale University. Unpublished doctorial thesis.

Fassler D (1980) Reducing pre-operative anxiety in children – Information versus emotional support. *Patient Counselling & Health Education*, January.

Harris P J (1981) Children in hospital. Preparation of parents and their children for a planned hospital admission. *Nursing Times*, **17**, 7 October, 44–6.

Jones P (1988) Determining the need for a preadmission programme in Southampton. Unpublished undergraduate nursing research project. University of Southampton.

Maddison M (1977) Consumer survey of paediatric wards. *Australian Nurses Journal*, **6**(1), 27–8.

Mahaffy P R (1965) The effects of hospitalisation on children admitted for tonsillectomy and adenoidectomy. *Nursing Research*, **14**(1), 12–19.

Mellish P W R (1969) Preparation of a child for hospitalisation and surgery. *Pediatric Clinics of North America*, **16**(3), August.

Meng A and Zastowny T (1981) Preparation for hospitalisation: A stress inoculation training program for parents and children. *Maternal–Child Nursing Journal*, 87–94.

Miller S (1979) Children's fears – A review of the literature with implications for nursing research and practice. *Nursing Research*, **28**(4), July/August.

Nicoll J H (1909) *British Medical Journal*, **2**, 753.

Rodin J (1983) *Will this Hurt?* London: Royal College of Nursing.

Smith R M (1986) *Anesthesia for Infants and Children*. 3rd edition. St Louis: C V Mosby.

Vernon D T A *et al.* (1960) Changes in children's behaviour after hospitalisation. *American Journal of Diseases of Children*, **111**, June.

21

The Development of a Paediatric Community Service

Peggy Gow and Grethe Ridgway

'If you take away a sick child from its parent you break its heart immediately'.
(George Armstrong, Proprietor of a London Dispensary for the Infant Poor in 1777)
(Lightwood, 1956)

The first paediatric home nursing scheme, as it might be recognised today, was introduced in Rotherham in 1949. Following a particularly severe winter in 1947, with a high death toll among infants, two Queen's Nurses were appointed to set up a home nursing service. Working with General Practitioners they set out to nurse children who it was considered could be nursed at home. These numbered 455 babies and children and resulted in 4,151 visits in all (Gillet, 1954). The marked reduction in infant deaths from gastroenteritis was attributed to this new service.

Further schemes followed, the two most notable being set up in 1954 in Paddington and in Birmingham. In 1959 the Platt Report advocated the care of sick children at home wherever possible, pointing out the potential adverse psychological effects on children of hospital admissions. A common aim of these early schemes was to prevent hospital admission whenever possible, facilitate early discharge and to support, advise and teach parents. Muriel Campbell, a member of the 1968 Edinburgh Home Care Programme, stated that she has 'the best job in the National Health Service' (Campbell, 1986).

Since the sweeping changes in the care and management of sick children recommended by Platt, the cumulative effect of the Court Report in 1974, the Cumberlege Report of 1986 and the sterling work of the National Association for the Welfare of Children in Hospital (NAWCH) now known as Action for Sick Children, have all contributed towards a growing interest in Paediatric Community Nursing Services.

However, despite the pioneers of such services, it is only in the last ten years that we have seen much growth in their introduction and development on a national basis. Mark Whiting's study in 1988 (Whiting, 1988) demonstrated that over forty District Health Authorities had some sort of Paediatric Community Service.

More recently, the recognition being afforded to paediatric community nurses has been reflected in the English National Board's validation of District Nursing Courses (Langlands, 1990) and in the Department of Health's Report on Nurse Prescribing (DoH, 1989).

These developments represent a major step forward in the widely-held belief that children should have the right to be cared for at home by an appropriately trained nurse, thereby ensuring that the individual needs of each child can be met.

An example of the way in which a community paediatric nursing service has developed is described below.

SOUTHAMPTON PAEDIATRIC SERVICE

The idea for the service was formed jointly by John Atwell, Paediatric Surgical Consultant, Ian MacGregor, Medical Officer of Health, and Isobel Ames, Senior Nursing Officer Community.

The original concept of the Southampton Service which was set up in 1969 by Mr Atwell (Atwell and Gow, 1985) was to care for children in the post-operative period following day surgery as initially the scheme was linked to the development of a day Surgical Unit.

Today's team, which consists of six sisters and a diabetic sister, provides care across a wide spectrum of conditions from birth to 16 years. The team is based at Southampton General Hospital but funded by the Community Health Services.

The Paediatric Service covers an area within approximately a 15 mile radius of the hospital, with a child population of 77,460 (0–16). 202 General Practitioners, 94 health visitors and 69 general trained district nurses work within the District. Southampton and its environs include both urban and rural settings, ranging from bed and breakfast accommodation to the large detached properties of the affluent.

Day Surgery

Southampton General Hospital has a purpose-built paediatric day unit catering for a wide range of surgical specialities. The majority of children are admitted and discharged between 8.30 a.m. and 6.30 p.m., the day being divided into two operating lists. For a day unit to run successfully, good communication networks are essential. Candidates for day surgery are carefully selected and always after discussion with parents. The very success of day care surgery, which includes orchidopexies, herniotomies, circumcisions, endoscopies and minor orthopaedic cases, is dependent on the support of the Community Nursing Team. Following a pre-discharge examination by medical staff, information from the ward, along with written guidelines for the post-operative period and a contact telephone number, children are discharged home. Every child who has had a general anaesthetic is visited the following day. Nursing care, advice and support to the family are given according to the individual needs of their condition. This may include a change of dressings, removal of steristrips or sutures, advice on pain control, diet and when the child can be expected to return to school.

The children's unit is visited daily by a member of the team; other areas are visited weekly. These include ENT, the Cardiac Units, and the Special Care Baby Unit. These visits enable the concept of holistic care to be implemented, providing opportunities for the staff to meet the child and family and prepare for early discharge plans.

In 1989, improved discharge slips were developed, which include both medical and surgical patients and which will link up with Personal Child Health record books held by parents. This record book was developed for parents by the Community Unit as a multi-discipline initiative.

In Southampton, community staff carry radio telephones which link into the General Hospital and a base Health Centre. Although not able to contact members of the team directly, parents can request a message relay by telephoning the Community Nursing Office. In this way parents are able to obtain help should they be concerned about their child in between planned contacts.

An important aspect of the paediatric community nurses' role is the ability to arrange for readmission to hospital should this prove necessary.

Children with Medical Conditions

Following the success of early surgical discharge, the team have progressed to providing care to almost all sick children in their homes.

It has proved possible to reduce the hospital stay of countless sick children suffering from conditions traditionally requiring considerable periods of hospitalisation. Diverse illnesses such as diabetes and cystic fibrosis can be successfully managed at home provided sufficient support can be planned and provided. In some instances, hospital admissions can be avoided completely and most General Practitioners welcome the opportunity to provide care for children in the primary health care setting.

Although many parents provide excellent caring environments for their sick children it is recognised that some may not be physically and emotionally capable of providing all the necessary care for their child. Nurses in hospital are not expected to provide all the care themselves without help and it would be wrong to expect parents to do so. The paediatric community sister, by providing support several times a week, or even several times a day, if necessary, may enable parents to keep their child at home and be happy to do so rather than having the child admitted to a long-stay Paediatric Unit.

Within Southampton the Community Nursing Team have developed expertise in five specialist areas. These are:

1. Support to parents giving intravenous antibiotic therapy at home for children with cystic fibrosis.
2. Oxygen therapy for babies with broncho-pulmonary dysplasia.
3. Continuous enteral feeding.
4. Care of children with tracheostomies – earlier discharge of such children into the community has increased considerably.
5. Care and support to children with some form of malignancy, along with the administration of platelets and support at home for children in the terminal phase of such illnesses.

One example of the type of support provided to families is in the management of cystic fibrosis. The long-term survival rate depends on the quality of care children receive both at home and in hospital. In many long-term patients, once the lungs have become colonised with pseudomonas, regular intravenous treatment is necessary in order to reduce symptoms.

The instigation of a Portacath or vascuport providing immediate access to the intravenous administration of drugs has completely changed the lives of cystic fibrosis sufferers. A child with a vascuport can lead a near-normal life, swimming and playing games (Sidey, 1989).

Long-term maintenance care for a child with a vascuport is very simple with either the nurse or parent flushing the reservoir with a heparin solution monthly. These patients do need long-term support, but periods of hospitalisation can be drastically reduced.

Premature Infants

Following a review of medical practice in several Special Care Baby Units throughout the United Kingdom it became clear that with adequate support and supervision, early discharge could be safely and easily achieved. From the point of view of both convenience and the development of mother–child relationship, such a change clearly has advantages. (Sleath, 1989).

Along with the improved survival of prematurely-born infants there is a corresponding increasing incidence of the chronic lung disease broncho-pulmonary dysplasia. Between the ages of 6 and 18 months these babies may require supplementary oxygen in order to reach their optimum in both social and mental development. By discharging them home where the possibility of cross-infection is reduced, much can be done to alleviate stress on the family and promote normal development in the child.

Babies are discharged home with oxygen concentrators prescribed by the General Practitioner. Nasal canulae are worn which are changed weekly. A teaching programme with the family is set up before discharge. This gives parents confidence in changing the nasal canulae, passing a nasogastric tube and using the suction machine should it be required.

The safe storage, handling and refilling of the portable oxygen unit is explained, checked and reinforced by the Paediatric Community Nurses. The use of an apnoea monitor may be required, and before discharge the parents are taught how to carry out resuscitation. In the planning of a programme for discharge, a phone in the home in this instance is essential. If necessary the local Social Services Department can give assistance in providing this.

On discharge from hospital babies are followed up daily, primarily to monitor oxygen saturation levels and to check on feeding. If a steady weight increase is not maintained nasogastric feeding is commenced. Good liaison between health visitors and General Practitioners is essential and for all these babies the paediatric community sister provides the vital link between the Special Care Baby Unit and the Primary Health Care Team.

Nasogastric feeding at home is a relatively commonplace occurrence. As parents achieve competence in replacing nasogastric tubes, not only in very young children but also in small babies, some children are able to have enteral feeding at home (Holden, 1990). This is particularly important, for children with cystic fibrosis, children who fail to thrive, children undergoing intensive chemotherapy for malignant disease, and those awaiting liver transplantation.

The use of polyurethane silk (Merle) nasogastric tubes, which are changed monthly and connected to a feeding pump, is very costly. Although the feeds are prescribed by the General Practitioner, the actual cost of the pumps and the giving sets are a constant drain on Community budgets, which tend not to have been allocated the extra money required to fund these developments in the Paediatric Community Nursing Service.

Tracheostomy

For whatever reason, whether it be acute sub-glottis obstruction due to congenital abnormality or acute infection, children may need a tracheostomy.

Over the past three years many more children with tracheostomies have been discharged into the Community at a much younger age than was previously felt to be safe.

As with oxygen-dependent children, full support at home, adequate equipment and careful preparation of the family are essential. Discharge cannot take place until parents feel confident to provide 24-hour cover in care of the child. The local ambulance station is alerted and made aware of these children in case their urgent assistance is required.

The family of each 'trachy' child is provided with two suckers (one portable and one electric). They are advised to buy a listening alarm. Very young babies may at times require a more humid atmosphere than is normally found at home and provision may have to be made for this.

Parents involved in the care of a child with a tracheostomy tube are going to need support for long periods of time. Thought and planning must be given to the child with a tracheostomy in situ, starting at playschool and later school. Thankfully, many babies are extubated before reaching this age.

It is important to bear in mind that the care of a child with a tracheostomy will have a profound effect, not only on the child and its parents, but also on siblings and a sympathetic approach to the whole family is essential. (Jennings, 1989).

Care of Patients with Malignant Disease

Many different types of malignant diseases can affect children. Following brief hospital admissions, maintenance therapy can be adequately administered at home on a daily basis. A multi-disciplinary approach is maintained in Southampton through weekly meetings of community staff, social workers and playleaders with staff working in the Oncology Day Unit.

Paediatric community nurses play a vital role in caring for oncology children, both during the aggressive stage of treatment and in the terminal stage when palliative therapy is implemented. This is obviously a distressing time for all concerned and particularly so when the decision has to be taken to abandon active treatment. The support parents need at this time is immense.

Many parents now elect to nurse their children with oncological diseases at home. The aim of the paediatric community nurse at this time is not only to support the family but to enable the child to have as near normal a lifestyle as possible within the limitations of the illness. As far as possible pain is eliminated and the remaining time spent together produces a quality of life which in retrospect may cause sadness in parents but creates a sense of achievement in that they were able to care for their child at home.

In the past, a number of children had to be readmitted to hospital because of distressing bleeding. Nowadays, during the terminal phase, platelet infusions can be administered at home with a 'piriton and hydrocortisone cover', thus avoiding the need for readmission.

Before this type of treatment can be given, further training is required. In addition, the District drug policy provides guidelines on the carrying of drugs and blood products. The care of the dying child at home is only possible with full GP involvement and adequate support for the family, which will include the availability of night sitters if required, support from health visitors, social workers and other members of the family.

It is the aim of paediatric staff who are caring for a terminally ill child at home to ensure the child's death should be peaceful and within the family unit. Such an achievement is coupled with sadness and a deep sense of privilege in being able to care for that child. (BPA King's Fund, 1988).

Bereavement visits continue as long as the parents require such support, and are an essential part of the follow-up for terminal care.

Long-term Problems

Children with asthma, skin problems or severe handicap also form part of the paediatric community team's caseload. These conditions often present the greatest hardship because of the necessity for long-term commitment on the part of parents, frequently with very little help or prospect of respite care.

AN EXPANDING SERVICE

The past ten years have seen many changes and developments within paediatric community care. Possibly the greatest change has been in the amount of equipment needed to support families. An example of this is shown below:

Equipment provided for the 1949 Rotherham scheme

4 treasure cots	6 wash bowls
1 dozen sheets	6 Enamel trays 6 × 4 in
2 pillows	6 Stay-bright measures.
3 enamel pails	6 Receivers and 6 gallipots

Thermometers, rubber gloves, masks, gowns.

1989 Southampton Paediatric Community Service equipment

Radiotelephones

14 Laerdal portable suckers	3 humidifiers
3 sheepskins	12 electric suckers
2 intravenous stands	Polycare mattresses
3 Gravesby syringe drivers	2 IV IVAC syringe drivers
2 respiratory monitors	2 nebulisers
3 portable oxygen cylinders	Resuscitation Bags
Continuous feeding pumps	1/2 giving sets
Tracheostomy tubes	Suction tubes
Feeding tubes	1 pulse oximeter

Low-flow adaptor for concentrator.

Clearly, what is needed now is a more realistic approach to the funding of community nursing schemes if children with varied and complex conditions are to continue to be nursed at home with their families.

THE FUTURE

Changes in nurse education with the advent of Project 2000 Nursing Diploma Courses and technological advances in medicine, together with a rapidly changing National Health Service, are resulting in a noticeable shift towards more acutely dependent patients receiving care in their own homes.

The service provided by the Southampton community paediatric nurses is demonstrating that the majority of children's illnesses can be managed at home. The advantages for the child and family have been shown time after time.

With the increasing emphasis on the identification of health need by purchasing authorities and in the quality of health care by the Department of Health, research is now required to show whether the commonly-held belief that home care is best can be justified. The experience of the Southampton Team and the families they work with and the recent report produced by Action For Sick Children (Thornes, 1993) indicate it must be the way forward.

From a philosophical and ethical point of view, the time is now right to state positively and unequivocally that children have the right to care from a paediatric nurse at home as well as in hospital.

'What a Paediatric Community Service does is to give back to the parents, control of the care of their children and improve the quality of that care so that children and families maintain as normal a life style as possible'. (Dryden, 1989)

The need to provide equity of care for children in community services is the challenge for the future.

REFERENCES

Atwell J D and Gow M A (1985) Paediatric trained district nurse in the community: expensive luxury or economic necessity. *British Medical Journal,* **291,** 227–9.

BPA King's Fund (1988) *The Care of Dying Children and Their Families.* London: NAHA.

Campbell M (1986) Community nurse. *The British Journal of Nurses in Child Health,* **1**(10).

Department of Health (1989) *Report of the Advisory Group on Nurse Prescribing.* London: HMSO.

Dryden S (1989) Paediatric medicine in the community. *Paediatric Nursing,* November, 17–18.

Gillet J (1954) Domiciliary treatment of sick children. *Practitioner,* **172,** 281.

Holden C (1990) Home enteral feeding. *Paediatric Nursing,* July, 14.

Jennings P (1989) *Tracheostomy Care, Learning to Cope,* **1,** 13–15.

Langlands T (1990) Meeting future needs. *Paediatric Nursing,* April, 9.

Lightwood R (1956) The home care of sick children. *Practitioner,* **177,** 10.

Sidey A (1989) Intravenous home care. *Paediatric Nursing,* May, 14–15.

Sleath K (1989) Breath of life. *Nursing Times,* **85,** 44.

Thornes R (1993) *Caring for Children in the Health Services. Bridging the Gap,* **4,** 21.

Whiting M (1988) Community Paediatric Nursing in England. Unpublished MSc thesis. University of London.

Index

Page numbers printed in *italics* refer to the addresses of the organisations concerned.

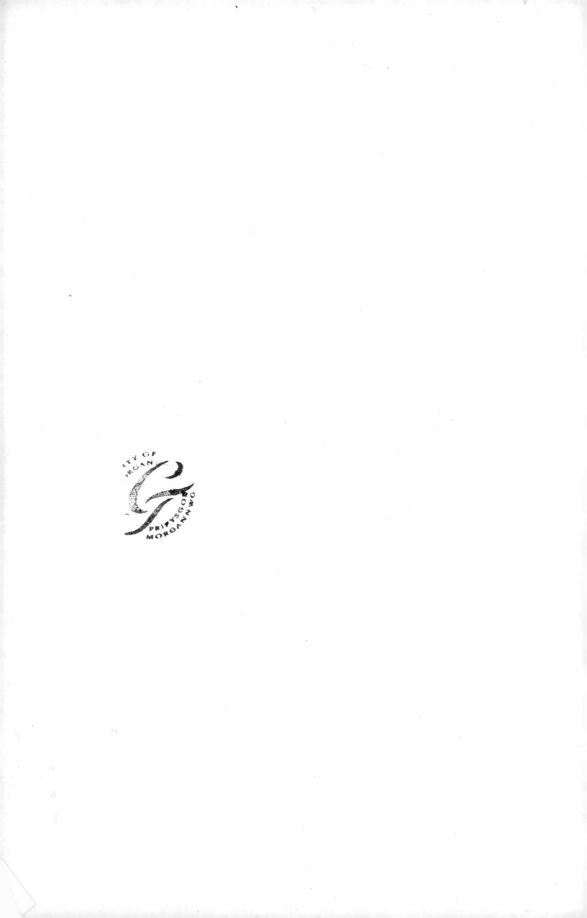